Grandparents Raising Grandchildren

Theoretical, Empirical, and Clinical Perspectives

Bert Hayslip Jr., PhD, is Regents Professor of Psychology at the University of North Texas, having joined the faculty in 1978. He teaches both undergraduate and graduate courses in Human Development, Psychology of Aging, Gerontological Counseling, and Death and Dying. He received his doctorate in Experimental Developmental Psychology from the University of Akron in 1975 and subsequently was on the Psychology faculty at Hood College in Frederick, Maryland. He has held grants from the National Endowment for the Humanities, the National Institute on Aging, and the Hilgenfeld Foundation. His research on the many facets of adult development and aging has appeared in such journals as *Psychology and Aging, The Gerontologist, The Journal of Gerontology, Experimental Aging Research, Research on Aging, The Journal of Applied Gerontology, The International Journal of Aging and Human Development, Educational Gerontology, Death Studies,* and *Omega: Journal of Death and Dying.* He is coauthor of *Adult Development and Aging* (2000, 3rd edition), *Hospice Care* (1992), and *Psychology of Aging: An Annotated Bibliography* (1995). He is currently Associate Editor of *Experimental Aging Research* and editor of *The International Journal of Aging and Human Development.* He is married and has two sons.

Robin S. Goldberg-Glen, PhD, MSW, is an Associate Professor in the School of Human Services, Center for Social Work Education, at Widener University in Chester, Pennsylvania. She received her MSW and PhD from the University of Chicago, School of Social Service Administration. She teaches courses in gerontology, human behavior, research, and cultural awareness/diversity. Her research interests include intergenerational family caregiving, Asian elderly, and practice evaluation. She is presently vice president of the Association for Geriatric Education in Social Work (AGE-SW). Her most recent publications on grandparent-headed families appear in *Family Relations, Families in Society,* the *Journal on Women and Aging,* and the *Journal of Social Service Research.*

Grandparents Raising Grandchildren

Theoretical, Empirical, and Clinical Perspectives

Bert Hayslip Jr., PhD
Robin Goldberg-Glen, PhD
Editors

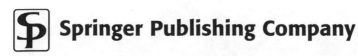 Springer Publishing Company

Copyright © 2000 by Springer Publishing Company, Inc.

All rights reserved

No part of this publication may be reproduced, stored in a retrieval system, or transmitted in any form or by any means, electronic, mechanical, photocopying, recording, or otherwise, without the prior permission of Springer Publishing Company, Inc.

Springer Publishing Company, Inc.
536 Broadway
New York, NY 10012-3955

Acquisitions Editor: Helvi Gold
Production Editor: J. Hurkin-Torres
Cover design by Susan Hauley

00 01 02 03 04 / 5 4 3 2

Library of Congress Cataloging-in-Publication Data

Grandparents raising grandchildren : theoretical, empirical, and
  clinical perspectives / Bert Hayslip, Jr. and Robin S.
  Goldberg-Glen, editors.
      p. cm.
    Includes bibliographical references and index.
    ISBN 0-8261-1336-2
    1. Grandparents as parents—United States. 2. Grandpar-
enting—United States. 3. Grandparents—United
States Psychology. 4. Grandparent and child—United States.
5. Grandchildren—Care—United States. I. Hayslip, Bert.
II. Goldberg-Glen, Robin S., 1958–
HQ759.9 .G7364 2000
306.874'5—dc21   00-021540
                                                                             CIP

Printed in the United States of America

Contents

Contributors

Raymond Albert, PhD
Graduate School of Social
   Work and Social Research
Law and Social Policy Program
Bryn Mawr College
Bryn Mawr, PA

Annabel Baird, MA
Department of Applied
   Gerontology
University of North Texas
Denton, TX

David B. Baker, PhD
Department of Psychology
The University of Akron
Akron, OH

Diana R. Brown, PhD
College of Labor and
   Metropolitan Affairs
Wayne State University
Detroit, MI

Donna M. Butts, BA
Executive Director
Generations United
Washington, DC

Richard K. Caputo, PhD
Wurzweiler School of Social
   Work
Yeshiva University
New York, NY

Lillian Chenoweth, PhD
Department of Family Sciences
Texas Woman's University
Denton, TX

Margaret Connealy, MSW
Mesilla Valley Hospice
Las Cruces, NM

Yosikazu DeRoos, PhD
School of Social Work
New Mexico State University
Las Cruces, NM

Diane D. Driver, MSW
Center on Aging
University of California-
   Berkeley
Berkeley, CA

Sarah L. Durant, MA
Department of Psychology
University of North Texas
Denton, TX

Michelle A. Emick, PhD
Department of Psychology
University of North Texas
Denton, TX

Esme Fuller-Thomson, MSW, PhD
Faculty of Social Work
University of Toronto
Toronto, Ontario

Robin S. Goldberg-Glen, PhD
Center for Social Work
   Education
Widener University
Chester, PA

Bert Hayslip Jr., PhD
Department of Psychology
University of North Texas
Denton, TX

Craig E. Henderson, MA
Department of Psychology
University of North Texas
Denton, TX

Nancy Henkin, PhD
Institute for Intergenerational
   Learning
Temple University
Philadelphia, PA

Barbara Hirshorn, PhD
Institute for Families in Society
University of South Carolina
Columbia, SC

Robert John, PhD
Department of Gerontology
University of Louisiana at
   Monroe
Monroe, LA

Daphne Joslin, PhD
Department of Community
   Health
William Patterson College
Wayne, NJ

Steve Kaufman, PhD
Center for Social Work
   Education
Widener University
Chester, PA

Karen Kopera-Frye, PhD
Department of Psychology
The University of Akron
Akron, OH

Jonathan Marx, PhD
Department of Sociology
Winthrop University
Rockhill, SC

Doriane Miller, MD
Robert Wood Johnson
   Foundation
Princeton, NJ

Meredith Minkler, PhD
School of Public Health
University of California-
  Berkeley
Berkeley, CA

Anita Rogers, PhD
Institute for Intergenerational
  Learning
Temple University
Philadelphia, PA

Roberta G. Sands, PhD
School of Social Work
University of Pennsylvania
Philadelphia, PA

R. Jerald Shore, PhD
Department of Psychology
University of North Texas
Denton, TX

Persephanie Silverthorn, PhD
Department of Psychology
University of New Orleans
New Orleans, LA

Jennifer C. Solomon, PhD
Department of Sociology
Withrop University
Rockhill, SC

Robert D. Strom, PhD
Division of Psychology in
  Education
Arizona State University
Tempe, AZ

Shirley K. Strom, PhD
Division of Psychology in
  Education
Arizona State University
Tempe, AZ

Cecilia Toledo, BA
Department of Psychology
University of North Texas
Denton, TX

J. Rafael Toledo, MD
Department of Psychology
University of North Texas
Denton, TX

Mary Jane Van Meter, PhD
Department of Sociology
Wayne State University
Detroit, MI

Richard Wiscott, MA
Department of Psychology
The University of Akron
Akron, OH

Foreword

In the early 1980s a group of researchers interested in grandparenthood gathered for the Wingspread Conference in Racine, Wisconsin. This conference was sponsored by religious organizations whose members were concerned about the transmission of family values. Recently, leafing through the collection of papers stemming from this conference, I noted that a great emphasis at that time lay in the symbols and meanings of grandparenthood, such as "being there" or being the "family watchdog." The content of the role was mainly discussed as a matter of styles of grandparenting, such as the "fun seeker," the "formal," or the "distant" grandparent (Bengtson & Robertson, 1985). Such depictions were usually traced in a large part to the fact that grandparents performed few basic functions of child rearing on a regular basis. Additionally, being a grandparent was not associated with life satisfaction, and grandchildren were not a source of support to older grandparents. A common saying at that time was "When in need of help, one good friend is better to have than a dozen grandchildren" (Wood & Robertson, 1976). In other words, consensus was that the role had little content and was not the most important dimension of one's life.

Lurking behind this lighthearted approach were a few family advocates, who expressed the hope or the wish that grandparents could perform more important functions in the American family (Kornhaber & Woodward, 1981). One particular area of interest was the potential helping role that grandparents could perform during the divorce processes of their children. My own research from 1981 to 1987 focused on that subject in the White middle-class and upper-middle-class suburbs in northern California, where divorce was rampant and serial monogamy was the norm rather than the exception.

Interviews with the divorcing parents indicated that they were reorganizing their lives on the basis of personal choices as they searched for happiness and self-actualization. Namely, they were organizing their postdivorce families in a postmodern world, where personal needs dominated over family needs. The grandmothers were more traditional in their values, but they preferred an "Auntie Mame" image to that of a cookie-baking, gray-haired woman. The fun-loving, friendlike relationship with grandchildren was still preferred. Because they felt it would be undermined if they had to act like parents, they avoided child-rearing functions if possible. Nevertheless, some had to become surrogate parents, usually with resistance and mostly on a temporary basis. Over 3 years later, the help they extended to children and grandchildren declined significantly.

Since the early 1980s, demographic findings have indicated dramatic family changes that have alarmed practitioners and researchers alike (Poponoe, 1993). In fact, such alterations in family structure make the marital changes of the previous decade seem like a minor problem. One area of particular concern is the rise in one-parent households and unwed teenage mothers. At the theoretical level, Aerts (1993) suggests that increased acceptance of the optional status of marriage and the erosion of fatherhood suggest a lack of institutional reinforcement of the nuclear family. In contrast to the worries of the family preservationists, the theme "good riddance to the family" suggests that it is time to search for alternatives to the much maligned nuclear family (Stacey, 1993). At the same time and more quietly, family therapists began to note the increasing numbers of grandmothers who were becoming surrogate parents to grandchildren whose parents had died or become incapable of caring for their children.

In view of these changes in the American family, the appearance of Hayslip and Goldberg-Glen's book *Grandparents Raising Grandchildren* is particularly timely. It is the first book to appear that is geared to family researchers and practitioners who are working with such grandparents and grandchildren. The breadth of the coverage is impressive, ranging from demographic chapters to legal issues to intervention techniques. This collection also reflects the cultural diversity in grandparenting, unlike the works in the early 1980s, when most studies dealt with White middle-class grandparents.

Emerging findings from my current work with Black families in middle age and old age reflects this diversity, which was often overlooked in the past. If grandparenthood in times of need seems to reflect the family organization in normal times, the new cohorts of California grandmothers are still resisting becoming parents to grandchildren. In contrast, Black families have always had flexible boundaries, unlike the relatively isolated White nuclear family, so single parents and children tend to have help from their extended families, in which grandmothers are particularly likely to take care of grandchildren. Today Black grandmothers are bearing the brunt of problems identified when grandmothers become parents. Those of us who are interested in such issues are fortunate to have this book available that brings to the reader the most up-to-date thinking on the many dimensions of this subject.

COLLEEN L. JOHNSON, PhD
University of California–San Francisco

REFERENCES

Aerts, E. (1993). Bringing the institution back in. In P.A. Cowan, D. Field, D. A. Hansen, A. Sholnick, & G. E. Swanson (Eds.), *Family, self and society: Toward a new agenda for family research* (pp. 3–48). Hillsdale, NJ: Lawrence Erlbaum.

Bengtson, V. L., & Robertson, J. F. (Eds.). (1985). *Grandparenthood.* Beverly Hills, CA: Sage.

Kornhaber, A., & Woodward, K. L. (1981). *Grandparents/grandchild: The vital connection.* Garden City, NY: Anchor.

Poponoe, D. (1993). American family decline, 1960–1990. *Journal of Marriage and the Family, 55,* 527–541.

Stacey, J. (1993). Good riddance to the family: A response to David Poponoe. *Journal of Marriage and the Family, 55,* 548–552.

Wood, V., & Robertson, J. F. (1976). Friendship and kinship interaction: Differential effects on the morale of the elderly. *Journal of Marriage and the Family, 40,* 367–375.

Preface

Grandparents Raising Grandchildren: Theoretical, Empirical, and Clinical Perspectives provides an overview of research and theoretically-based discussions of the emerging phenomenon of grandparents who raise their grandchildren to researchers and practitioners in the fields of psychology, social work, nursing, child welfare, human development, gerontology, counseling, and family studies. In this light, our text should be quite useful for teachers and nurses in school systems, lawyers, family therapists, and both self-help and community-based organizations providing services to kinship families, children, and grandparent support groups.

Recent census data (see Casper & Bryson, 1998) reveal the increasing numbers of grandparents who are called upon to become the parents of their grandchildren as a result of the death, divorce, or incapacitation of their adult children in their roles as parents due to drug abuse, child abuse, or incarceration. To date, although there are a number of popular press texts available, written specifically for grandparents who are raising their grandchildren, no text written for those in the above fields to guide research and clinical practice is currently available. The availability of such resources is critical not only to research on the many dimensions of what has been termed custodial grandparenting (Emick & Hayslip, 1996; Shore & Hayslip, 1994) but is also crucial to those who have direct hands-on experience with either custodial grandparents or the grandchildren that such middle-aged and older persons are raising. These professionals are often those whose programs and interventive efforts are the most crucial in the lives of the grandparents and grandchildren they serve.

Grandparents Raising Grandchildren explores the many dimensions of custodial grandparenting in discussing the cultural and historical antecedents of surrogate parenting in middle and later life, that is, what parenting and custodial grandparenting have in common, historical changes in the experience of custodial grandparenting, as well as the special difficulties grandparents face in dealing with grandchildren suffering from a variety of physical and psychological difficulties that may exacerbate the problems that custodial grandparents might otherwise face in raising their grandchildren. Moreover, many chapters present empirical data speaking to questions of cultural differences in custodial grandparenting, as well as discussing both clinical, legal, service-related, and policy-sensitive dimensions of surrogate parenting by grandparents. We hope that our text will serve as both a reference work and a guide to practice for professionals who work with either children or older adults. It also might be used as a text for courses in which students are trained to work with family forms of all types or do either social work, behavioral, policy-oriented, or legal research.

The chapters are organized to reflect the fact that (1) grandparents who parent their grandchildren were at one time both parents and grandparents, and consequently their experiences as parents and grandparents can help us understand their newly acquired roles as custodial grandparents; (2) that the experience of raising a grandchild is unique and consequently variable across persons, based on race, ethnicity, culture, or the particular demands that raising a grandchild makes on such grandparents; (3) that the difficulties (and benefits) of raising a grandchild can be better appreciated and indeed lessened (hence enhancing the benefits) by therapeutic efforts with custodial grandparents that are either preventive or ameliorative in nature; and (4) that custodial grandparenting must be understood in the larger context of the legal, service-related, educational, and policy-oriented dimensions that can affect the health and well-being of both grandparent and grandchild.

For these reasons, *Grandparents Raising Grandchildren* is organized into four sections: a first section labeled "Theoretical and Historical Perspectives on Custodial Grandparenting," a second section entitled "Variations in Surrogate Parenting in Middle and Late Life," a third section examining "Clinical Perspectives on Grandparents Who Raise Their Grandchildren," and a fourth section, dealing with "Service Delivery and Public Policy Implications of Custodial Grandparenting." Each chapter in some measure speaks to either the clinical, service, or policy-oriented implications of its content.

REFERENCES

Casper, L. M., & Bryson, K. R. (1998). Co-resident grandparents and their grandchildren: Grandparent maintained families. *Population Division Working Paper No. 26*. Washington, DC: U.S. Bureau of the Census.

Emick, M., & Hayslip, B. (1996). Custodial grandparenting: New roles for middle-aged and older adults. *International Journal of Aging and Human Development, 43*, 135–154.

Shore, R. J., & Hayslip, B. (1994). Custodial grandparenting: Implications for children's development. In A. E. Gottfried & A. W. Gottfried (Eds.), *Redefining families: Implications for children's development* (pp. 171–218). New York: Plenum Press.

Theoretical and Historical Perspectives on Custodial Grandparenting

CHAPTER 1

America's Grandparent Caregivers: Who Are They?

Esme Fuller-Thomson and Meredith Minkler

One of the most dramatic findings of the 1990 census was that of nearly a 44% increase over the preceding decade in the number of children living with their grandparents or other relatives. In a third of these homes, neither parent was present (Saluter, 1992), often making the grandparent the sole or primary caregiver. By 1997 approximately 4 million children, or 5.5% of all children under 18, lived in homes maintained by their grandparents (Lugailia, 1998). The most rapid growth during the 1990s occurred in those "skipped generation" families in which neither of a grandchild's biological parents was present (Bryson & Casper, 1999).

Who are America's grandparent caregivers, and what do we know about their life circumstances and the contexts in which care is provided? This introductory chapter will present a broad overview of the nation's intergenerational families headed by grandparents. Drawing on our own research and that of other scholars, we discuss the lifetime prevalence of grandparent caregiving and provide a profile of grandparent caregivers in the United States. Key factors contributing to the increase in intergenerational households headed by grandparents will be discussed, as will those personal and contextual variables that may help explain why some grandparents assume caregiving responsibility for grandchildren and others do not.

Although other chapters discuss in detail the clinical and policy implications of the growth of grandparent caregiving, we will close by highlighting several key areas in need of increased attention by clinicians, researchers, and policy makers if we are to better understand and address the strengths and needs of the growing number of intergenerational grandparent-headed families in the 21st century.

LIFETIME PREVALENCE OF GRANDPARENTS RAISING GRANDCHILDREN

As noted above, almost 6% of American children were living in households maintained by a grandparent by the late 1990s. Census data also revealed significant variations by race/ethnicity, with 4.1% of White children, 6.5% of Hispanic children, and 13.5% of African American children living with grandparents or other relatives (Lugaila, 1998).

Yet as Szinovacz (1998) has pointed out, census reports of the total population "considerably underestimate" the phenomenon of surrogate parenting by grandparents, because they "are limited to 'current' households among the population at large" (p. 37). The census data thus fail to address the lifetime prevalence of becoming a primary caregiver for one's grandchildren—a statistic that may present a very different picture.

To better gauge the lifetime prevalence of grandparent caregiving, we utilized data from a large, nationally representative longitudinal study, the National Survey of Families and Households (NSFH), undertaken by the Center for Demography and Ecology at the University of Wisconsin-Madison. In the most recent wave of the NSFH, conducted during 1992, 1993, and 1994, a probability sample of 10,008 respondents was interviewed. (For a more detailed summary of study design and questions, see Sweet, Bumpass, & Call, 1988.)

Our study's subsample consists of the 3,477 respondents to the 1992–1994 NSFH who reported having one or more grandchildren. Lifetime prevalence of grandparent caregiving was determined by calculating the proportion of grandparents who replied in the affirmative to the question "For various reasons, grandparents sometimes take on the primary responsibility for raising a grandchild. Have you ever had the primary responsibility for any of your grandchildren for six months or more?" Of the 3,477 grandparents in this study, 380 (10.9%) reported having had primary responsibility for raising a grandchild for a period of 6 months or more at some point in their lives. In other words, more than 1 in 10 grandparents had raised a grandchild for at least 6 months. Nearly half (44%) of the grandparents who had been primary caregivers for a grandchild took over parenting responsibilities when their grandchild was still an infant. An additional 28% became custodial grandparents when their grandchild was 1 to 4 years old. Close to three-quarters (72%) began caregiving before the child turned 5. Two thirds (69%) of the grandparents were raising the child of a daughter, and one third (31%) were raising a son's child.

Our study also revealed that for many caregiving grandparents, this role did not represent a short-term commitment. Indeed more than half (56%) of the caregiving grandparents had given care for a period of at least 3 years, and one in five had done so for 10 or more years.

A PROFILE OF AMERICA'S GRANDPARENT CAREGIVERS

To develop a national profile of America's grandparent caregivers, we examined in detail the characteristics of grandparents who reported that they had raised a grandchild for at least 6 months during the 1990s and contrasted them with the characteristics of noncaregiving grandparents. As Table 1.1 suggests, we learned that slightly over half (54%) of custodial grandparents in the United States were married, that more than three quarters (77%) of all caregiving grandparents were women, and that the majority (62%) of caregivers were non-Hispanic White. Custodial grandparents had a mean age of 59.4 years. Three quarters (74%) of recent custodial grandparents lived

**TABLE 1.1   Comparative Profile of Custodial Grandparents vs. Noncusto-
dial Grandparents of the 1990s**

Variable	% Noncaregiving Grandparents (n = 3304)	% Caregiving Grandparents (n = 173)
Marital status in 1993		
Widowed/divorced/separated/never married	32%	46%***
Married	68%	54%
Mean age in 1993	62.3 years	59.4 years**
Race		
Black	10%	27%***
White, non-Hispanic	84%	62%
Hispanic	6%	10%
Other	0%	1%
Gender		
Male	44%	23%***
Female	56%	77%
Education level in 1993		
Grade 11 or less	29%	43%***
Grade 12 or higher	71%	57%
Geographic region in 1988		
South	34.8%	42.5%*
Elsewhere	65.2%	57.5%
Urban/rural status in 1988		
Nonstandard metropolitan area (rural)	27%	26%
Standard metropolitan areas (urban)	73%	74%
Income in 1993		
Mean income	$37,814	$31,643*
Median income	$29,000	$22,176
Families below poverty line	13.7%	22.9%**
Families above poverty line	86.3%	77.1%
Offspring		
Total number of children	3.25	3.94***
One or more coresident children	30.4%	52.8%***
One or more non-coresident children within 20 miles	69%	76%*
Total number of grandchildren	5.39	7.29***
Child died in past 5 years	2.7%	6.5%**

p-values are based on the chi-square statistic for proportions and t-test statistic for means.
*p < .05.
**p < .01.
***p < .001.

in urban areas, and more than half (57.5%) of caregivers had completed high school.

Custodial grandparents of the 1990s differed markedly from noncustodial grandparents on several key demographic variables. The caregivers were significantly more likely to be unmarried, to be African American or Hispanic, to be female, and to have not completed high school. Custodial grandparents were also, on average, 3 years younger than noncaregiving grandparents. Compared to noncaregiving grandparents, those who were primary caregivers to a grandchild had lower mean incomes ($31,643 vs. $37, 814). In fact, caregiving grandparents were 60% more likely than noncustodial grandparents to report incomes below the poverty line (23% vs. 14%). Finally, although caregiving grandparents did not differ significantly from their noncaregiving peers with respect to urban/rural status, they were significantly more likely to have lived in the South (43% vs. 35%). Furthermore, caregivers had a higher mean number of offspring (3.9 vs. 3.3 children) and grandchildren (7.3 vs. 5.4 grandchildren). More than half (53%) of the caregiving grandparents had one or more of their offspring in their home, versus less than a third (30%) of the noncaregiving grandparents. Caregivers were also more likely than noncaregiving grandparents to have children living within 20 miles (76% vs. 69%). Finally, caregiving grandparents were much more likely than noncaregivers to have had a child die in the preceding 5 years (6.5% vs. 2.7%).

A logistic regression was run to verify which factors help predict caregiving status, while controlling for other variables (see Table 1.2). In general, these findings were similar to the results of the bivariate analyses. The results shown in Table 1.2 indicate that the odds of being a caregiving grandparent were more than twice as high for females (O.R. = 2.18) and for those who had experienced the death of a child in the previous five years (O.R. = 2.16). African Americans had 83% higher odds of being grandparent caregivers than did respondents from other races. For every decade of age, the odds of being a custodial grandparent decreased 25%. There was a trend ($p < .10$) indicating that those with a high school diploma had somewhat lower odds of being a caregiver; however, this trend did not reach the level of significance it had achieved in the bivariate analyses. Family size and structure also played significant roles. Although, in contrast to the findings of the bivariate analyses, overall

TABLE 1.2 Logistic Regression of Custodial Grandparents vs. Noncustodial Grandparents of the 1990s

Variable	Odds Ratio	(95% Confidence Interval)
Marital status in 1993 (married = 1)[a]	0.76	(0.53, 1.10)
Age in 1993 (by decade)	0.75***	(0.63, 0.89)
Race (Black = 1)[b]	1.83**	(1.19, 2.81)
Gender (female = 1)	2.18***	(1.47, 3.22)
Education (high school graduate = 1)[c]	0.72+	(0.50, 1.03)
Geographic region in 1988 (South = 1)[d]	1.17	(0.84, 1.66)
Urban status in 1988 (urban = 1)	0.99	(0.69, 1.44)
Poverty level (families below poverty line = 1)	1.08	(0.71, 1.65)
Total number of children	0.98	(0.88, 1.09)
Number of coresident children	1.23*	(1.02, 1.49)
Total number of grandchildren	1.08***	(1.03, 1.12)
Parental bereavement (child died in past 5 years = 1)	2.16*	(1.06, 4.38)

+$p < .10$.
*$p < .05$.
**$p < .01$.
***$p < .001$.
[a]Reference category includes all people not currently married—widowed, divorced, separated, never married.
[b]Reference category includes all non-Blacks.
[c]Reference category is 11 or fewer years of education.
[d]Reference category is all other areas of United States.

number of children was not significantly associated with caregiving status in the multivariate analysis, number of coresident children (O.R. = 1.23) and number of grandchildren (O.R. = 1.08) remained a significant factor. Unlike the bivariate analyses, marital status, living in the South, and living below the poverty line were not statistically significant in the multivariate analysis.

In sum, the results of our study, like that of other researchers (Chalfie, 1994; Harden, Clark, & Maguire, 1997), suggest a number of "vulnerability factors" for becoming a caregiver to one's grandchild, key among them being a woman, being African American, being younger, having more coresident children, and having experienced the loss of a child. Other studies, based on census data, add to this list being single, living in the South, and/or having a low income (Chalfie, 1994; Harden et al., 1997).

Such information is important in what it tells us about why some people are more likely to become caregivers to their grandchildren while others are not. Yet it does not explain the reasons for the dramatic increase in grandparent-headed households over the past two decades. It is to this topic that we now turn.

CAUSES OF THE INCREASE IN GRANDPARENT HEADED HOUSEHOLDS

To fully understand the trend toward intergenerational households headed by grandparents, one must look to a wide range of social factors. The increase in drug abuse, for example, has been cited as perhaps the most dramatic and immediate causal factor, with the crack cocaine epidemic of the 1980s playing a particularly pronounced role (Barth, 1991; Feig, 1990). It is likely that drug and alcohol abuse will continue to be an important contributor to the formation of grandparent-headed households in the 21st century.

A dramatic drop in the number of children living in two-parent households—from over 86% in 1950 to about 70% by the mid-1990s—as a consequence of divorce, teen pregnancy, and other factors also appears to be contributing to the increase in grandparental care (Harden et al., 1997). Similarly, dramatic increases in the number of incarcerated women, which grew sixfold over the past decade and a half (U.S. Department of Justice, 1997) as a result of stiffer sentencing and the like, also contributes to the rise in grandparent caregiving, because grandparents are primary caretakers to well over half of the children of imprisoned mothers in the United States (Greenfield & Minor-Harper, 1991).

As noted above, the death of an adult child significantly increases a grandparent's chances of becoming a caregiver to her grandchild, and in recent years both violence and AIDS have played a role in the death of young people, particularly in low-income inner-city communities. Projections by the Centers for Disease Prevention and Control suggest that between 125,000 and 150,000 children and teenagers will have lost their mothers to AIDS by the year 2000 (Geballe, Gruendel, & Andiman, 1995), and the great majority of these children are cared for by grandparents. Particularly in the African American community, where AIDS is the leading cause of death in the 15–44 age group, the importance of this tragic contributor to grandparent caregiving should not be overlooked.

It should be stressed that most of the factors discussed above are tied in fundamental ways to the continued problem of poverty in our nation, which itself remains a significant vulnerability factor for grandparent caregiving (Burnette, 1997; Minkler, 1999). Ironically, however, another major cause of the increase in grandparent-headed households was related, in part, to legislative efforts to assist low-income custodial grandparents, for whom historic inequities in the child welfare system had often translated into far less generous benefits than were received by foster care parents unrelated to the children in their care.

The 1979 Supreme Court case, *Youakim v. Miller*, for example, gave a major boast to "kinship care," or the formal placement of children with relatives, when it upheld a lower court's decision that federal foster care benefits could not be denied to relatives who were otherwise eligible (e.g., if children were removed formally from an AFDC-eligible family and entered care by court order or voluntary placement). By the late 1980s close to a third (31%) of the foster care children in the legal custody of the 20 states able to track such developments had in fact been placed with grandparents or other relatives (Kusserow, 1991). States that implemented the most liberal policies toward kinship care (e.g., New York, Illinois, and California), moreover, experienced the most rapid growth in such placements (Goerge, Wulczyn, & Harden, 1995). The contribution of changing federal and state laws and policies promoting formal kinship care to the increase in this phenomenon, in short, should not be underestimated (Berrick & Needell, in press). Yet as Harden et al. (1997) have pointed out, such policy changes do not explain the sizable concomitant growth in the number of children who have informally come into the care of grandparents, for many of the reasons discussed above.

SPECIAL AREAS OF CONCERN FOR RESEARCH, POLICY, AND PRACTICE

This chapter has examined the demographics of grandparent caregiving in America, as well as the causal factors that help explain the significant increase in intergenerational households headed by grandparents over the past two decades. Although many of the factors discussed in this overview chapter will be examined in greater detail in subsequent chapters, we turn now to several of the areas that, we believe, merit particular attention by researchers, clinicians, and policy makers if we are to better understand and address the strengths and needs of America's grandparent caregivers and their families.

Health

Clinicians should be attentive to the potential for health problems and to delayed help seeking for such problems by grandparents raising grandchildren. High rates of depression, poor self-rated health, and/or the frequent presence of multiple chronic health problems have been reported in both local and national studies (Burnette, in press; Dowdell, 1995; Minkler & Roe, 1993; Minkler, Fuller-Thomson, Miller, & Driver, 1997; Roe et al., 1996). Our own national study (Minkler et al., 1997), for example, demonstrated that grandparent caregivers have close to twice the rates of depression of other grandparents (25.1% vs. 14.5%). That grandparents who are in the poorest health (Burnette, in press) and those raising children they perceive as having neurological, physical, emotional, or behavioral problems (Shore & Hayslip, 1990, 1994) may be among the least likely to seek and receive counseling and other help for themselves also suggests an area in need of special attention by clinicians and researchers. High-quality psychotherapeutic interventions, support groups, respite care, and other programmatic responses should be developed and carefully evaluated in efforts to improve and maintain the emotional health of grandparents raising grandchildren. Further, policies and programs supporting diligent outreach to such grandparents should be developed, as well as the creation of "one-stop shopping" centers where they can receive health care and services for their grandchildren and themselves under one roof (Minkler, 1999). Finally, access to health insurance should be assured for both grandparents and the grandchildren in their care.

From the perspective of research, additional longitudinal and other studies on the health of grandparent caregivers are needed to better determine baseline physical and mental health, the impacts of caregiving on health status, and the role of health-promoting programs and interventions in facilitating health maintenance and improvement. In addition, however, greatly increased attention should be directed to the health status of the children in their grandparents' care, particularly because the current literature is contradictory in this area (Dowdell, 1995; Emick & Hayslip, 1996; Minkler & Roe, 1996; Solomon & Marx, 1995). While one national study suggests that children reared by grandparents fare no worse in terms of health than those in traditional two-parent families, for example (Solomon & Marx, 1995), several smaller scale studies have pointed to a host of health problems common among these children, including respiratory ailments, hyperactivity and other behavioral problems, and the health aftereffects of prenatal drug and alcohol exposure (Dowdell, 1995; Minkler & Roe, 1996; Shore & Hayslip, 1990). Wherever possible, the family health of intergenerational grandparent-headed households, rather than solely the health of individual members, should be assessed and approached through family-centered intervention efforts.

Social Isolation

Decreased socialization with friends and/or family as a consequence of grandparent caregiving has been observed by several investigators (Burton, 1992, in press; Jendrek, 1993, 1994; Minkler & Roe, 1993; Poe, 1992), with Shore and Hayslip's (1990) Texas-based study revealing that almost 40% of custodial grandparents felt isolated from friends as a consequence of this role. Similarly, Jendrek (1993) found that declines in marital satisfaction were four times more likely among the grandparent caregivers in her study than in the two comparison groups of noncustodial grandparents examined.

Not infrequently, social isolation is exacerbated by feelings of shame and alienation as a consequence of the nature of the intrafamily problems that lead to the assumption of caregiving. The stigma attached to parental AIDS or drug use, for example, particularly among communities that have failed to acknowledge the extent of these problems, leads some grandparents to experience feelings of alienation from churches and other social networks and mediating structures that previously had provided important sources of support for coping with life's problems (Campbell-Jackson, 1997; Minkler & Roe, 1993).

To combat the social isolation and alienation frequently experienced by grandparent caregivers and their families, more than 500 support groups (M. Hollidge, personal communication, July 1, 1999) have been developed in all 50 states. Organizations like the Brookdale Foundation in New York and AARP's Grandparent Information Center in Washington, DC, are doing an excellent job of encouraging the formation of such groups and, in the latter case, helping grandparents and professionals alike to identify and connect with preexisting groups and services in their geographic areas. However, the sheer numbers of relative caregivers, the informality of most support groups, and the short life expectancy of many such groups and service programs constitute real barriers to meeting the demand.

Several investigators (Burnette, 1998; Burton, 1992; Dressel & Barnhill, 1994; Miller, 1991; Minkler & Roe, 1993; Poe, 1992) have underscored the important role that support groups and similar interventions may play in helping to reduce feelings of social isolation while providing both tangible and intangible assistance in coping with the new role. As Strom and Strom (1993) and Emick and Hayslip (1996) have indicated, however, and with few exceptions (see Burnette, 1998) the effectiveness of such groups has not been well documented. As noted above, the role of support groups and more formal psychotherapeutic interventions should be carefully examined, particularly in relation to helping address the social isolation and related problems faced by many grandparents raising grandchildren.

Economic Insecurity

One of the most striking findings of the national studies of grandparent-headed households to date involves their disproportionately high poverty rates. The findings that 41% of skipped-generation families live in or near poverty (Chalfie, 1994) and that almost a quarter of the larger universe of intergenerational households headed by grandparents live below the poverty line (Fuller-Thomson, Minkler, & Driver, 1997) suggest that poor economic health may well compound the other difficulties faced by such families.

The high costs of caring, moreover, may be particularly pronounced in communities where economic vulnerability is already endemic. As Harden et al. (1997) have pointed out, children in kinship care families in 1992–1994 were more than twice as likely as other children to be living in families receiving public assistance or welfare benefits and almost five times more likely to be living in a family in which at least one member received Supplemental Security Income (SSI), a government program assistance for the elderly and disabled poor. For many low-income grandparents, taking in grandchildren means stretching still further an already inadequate SSI check and/or facing the indignity of "going on welfare" to receive a monthly allotment that typically is insufficient to meet the need. For younger grandparents, taking in one's grandchildren may mean quitting a job or making other job related sacrifices that may put their own future economic well being at risk. Retired or non working caregivers also frequently suffer financially, and sometimes report spending their life savings, and cashing in life insurance policies to cope financially (Minkler & Roe, 1993, 1996).

As noted above, legal challenges and other factors have resulted in increasing numbers of grandparent caregivers becoming eligible for kinship care payments, which can be two or three times higher than rock bottom Temporary Assistance to Needy Families (TANF, formerly AFDC) rates. For the many relative caregivers without formal custody arrangements, however, and for others in states that fail to inform them about their eligibility for higher foster care payments and other benefits, low-income grandparent caregivers continue to receive no assistance or low and stigmatizing TANF benefits. Finally, and regardless of the state in which they are living, many grandparent caregivers report experiencing considerable delay, eligibility problems, and other difficulties in trying to access needed financial assistance (Chalfie, 1994; Minkler & Roe, 1996; Mullen, 1997; Poe, 1992). A strong political commitment is needed to ensure that the increasing number of low-income intergenerational families headed by grandparents receive, without stigma or delay, financial support and related services at a level that will enable them to adequately provide for their new families. At minimum, kinship care providers should receive full foster care rates as a matter of equity, as well as access to other benefits accorded to nonrelative foster parents.

Strengths and Needs of Diverse Groups of Grandparent Caregivers

As noted above, although the majority of intergenerational households headed by grandparents are White, the disproportionate representation of Hispanics and particularly of African Americans is noteworthy. The fact that African Americans have almost twice the odds of becoming caregivers to their grandchildren reflects, in part, a long history of caregiving across generations in Black families, with roots in West African culture and tradition (Sudarkasa, 1981; Wilson, 1986). Yet as Burton and Dilworth-Anderson (1991) suggest, the experience of many of today's African American grandparents, who assume the role of caregiver as a result of a child's drug addiction, incarceration, teen pregnancy, death, or incapacitation due to AIDS, may vary dramatically from that of their foremothers and fathers who took on a caregiving role under very different sociohistorical circumstances. Resentment, shame, perceived social isolation, severe financial strain, and depression are among the adverse outcomes that have been identified among such caregivers. Although positive outcomes, including relief at being able to "keep the family together" and a renewed sense of purpose in life also frequently are observed (Burton, 1992; Campbell-Jackson, 1997; Jendrek, 1994; Minkler & Roe, 1993; Poe, 1992), the former deleterious factors are cause for concern.

While not as prevalent as in African American families, the increase in grandparent-headed households among Hispanics also merits special consideration, especially given the rapid growth of this population group. Latinos made up fully 10% of the relative caregivers in Chalfie's (1994) national study of skipped-generation families, as well as in our NSFH study (Fuller-Thomson et al., 1997). Census data further have revealed a significant difference between Hispanic and non-Hispanic skipped-generation households in that aunts, godparents, and others, rather than biological grandparents, are more likely to be the primary caregivers in the former (Harden et al., 1997). This difference alone suggests that the experience of Hispanic relative caregivers may be qualitatively different from that of the majority of non-Hispanic surrogate parents, who typically are the grandparents of the children in their care.

To date, however, only one investigator has looked in depth at intergenerational Hispanic households headed by relatives, and her work explores primarily the experience of Puerto Ricans in New York City (Burnette, in press). As Burnette's work makes clear, however, the experience of Hispanic caregivers takes on special relevance in the light of language barriers; traditional cultural values, such as familism; the impacts of acculturation on such values and their expression; and recent antiimmigration sentiments and their legal manifestations. In the latter regard, efforts to deny health and social services to undocumented and in some cases even legal immigrants may have an especially pronounced effect on first-generation relative caregivers who may be even more reluctant to seek needed help within the current political and social milieu.

The special issues facing the disproportionate number of African American and Hispanic intergenerational households headed by relatives must be taken into account in the crafting of culturally sensitive and appropriate policies, programs, and outreach efforts. Efforts like Philadelphia's Project GUIDE, which focuses on building cultural pride and self-esteem among intergenerational households headed by African-American grandparents, can help meet the psychosocial needs of such families. Efforts are needed to create and support similar programs, to more effectively involve churches, and to link clinical supports with these and other preexisting cultural institutions in an attempt to better address the needs of diverse groups.

As a basis for effective clinical interventions and sound policies, further research is needed on the meaning and significance of relative caregiving for different racial and ethnic groups, with particular attention to these two overrepresented groups: Native Americans, with their rich tradition of grandparent caregiving (Emick & Hayslip, 1996; John, Blanchard, & Hennessey, 1998), and the many Asian Pacific Islander groups on whom little or no research exists in this area. The racial and ethnic diversity of America's grandparent caregivers and their families, in short, underscores the need for better understanding of the sociocultural variations in surrogate parenting by grandparents and other relatives and the implications of these differences for effective practice and policy.

CONCLUSION

Intergenerational households headed by grandparents exhibit many strengths, with grandparents who assume caregiving often doing so willingly and with relief that they can "be there for the grandchildren." A renewed sense of purpose and the sheer fun that children can bring into a household are among the benefits cited by grandparent caregivers (Minkler & Roe, 1993). At the same time, as Shore and Hayslip (1994) have noted, "If grandparents have to assume full time parenting, it is most likely to occur in the context of family trauma" (p. 184) and can, consequently, be a highly stressful process.

Clinicians working with midlife and older clients, particularly if they are low-income women, African Americans, or Hispanics or parents of teenage mothers need to be alert to the possibility of the sudden assumption of caregiving for one's grandchildren and its health and social impacts. Similarly, policy makers need to examine current and proposed policies in terms of their real and potential impacts on intergenerational families headed by grandparents. As Faith Mullen (1997) has pointed out, for example, the dramatic new welfare reform changes that became law in 1996 and that imposed work requirements, time limits, and other restrictions on the receipt of aid, "were not made with grandparent headed households in mind, and by and large they do not help these households." The special circumstances faced by many grandparents raising grandchildren should be stressed in the analyses of such legislative measures and serious efforts made to uncover and redress problematic unintended consequences of the legislation for intergenerational households headed by grandparents.

Although the focus of this chapter and this volume is on grandparents and the grandchildren in their care, the importance of broadening our gaze to the entire family unit (including, importantly, the living biological parents who may be physically missing from the household) should be underscored (Minkler, 1999). In particular, national surveys, including the census, should contain questions that permit the more accurate assessment of all members of complex households and their relationships to one another.

Qualitative research also should pay more attention to the "invisible" middle generation of parents who are unwilling or unable to care for their children. As Dressel and Kelly (1996) have noted, only by exploring the needs and perspectives of *all* generations and across family members will we be in a position to understand and hence better confront the issues facing growing numbers of intergenerational households headed by grandparents.

ACKNOWLEDGMENTS

The authors gratefully acknowledge the Commonwealth Fund for its support of this research. The Commonwealth Fund is a New York City–based national foundation that undertakes independent research on health and social issues. This chapter is based on two earlier publications: E. Fuller-Thomson, M. Minkler, & D. Driver, "A Profile of Grandparents Raising Grandchildren in the United States," published in *The Gerontologist*, 37(3), p. 406–411, and Minkler, M. (1999) Intergenerational households headed by grandparents: Contexts, realities and implications for policy. *Journal of Aging Studies* 13(2), 199–218. Reprinted with permission.

REFERENCES

Barth, R. (1991). Educational implications of prenatally drug-exposed children. *Social Work in Education, 13*, 130–136.

Berrick, J. D., & Needell, B. (in press). Recent trends in kinship care: Public policy, payments and outcomes for children. In P. A. Curtis & D. Grady (Eds.), *The foster care crisis: Translating research into policy and practice.* Washington, DC: Child Welfare League of America and the University of Nebraska Press.

Bryson, K., & Casper, L. (1999). Co-resident grandparents and their grandchildren. In *Current population reports* (P-23 198 [May] pp. 1–11). Washington, DC: U.S. Department of Commerce.

Burnette, D. (1997). Grandparents raising grandchildren in the inner city: Families in society. *Journal of Contemporary Human Services*, Sept./Oct., 489–499.

Burnette, D. (1998). Grandparents rearing grandchildren: A school-based small group intervention. *Research on Social Work Practice, 8*, 1–27.

Burnette, D. (1999). Custodial grandparents in Latino families: Patterns of service utilization and predictors of unmet needs. *Social Work, 44*, 22–34.

Burnette, D. (in press). *Latino grandparent caregivers.* New York: Columbia University Press.

Burton, L. (1992). Black grandmothers rearing children of drug-addicted parents: Stressors, outcomes and social service needs. *Gerontologist, 32,* 744–751.

Burton, L. M., & Dilworth-Anderson, P. (1991). The intergenerational roles of aged Black Americans. *Marriage and Family Review, 16,* 311–330.

Campbell-Jackson, S. (1997, October). Supportive services for kinship care families. Paper presented at the Generations United/AARP Symposium on Grandparents and Other Relatives Raising Children, Washington DC.

Chalfie, D. (1994). *Going it alone: A closer look at grandparents parenting grandchildren.* Washington, DC: American Association of Retired Persons.

Dowdell, E. B. (1995). Caregiver burden: Grandparents raising their high risk children. *Journal of Psychosocial Nursing, 33*(3), 27–30.

Dressel, P., & Barnhill, S. (1994). Reframing gerontological thought and practice: The case of grandmothers with daughters in prison. *Gerontologist, 34,* 685–690.

Dressel, P., & Kelly, S. (1996, November). *Grandparent caregivers: Expanding the agenda.* Paper presented at the annual meeting of the Gerontological Society of America, Washington DC.

Emick, M., & Hayslip, B. (1996). Custodial grandparenting: New roles for middle aged and older adults. *International Journal of Aging and Human Development, 43,* 135–154.

Feig, L. (1990). *Drug exposed infants and children: Service needs and policy questions.* Washington, DC: Department of Health and Human Services.

Fuller-Thomson, E., Minkler, M., & Driver, D. (1997). A profile of grandparents raising grandchildren in the United States. *Gerontologist, 37,* 406–411.

Geballe, S., Gruendel, J., & Andiman, W. (1995). *Forgotten children of the AIDS epidemic.* New York: Yale University Press.

Goerge, R. M., Wulczyn, F. H., & Harden, A. (1995). *Foster care dynamics, 1988–1993: An update from the multistate foster care data archive.* Chicago, IL: Chapin Hall Center for Children.

Greenfield, L. A., & Minor-Harper, S. (1991). *Women in prison.* Washington, DC: Bureau of Justice Statistics.

Harden, A. W., Clark, R. L., & Maguire, K. (1997). *Informal and formal kinship care.* Washington, DC: U.S. Department of Health and Human Services.

Jendrek, M. P. (1994). Grandparents who parent their grandchildren: Circumstances and decisions. *Gerontologist, 34,* 206–216.

Jendrek, M. P. (1993). Grandparents who parent their grandchildren: Effects on lifestyle. *Journal of Marriage and Family, 55,* 609–621.

John, R., Blanchard, P., & Hennessey, C. H. (1998). Hidden lives: Aging and contemporary Indian women. In J. Coyle (Ed.), *Women and aging: A research guide.* Westport, CT: Greenwood Press.

Kusserow, R. P. (1991). *Issues in relative foster care.* Washington, DC: Department of Health and Human Services, Office of the Inspector General.

Lugaila, T. (in press). *Marital status and living arrangements: March 1997.* In *Current population reports.* Washington, DC: U.S. Bureau of the Census.

Miller, D. (1991, November). The "grandparents who care" support project of San Francisco. Presentatio, the Annual Meeting of the Gerontological Society of America, San Francisco, CA.

Minkler, M., Fuller-Thomson, E., Miller, D., & Driver, D. (1997). Depression in grandparents raising grandchildren. *Archives of Family Medicine, 6,* 445–452.

Minkler, M., & Roe, K. M. (1993). *Grandmothers as caregivers: Raising children of the crack cocaine epidemic.* Newbury Park, CA: Sage.

Minkler, M., & Roe, K. (1996). Grandparents as surrogate parents. *Generations, 1*(spring), 34–38.

Minkler, M. (1999). Intergenerational households headed by grandparents: Contexts, realities and implications for policy. *Journal of Aging Studies, 13*(2), 199–218.

Mullen, F. (1997, October). *Grandparents raising grandchildren: Public benefits and programs.* Paper presented at the Generations United/AARP Symposium on Grandparents and Other Relatives Raising Children, Washington DC.

Poe, L. (1992). *Black grandparents as caregivers.* Unpublished manuscript.

Roe, K. M., & Minkler, M. (in press). Grandparents raising grandchildren: Challenges and responses. *Generations.*

Roe, K. M., Minkler, M., Saunders, F. F., & Thompson, G. (1996). Health of grandmothers raising children of the crack cocaine epidemic. *Medical Care, 34,* 1072–1084.

Saluter, A. F. (1992). Marital status and living arrangements: March 1991. In *Current population reports* (Series P-20 No. 461). Washington, DC: U.S. Government Printing Office.

Shore, R. J., & Hayslip, B. (1990, November). *Comparisons of custodial and non custodial grandparents.* Paper presented at the annual scientific meeting of the Gerontological Society of America, Boston.

Shore, R. J., & Hayslip, B. (1994). Custodial grandparenting: Implications for children's development. In A. Godfried & A. Godfried (Eds.), *Redefining families: Implications for children's development.* New York: Plenum.

Solomon, J. C., & Marx, J. (1995). "To grandmother's house we go": Health and school adjustment of children raised solely by grandparents. *Gerontologist, 35,* 386–394.

Strom, R. D., & Strom, S. K. (1993). Grandparents raising grandchildren: Goals and support groups. *Educational Gerontology, 19,* 705–715.

Sudarkasa, N. (1981). Interpreting the African heritage in Afro-American family organization. In H. P. McAdoo (Ed.), *Black families* (pp. 37–53). Beverly Hills, CA: Sage.

Sweet, J., Bumpass, L., & Call, V. (1988). *The design and content of the national survey of families and households* (NSFH working paper no. 1). Madison: University of Wisconsin, Center for Demography and Ecology.

Szinovacz, M. E. (1998). Grandparents today: A demographic profile. *Gerontologist, 38,* 37–52.

U.S. Department of Justice. (1997). *Prisoners in 1996* (Report No. NCJ 164619). Washington, DC: Bureau of Justice Statistics.

Wilson, M. N. (1986). The Black extended family: An analytical consideration. *Developmental Psychology, 22,* 246–259.

CHAPTER 2

Grandparenting and Family Preservation

Margaret Connealy and Yosikazu DeRoos

BACKGROUND

This book is testament to the increasing awareness of and concern about grandparents raising grandchildren. Because of the significant increase in the number of children living with grandparents, family preservation workers are faced with developing and improving theories and practice methods to maximize family functioning.

Family instability may be triggered by a variety of circumstances, and families may be more vulnerable than in years past. Unwed motherhood, single-parent families, diseases such as AIDS and death by other means, substance abuse epidemics, and children whose parents are incarcerated affect the structure and functioning of the family. Complementary to these family configurations is the grandparent-headed household—complementary because as a woman becomes a single parent, a parent divorces, becomes a substance user, is placed in prison, suffers a debilitating disease, or dies, the likelihood of grandparental involvement increases, as does the likelihood that the grandparents will gain formal or informal custody of the grandchildren. Thus, those of us involved in family preservation practice and research believe that custodial grandparenting is one of the family types in which family preservation must play a role.

FAMILY PRESERVATION

Family preservation practice varies by duration and intensity of service. Intensive family preservation practice has been steadily gaining acceptance in child welfare service systems. It is characterized primarily by short-term, intensive, family-focused, in-home services provided to families who are at risk of child placement. The goals of intensive family preservation are to protect children; prevent out-of-home placement into either foster care or institutional care, if possible; and strengthen and support the functioning of the family (Berry, 1992). Sometimes, for the benefit of children and parents, particularly when safety is involved, children are placed with those offering temporary custodial care. However, family preservation practitioners acknowledge that not all families can be maintained and that the configuration of a family may be permanently altered, such as with the death of a parent or with severe family conditions that cannot be sufficiently ameliorated. Although most family preservation programs are characterized by their intensive, short-term, crisis-oriented intervention and focus on reducing outplacement of and reducing risk to children, family preservation can be characterized more broadly as a program in which the goal is to enhance family development and functioning, regardless of whether the family is experiencing a crisis.

In the past, when outplacing a child because of abuse, neglect, or other problem condition in the family, foster parents were a primary option for custodial care. However, in reaction to the troubling history of foster care, in which children were often allowed to languish in foster placements for many months and in some cases, given serial placement of children in consecutive foster placements, for years, and in which family ties were sometimes irrevocably broken, an alternative philosophy and practice emerged, arguing for maintaining family contact and ties and reducing outplacement of children as much as possible.

From this position, one argues that the best setting for developing more effective family functioning and resolving family problems—whether in regard to parental abuse or neglect, substance use by parents, situations in which the parent may have an illness, or numerous other situations—is in the family in which the children are reared and in which emotional and supportive ties exist. Given this, one recognizes that a family can consist of more than or other than parents and children and allows for the possibility that a family may consist solely of grandparents and grandchildren, a family configuration we will refer to as custodial grandparenting. Thus, from a family preservation perspective, under certain conditions, either temporary or permanent, custodial grandparenting may be seen as the best available alternative, certainly for grandchildren, and a very positive one for grandparents, one that can be a strong, nurturing environment for all family members.

In family preservation, *family* is defined as two or more individuals who have emotional bonds and commitments to one another, which are reflected in an ongoing pattern of interaction that provides care, concern, and nurturance and which influence and shape the development and maintenance of norms, roles, and rules. The expectation is that the commitment is long-term. In simpler terms, a family is two or more people who love and care for one another and are committed to and support one another's well-being. *Preservation* is defined as a process of using individual, family, and community strengths and resources to enhance, improve, and support family functioning over the short and long term, working primarily from the needs, goals, and values of the family. In simpler terms, preservation is a process in which the family is strengthened.

Both custodial grandparenting and family preservation programs have increased in the past 20 years. Both are a result of social, political, economic, and ideological changes addressing child welfare, including those noted earlier. The change in child welfare ideology has centered on who or what is to take primacy. For most of the history of American child welfare, the leading argument and action focused on placing the welfare of children first. The position was understandable, given the condition and status of children in society and the lack of significant services or supports to ameliorate or prevent abuse and neglect. However, by focusing primarily on children and their welfare, the effect was to view children and their families as adversaries. A child welfare worker, often called a child protection worker, saw his or her role as that of protecting the child from adverse conditions or situations and from those assumed to be responsible for creating such adversity, usually the parents. Given this adversarial view, removing a child from a family often clearly seemed to be in the child's best interest.

The ideological change began when greater account was given to the role of social, political, and economic forces and conditions and to a systemic view that conceptualized family functioning, including adverse functioning, as related in significant part to factors outside the family. By reducing family blameworthiness, it became possible to view the family, in relation to a child, less adversarially and as more central to a child's well-being even under conditions of adversity. This more balanced view allowed for the assumption that solutions as well as problems may lie with the family, that resources as well as needs may be found in the family, and that strengths as well as deficits may be possessed by the family. The recognition that external factors play a role in family functioning, including adversities being experienced by the family, furthered the idea that the solution lay not in removing a child from a family but in mobilizing strengths and resources, both internal and external, to address problems experienced by the family and to develop family skills and strategies to buffer the family from external conditions that might adversely affect problem resolution. Supporting this view was evidence that, in many cases, removing a child from a family created as many problems, although different ones, as it was meant to alleviate (Swift, 1995).

Therefore, the new ideology, family preservation, with its focus on mobilizing strengths and resources and on developing solutions from within the family became increasingly preferred as a mode for addressing concerns related to child well-being. The change from a child to a family focus also broadened welfare concerns to include . other family members' well-being and lessened the adversarial nature of formal child welfare activity.

With the focus on mobilizing strengths and resources, the family became the locus of activity and family members the most active players in problem resolution and family enhancement. Today, family preservation continues to develop as an approach to child and family practice. It is seen as both more humane than focusing on just the child and more efficient and effective than services directed at just individuals (Berry, 1997). Although often not recognized, much of child welfare practice has moved in the direction of infusing both the ideology and practice of family preservation (J. Rycraft, personal communication, 1995).

One of the most important concepts underlying family preservation practice, which argues for the viability of custodial grandparenting, is the concept of *strengths*. More correctly thought of as the strengths metaphor, it focuses on the abilities and capacities of individuals, groups, and families to think and act in ways that promote growth and well-being (Goldstein, 1992). The history of child and family practice has portrayed individuals and families as deficit-ridden and in need of intervention by experts considered as more knowledgeable than those being served.

Historically, despite the norm that relatives were expected to care for kin, particularly minors, when needed and despite evidence that kin did exactly that, when child and family service staff worked with families, including custodial grandparenting families, they employed various explanatory theories to focus on families' and their members' deficits and limitations. Issues raised about grandparents included limited life span, physical limitations, mental incapacity, financial restrictions, emotional attachment, and even child-rearing ability. Concerns about grandchildren being raised by grandparents included proper ego development, socialization, and role model availability (Smith & Merkel-Holguin, 1995).

Such theory-based models of intervention, often lacking sound empirical foundation, typically approached assessment in terms of limitations and deficits (Cowger, 1992). Such models focused on identifying and correcting deficiencies found in families, usually by restructuring membership or restructuring relationships. Inherent, albeit often implicit, in almost every theory-based model of intervention used in child welfare was a deficit perspective of family functioning and often of individual functioning.

In contrast, the strengths perspective accepts and permits individuals and families to be experts about their own life situation, to portray their lives from their own perspective, and to have opportunities to initiate action designed to improve that life situation. Family preservation practice focuses on strengths found in families, whatever the state of a family and whatever issues or problems need to be addressed by the family.

The strengths perspective begins from an empirical rather than a theoretical base and assumes that the family has the capacity and desire to direct action toward goal attainment. Whatever the limitations or incapacities of a family, recognizing that change can occur only when one addresses, focuses on, and mobilizes strengths, results in a perspective that refocuses assessment from being the purview of the worker to being a joint activity of worker and family and moves the locus of action from the worker to the family. It also reorients the interpretive activity, that is, the purveying of meaning about the significance, the relevance, the purpose of a family's actions and goal attainment from the worker to the family.

This interpretive activity is among a family's most important activities. Rather than having a worker provide a theory-laden interpretation of reasons that a family is experiencing a problem, why it should choose a particular course of action, and the significance of an outcome, from a strengths perspective a family develops its own understanding from its own perspective of the problem, of action to be taken and the significance of an outcome. A family's interpretive framing of facts and events serves as the process through which its decisions are made as to actions taken and whether goals are fulfilled, and it serves as the basis for future action.

In the absence of a family-centered perspective, a worker maintains control of the interpretive process. The notion that a worker will reveal to a family what is wrong and what should be done to correct the problem and will determine when the problem is resolved is a powerful perspective inherent in the role of outside expert. Theories are useful to workers because they can dispute and undermine family-based interpretations and reorient a family's interpretations to be congruent with those of the worker's. Proponents of widely varying theories counter challenges to a theory's tenets by charging critics as being guilty of resistance (Freud) (Torrey, 1992), class consciousness (Marx) (Lukacs, 1923/1971), sabotage (Derrida) (Lehman, 1992), or whatever a theory allows an apologist to use to counter criticism of the theory by criticizing the critic. Theories, as interpretive schemes, are a powerful tool because they not only structure but also justify the thoughts and actions of a worker who invokes them and exonerate the worker of blame if a situation goes awry.

The implicit objection to a family-centered approach to interpretation is that it usurps the power of experts and social and legal institutions and undermines one of the primary roles of those sanctioned by social and legal institutions as experts. The idea that families may have the wisdom to understand and act to solve problems is contrary to deficit models used by many workers. That is why theory-based, deficit-oriented practice models clash with strengths-based practice. In the final analysis, it is an issue of who has the power and control, who will decide, and, ultimately, who will benefit.

Given family preservation's current state and what has been discussed above, the role family preservation practice can play in custodial grandparenting becomes more evident. Gottfried and Gottfried (1994) state, "The body of accumulating evidence across various types of non-traditional families shows no clear, consistent, or convincing evidence that alterations in family structure per se are detrimental to children's development." Grandparents have been termed "silent saviors of children from faltering families" (Robertson, 1995), the "second line of defense" (Kornhaber, 1996), and "stabilizers during divorce and remarriage" (Barranti, 1985). Grandparents provide a historical link that puts younger generations in touch with their family history and provides a sense of continuity (Robertson, 1995). In the absence of parents to pass on the culture and family heritage to children, grandparents are a excellent alternative. They will be biologically, historically, and most often culturally matched with their grandchildren. Because a family preservation perspective is respectful of a family's ethnic, cultural, and religious background and values and community ties, such a perspective holds many advantages for work in custodial grandparenting.

Grandparents vary in the degree to which they become involved in caring for grandchildren, the degree to which they desire such involvement, and the manner in which they help in raising their grandchildren. Neugarten and Weinstein's five grandparenting role categories (Crandall, 1991) of biological renewal, emotional fulfillment, resource person, vicarious achievement, and remote suggest the degree to which one might expect a grandparent to want and to be able to fulfill a custodial grandparenting role. Except for the last one, these roles characterize desirable qualities also found in parents. When these roles are fulfilled by grandparents, there is the added benefit of the knowledge and skill that grandparents have gained during the years subsequent to having raised their own children. They are able to bring such knowledge and skill to their grandchildren's lives and to impart understanding to grandchildren that only they, as grandparents, can.

From a family preservation perspective, one works, whenever possible, toward an inclusive model of parenting, in which grandparents and parents contribute, as they are able, to the support and nurture of the children. As problems get resolved and circumstances change, responsibilities for parenting also shift. However, when it is no longer possible for the children to be raised by their parents, the custodial grandparenting family ceases to be temporary or transitional.

Custodial grandparenting may be short- or long-term. A grandparent may have temporary custody while the parent or parents achieve economic stability, work through a substance abuse problem, serve time in incarceration, or work out an emotional difficulty. During these periods the parents may visit the child and perform some parental functions while the grandparents provide stability and consistency. When the custodial relationship becomes long-term, consideration of grandparents' well-being becomes especially important. Whereas in older approaches to child welfare the focus was on a child's well-being, family preservation focuses on the well-being of all family members. A long-term relationship cannot remain viable if a child is well cared for and nurtured but caregivers are experiencing distress.

Therefore, let us look at some negative effects of raising grandchildren, effects that would be positively addressed from a family preservation perspective. Roe, Minkler, and Saunders (1995) and Burton (1992) studied the experiences of Black grandmothers and great-grandmothers who were raising their grandchildren because of the drug dependence of the parents. Among the most commonly articulated experiences was high levels of stress. All the respondents in Burton's study indicated they experienced some form of stress in their current life situation. Eighty-six percent of the respondents reported feeling depressed or anxious most of the time; 61% noted that they were smoking more than they ever had in their lives. Central themes voiced by caregivers in the Roe, Minkler, and Saunders study were the significant loss of freedom, the feeling of being cheated out of the middle or later period of their lives, and the sense of having moved backward in time. Also, they worried about their ability to maintain the necessary physical and emotional stamina for at least another decade and expressed profound fear about what would happen to their grandchildren if something happened to them.

Kornhaber (1996) notes that caretaking grandparents frequently complain about the inadequacy of social agencies in dealing with their problems. Financial problems are often cited by grandparents raising grandchildren. More than two thirds of grandparents in the Roe, Minkler, and Saunders (1995) study reported that their income was inadequate to meet their grandchildren's needs. In Burton's study, 77% of respondents stated that they needed economic assistance to care for their grandchildren. The need for social support for grandparent caregivers was often mentioned. Because grandparenting one's grandchildren is an experience outside the normative life cycle (Merriwether-de Vries, Burton, & Eggletion, 1996), many grandparents expressed the need for support and appreciation for their efforts.

For custodial grandparenting to succeed, these issues must be addressed. Family preservation practice offers an approach to addressing such concerns because the focus is not solely on the child but on all members of the family, not only on individual well-being but on interpersonal well-being. A family preservation worker focuses on helping the entire family to meet its biopsychosocial needs. For grandparents, the biological and physiological concerns include overall health and health care, nutrition, physical strength, and stamina. Psychological and behavioral concerns include overall mental health, stress and anxiety, speed of behavior (i.e., how quickly one acts or reacts), and learning and memory. Social and environmental concerns include changes in social patterns (not just with the children and grandchildren but also with other family members and relatives, friends, and spouse), financial issues, shelter, mobility and transportation, social support, privacy, time for other activity, and autonomy.

Given two levels of family preservation practice—(1) intensive family preservation practice, designed primarily as a crisis-oriented intervention, and (2) midlevel family preservation practice, designed to address more directly long-term development and enrichment—a combination of the two is probably the most effective for custodial grandparenting families experiencing significant change or distress and in need of long-term stability and viability.

For grandparents, issues calling for immediate attention may include their health and stamina to care for grandchildren without undue stress or exertion. A family preservation worker will consider the needs of grandparents to maintain and care for the grandchild and also assess speed of behavior and learning and memory to determine if formal services are needed to complement grandparents' abilities to care for the grandchild. Knowing that social patterns will change in a custodial relationship and knowing that those relationships may be central to maintaining mental health and family viability, the family preservation worker will address how such social patterns with the grandparents' children and other family members and friends will be maintained. Concerns about the effect of the custodial relationship on the grandparent couple also must be addressed. It is not uncommon for one grandparent to be more enthusiastic than the other about creating and maintaining a custodial relationship with a grandchild. The emotional burden and differing workloads arising under such conditions may create significant stress that, if not resolved, may harm both the custodial relationship and the marital one. Custodial grandparenting may create financial hardship. At a time in one's life when one may be on fixed income, assistance programs may not suffice to meet the family's financial needs.

The family preservation worker is aware of the need to address all these and other issues and understands the need to determine how these various concerns may be interrelated. In family preservation practice, a partnership of family members and worker is created (Berry, 1997). The worker, acting primarily as a facilitator, assists the family, in this case the grandparents, grandchild, and others, to identify issues for work, to formulate problem-solving strategies, to initiate action to resolve problems, and to assess outcomes and the need for future action. This partnership is designed to allow grandparents and grandchild to meet needs and to continue to enrich the lives of family members through decisions and actions that are family-centered.

Custodial grandparenting requires considerable time, effort, and resources. Despite the impositions and difficulties of custodial grandparenting, there are also many rewards. In Merriwether-de Vries, Burton, and Eggletion (1996), the rewards were expressed as another chance to do it right, parenting with more effectiveness in part due to the lessons learned from the first experience; the ability to nurture family legacies and traditions through the lives of the grandchildren; and finally, the receipt of the unconditional love and supportive companionship of a child. In Minkler and Roe (1993) the custodial grandparents often remarked that the joy and reward of raising their grandchildren came from knowing that the grandchildren were safe and had been given a better chance to succeed. All the children in Minkler and Roe's study had parents who were crack-addicted and their lives before coming to live with grandparents had been precarious at best. After worrying about crack-addicted children, grandparents were often relieved and grateful at the chance to do something positive for the family.

Family preservation practice, whether intensive family preservation or practice designed to address issues over the long term, addresses the needs of all members of the family. Custodial grandparenting, even with its burdens, can be made more effective through involvement of family preservation workers who understand that a family's viability and continued growth and enrichment rests on having all family members nurtured and supported. Family preservation practice will continue to develop means to ensure the inclusion of all family members across the life span to enhance family viability and growth.

REFERENCES

Barranti, C. C. (1985). The grandparent-grandchild relationship: Family resource in an era of voluntary bonds. *Family Relations, 34,* 343–352.

Berry, M. (1992). An evaluation of family preservation services: Fitting agency services to family needs. *Social Work, 37,* 314–321.

Berry, M. (1997). *The family at risk.* Columbia: University of South Carolina Press.

Burton, L. (1992). Black grandparents rearing children of drug-addicted parents: Stressors, outcomes, and social service needs. *Gerontologist, 32,* 744–751.

Cowger, C. D. (1992). Assessment of client strengths. In D. Saleebey (Ed.), *The strengths perspective in social work practice* (pp. 139–147). White Plains, NY: Longman.

Crandall, R. C. (1991). *Gerontology: A behavioral science approach* (2nd ed.). New York: McGraw-Hill.

Goldstein, H. (1992). Victors or victims: Contrasting views of clients in social work practice. In D. Saleeby (Ed.), *The strengths perspective in social work practice* (pp. 27–38). White Plains, NY: Longman.

Gottfried, A. E., & Gottfried, A. W. (1994). *Redefining families: Implications for children's development.* New York: Plenum.

Kornhaber, A. (1996). *Contemporary grandparenting.* Newbury Park, CA: Sage Publications.

Lehman, D. (1992). *Signs of the times: Deconstruction and the fall of Paul de Man.* New York: Poseidon.

Lukacs, G. (1971). *History and class consciousness: Studies in Marxist dialectics* (Trans. R. Livingstone). Cambridge, MA: MIT Press. (Original work published 1923)

Merriwether-de Vries, M., Burton, L., & Eggletion, L. (1996). In J. Graber, J. Brooks-Gunn, & A. Petersen (Eds.), *Transitions through adolescence: Interpersonal domains and context* (pp. 7–31). Hightown, NJ: Erlbaum.

Minkler, M., & Roe, K. (1993). *Forgotten caregivers: Grandmothers raising children of the crack cocaine epidemic.* Newbury Park, CA: Sage.

Robertson, J. (1995). Grandparenting in an era of rapid change. In R. Bleiszner & V. H. Bedford (Eds.), *Handbook of aging and the family* (pp. 243–260). Westport, CT: Greenwood.

Roe, K., Minkler, M., & Saunders, F. (1995). Combining research, advocacy and education: The methods of the grandparent caregiver study. *Health Education Quarterly, 21,* 458–475.

Smith, E. P., & Merkel-Holguin, L. (Eds.). (1995). Lessons from the past: A history of child welfare [Special issue]. *Child Welfare, 74*(1).

Swift, K. J. (1995). An outrage to common decency: Historical perspectives on child neglect. *Child Welfare, 74*(1), 71–91.

Torrey, E. F. (1992). *Freudian fraud: The malignant effect of Freud's theory on American thought and culture.* New York: Harper Collins.

CHAPTER 3

Perceptions of Grandparents' Influence in the Lives of Their Grandchildren

Bert Hayslip Jr., R. Jerald Shore, and Craig E. Henderson

Relative to work on grandparenting in middle and later life, the topic of grandparent-grandchild relationships has historically not been the subject of intense empirical research, although there has been an increase in such work over the past decade (see Kornhaber, 1996). Despite the increase in research on grandparents' relationships with their grandchildren, most of what exists reflects data gathered from the grandparent's perspective; thus, comparatively few studies have specifically addressed perceptions of the grandchild-grandparent connection from the grandchild's viewpoint. For example, recent work by Bence and Blackburn (1992), Sanders and Trystad (1993), Stricker and Hillman (1994), Hodgson (1992), Roberto and Stroes (1992), and Kennedy (1990, 1992a, 1992b) suggests that perceptions of grandparents vary, mediated by both the *gender of the grandparent*, with grandmothers typically, but not always, being perceived more positively; *grandparent health*, favoring those in better health (see Greasey & Kahiler, 1994); *frequency of contact*, favoring those grandparents with whom the grandchild reported greater everyday contact (see Kivett, 1991); and the *presence of conflictual relationships within the family*, particularly regarding the quality of the marital relationship between the child's parents as well as that of the adult parent's relationship to his or her parent (see Cherlin & Furstenberg, 1986). These and other studies also suggest that perceptions of grandparents vary by grandchild characteristics such as age, gender, or lineage position of the child relative to the grandparent. Hoffman (1979–1980) found that maternal grandmothers were viewed most positively, while Tetrick (1990) found that grandmothers were preferred over grandfathers, irrespective of kinship position.

In contrast, Walther-Lee and Stricker (1998) found that when all four grandparents were known to the grandchildren, no differences in perceptions of closeness were observed in a sample of young adults. Grandparents to whom grandchildren felt close were, however, perceived as kinder, warmer, and gentler than those grandparents who were seen as less close. As perceptions of closeness are colored by familiarity and geographic proximity (Walter-Lee & Sticker, 1998), generalized perceptions of grandparents are also confounded by feelings of closeness (Emick & Hayslip, 1996). For this reason, variables other than closeness and positiveness of the relationship might be more desirable parameters of the quality of the bond between grandchild and grandparent.

These findings highlight the individualistic nature of perceptions of grandparenting by grandchildren. Thus, a relativistic, multidimensional approach to this issue may more realistically portray the role that grandparents play in their grandchildren's lives.

In light of the phenomenon of custodial grandparenting (Shore & Hayslip, 1994), it is important to note that positive perceptions of one's grandparents lay the groundwork for the transmission to younger generations of family values, culturally bound traditions and practices, and behavioral and vocational expectations, as well as facilitating identity development among children and adolescents. Relationships with grandparents that are perceived as valuable and beneficial are also highly relevant should the grandparent be asked to take on the responsibility of raising the grandchild in the event of a parent's death, divorce, incapacitation, or incarceration, or should questions regarding spousal abuse, or the physical, sexual, or emotional abuse of the child arise (Hayslip, Shore, Henderson, & Lambert, 1998).

As previous work suggests that perception of the quality of grandparenting may vary with both the age and gender of the grandchild (see Emick & Hayslip, 1996, 1999; Kornhaber, 1996), this chapter explores variations in the perceived influence of grandparents in the lives of their grandchildren.

METHOD

Participants

Participants for this study were 181 children (64 males, 117 females), who were recruited through junior high, high school, and college classes in the Dallas–Ft. Worth Metroplex. Sixty-nine adolescent grandchildren aged 14–18 and 112 young adult grandchildren aged 19–24 completed a battery of measures ascertaining five dimensions of perceptions of grandparenting.

Assessment

The first assessed the extent to which the grandparent engaged in parent-like behavior with the grandchild, such as giving advice on a variety of personal and vocational matters and meting out discipline, which was defined by 8 Likert-type items. The second measured the degree to which the grandparent had regular contact with the grandchild, in terms of the extent to which the grandparent was present at family functions or the frequency with which he or she interacted with the grandchild. This was defined by 5 items. The third defined the extent to which the grandparent helped the parent raise the grandchild, such as cooking for or dressing the grandchild, taking the child to the park or to church, assisting the child with his or her homework, or sharing child care responsibilities with the parent. This was defined by 6 items. The fourth measured the perceived degree of the grandparent's direct and positive influence on the grandchild's life, in terms of making vocational or educational choices, influencing religious values, shaping the use of the child's free time, helping in the learning of new skills, aiding the grandchild in problem solving, or passing on traits similar to those of the grandparent. This was assessed by 10 questions. The fifth dimension, defined in terms of 5 items, reflected the breadth of influence in the grandchild's family, such as being emotionally available, being consulted on family decisions, having authority in the family or in resolving family conflicts. Alpha coefficient estimates of each scale's internal consistency that were derived for both grandmothers and grandfathers for each kinship position (i.e., maternal and paternal) suggested that with the exception of grandparental contact, each scale was internally consistent, with alpha coefficients ranging from .77 to .92. for all subscales. For grandparental contact, alpha coefficients failed to exceed .50. Correlations among these five dimensions within kinship position ranged from .02 (Contact and Raise grandchild) to .78 (Parenting and Breadth).

Scoring

Separate scores in each of these five domains were derived from grandchildren's responses to the above dimensions, pertaining separately in a fixed order to the maternal grandmother, paternal grandfather, paternal grandmother, and paternal grandfather, wherein each child, adolescent, or young adult reported on each of four grandparents, to the extent that each was still living. In this sample, of the 181 participants, 116 were able to report on a paternal grandfather, 141 reported on a maternal grandfather, 150 discussed a paternal grandmother, and 156 discussed a maternal grandmother. All responses were gathered with reference to the respondent's biological parents.

RESULTS AND DISCUSSION

These data were first analyzed via a series of 2 (gender of grandchild) × 2 (age level: age 14–18 vs. age 19–24) MANOVAs. These analyses indicated that for each kinship/gender target combination (resulting in four separate analyses), there was neither a multivariate main effect for age nor a multivariate Gender × Age interaction on perceptions of grandparenting. Multivariate main effects for grandchild gender ($p < .01$) were, however, substantial in each case and were particular to grandparental help in raising the grandchild and breadth of grandparental influence. As Table 3.1 suggests, for all combinations of grandparent gender and kinship position (maternal vs. paternal), male grandchildren reported more grandparental involvement in their upbringing and greater breadth of influence in their everyday lives than did female grandchildren.

A supplementary MANOVA utilizing approximately half the sample ($n = 86$) who had complete data for all combinations of grandparent kinship position and grandparent gender was conducted, again varying grandchild gender and grandchild age. In this case, however, grandparent gender and kinship position were specifically incorporated as within-subject variables, wherein grandparent gender was nested within kinship position. This analysis yielded a statistically significant multivariate Grandchild gender × Grandparent gender interaction ($F_{6, 77} = 3.84$, $p < .01$). This was particular to the perception of the grandparents helping to raise the grandchild ($F_{1, 82} = 4.63$, $p < .05$) and grandparent contact ($F_{1, 82} = 5.27$, $p < .03$).

Ignoring the grandparent contact variable in light of its low internal consistency (see above), data indicated that although females attributed more parental salience to their relationships with their grandmothers, males saw grandmothers and grandfathers as equally involved in their upbringing (see Table 3.2), though means for males tended to favor grandmothers as well. Such effects generalized across kinship position of the grandparent, consistent with findings by Walther-Lee and Stricker (1998). This analysis also yielded a strong multivariate main effect for grandparent gender ($F_{6, 77} = 8.42$, $p < .01$), which generalized across all dimensions of grandparenting, where grandmothers were perceived as being more parental, were more directly involved in raising the child, had a more direct and positive influence on the child, exerted greater breadth of influence on the child, and interacted more frequently with the child than did grandfathers. The reduced sample analyses reflect the salience of grandmothers in the lives of grandchildren, especially for adolescent and young adult women, a finding that has been reported elsewhere a number of times (e.g., Kennedy, 1990; Roberto & Stroes, 1992). This may be due to the predisposition to see grandmothers as more nurturant, perhaps based on age and gender stereotypes, but it is

TABLE 3.1 Gender Effects in Perceptions of Grandparents

	Male Grandchildren								Female Grandchildren							
	PGF		MGF		PGM		MGM		PGF		MGF		PGM		MGM	
	M	SD	M	SD	M	SD	M	SD	M	SD	M	SD	M	SD	M	SD
Parental behaviors	19.91	8.05	19.33	8.04	19.58	8.28	19.31	7.53	18.39	7.75	18.53	7.44	18.90	7.52	18.90	7.82
Contact	15.41	3.38	15.41	3.51	15.10	3.39	15.18	3.31	15.32	2.51	15.31	2.59	15.31	2.58	15.20	2.58
Raise Gc	13.32	5.76	12.95	5.90	13.17	5.91	12.98	5.49	11.53	4.85	11.54	4.85	11.61	4.49	11.80	4.80
Direct influence	32.87	5.49	32.15	6.05	32.48	5.65	31.66	6.42	30.29	8.63	30.68	8.13	30.65	8.17	30.78	8.21
Breadth of influence	13.57	5.97	13.55	6.14	13.51	6.12	13.55	5.85	11.54	5.23	11.60	5.05	11.53	4.92	11.90	5.06

PGF = Paternal grandfather (n = 116).
MGF = Maternal grandfather (n = 141).
PGM = Paternal grandmother (n = 150).
MGM = Maternal grandmother (n = 156).
Gc = Grandchild.
M = Mean.
SD = Standard deviation.

TABLE 3.2   Perceptions of Grandparents by Gender of Grandchild
(*N* = 86)

	Female Gc				Male Gc			
	Female GP		Male GP		Female GP		Male GP	
	M	*SD*	*M*	*SD*	*M*	*SD*	*M*	*SD*
Parental behaviors	21.17	5.06	17.15	5.46	18.87	6.94	17.10	7.20
Contact	15.71	2.02	15.14	2.43	15.89	2.52	14.14	3.40
Raise Gc	12.42	2.97	10.58	3.20	13.12	4.17	11.34	4.60
Direct influence	33.03	5.01	30.18	6.12	33.07	4.12	32.44	4.16
Breadth of influence	12.38	3.86	11.52	4.39	12.75	4.89	11.62	5.79

Gc = Grandchild.
GP = Grandparent.
M = Mean.
SD = Standard deviation.

also a function of (female) grandchildren's greater contact with them. This hypothesis was confirmed in an analysis of the determinants of grandparental contact by Uhlenberg and Hammill (1998), utilizing data from the National Survey of Families and Households (*N* = 4629).

The findings here also suggest, of course, that grandfathers are less likely to be perceived as being salient in their grandchildren's lives. This poses both a challenge and an opportunity for grandfathers to reverse their grandchildren's stereotypic perceptions of them as distant or symbolic family figures, perhaps by becoming more assertively involved in their grandchildren's everyday lives. This may be especially true for grandfathers who are married, relative to grandfathers who are either divorced, remarried, or separated, who had greater contact with their grandchildren (Uhlenberg & Hammill, 1998). They therefore may serve as viable role models for their male grandchildren. This also may be true for such middle-aged and older men to whom being a positive grandparent is important.

In light of the relationship of geographical proximity to grandparent kinship position (e.g., Cherlin & Furstenberg, 1986; Hoffman, 1979–1980; Kennedy, 1990), as well as the relationship of geographical proximity and grandchild-grandparent closeness (e.g., Hodgson,

1992; Kennedy, 1992a & b), greater attention to the development of positive grandchild-grandparent relations might be paid to both male grandparents and those who live less close to their grandchildren, in the event that such grandparents are asked to raise their children's children. In such cases, realistic expectations about both generations' behavior are less likely to be in place, resulting in a more difficult adjustment for both grandchildren and grandparent. Moreover, as the quality of relationships between grandchild and grandparent are mediated by the middle-generation parent (see Shore & Hayslip, 1994; Somary & Stricker, 1998; Uhlenberg & Hammill, 1998), greater effort also might be invested by adult children and their parents into maintaining both frequency of contact and meaningful involvement in one another's lives, providing the grandchildren with varied opportunities to know their grandparents as individuals capable of behaving in many ways—as role models, advisors, mentors, and sources of emotional support.

The grandchild gender differences found here in perceptions of grandparenting suggest that, for both adolescent and young adult males, grandparents are seen as exerting a great deal of everyday influence in family decision making, in the resolution of conflict within the family, as sources of advice, and in influencing how the parent raises the grandchild. Moreover, such perceived influence is equally salient in the lives of both adolescent and young adult samples of grandchildren, wherein one might otherwise predict that as grandparents' health worsens and their grandchildren's lives diversify, the latter's perceptions of their grandparents would reflect lessened intergenerational influences in their everyday lives (Kahana & Kahana, 1970, 1971).

In contrast to the view of grandparenting as a role that carries with it little status, as Rosow (1985) has argued, especially as the grandchildren themselves grow older (see Kahana & Kahana, 1970, 1971), these findings highlight grandparents as both active role models for young males and pivotal figures in concert with parents in the extended family of many grandchildren, irrespective of the age of the grandchild. Such influence may be a function of the verticalization of the family (Hagestad, 1988), enhancing the likelihood of children's interacting with their grandparents in other than role-bound, symbolic ways, as well as reflecting the increased influence of grandparents in their grandchildren's lives in either the dual-income or single parent family situations that characterize American culture today (see Bengtson, Rosenthal, & Burton, 1990; Hagestad, 1988).

These findings are also especially significant in light of other research that we have recently published (Emick & Hayslip, 1999; Hayslip et al., 1998), which suggests that, in two independent samples of both traditional and custodial grandparents, male children are more likely to be exhibit a variety of problem behaviors as a consequence of either of those circumstances leading to their being raised by their grandparents or as a function of the interaction of preexisting difficulties attributed to dysfunction in their families of origin and either deficits in the grandparent's parenting skills or problems in relationships with grandparents who are now raising them. Significantly, such children may have enjoyed less confrontational relationships with these same grandparents prior to the death, divorce, or incapacitation of their parents. These data indicate that this may be true in certain cases. One might speculate on the fate of such grandchildren raised by their grandparents if such interpersonal resources had instead been utilized to improve grandchild-grandparent communication, rather than becoming a source of distress for custodial grandparents, perhaps in the context of intergenerational family therapy, parent training or retraining, or stress management programs targeting both grandchild and grandparent. Attention to the antecedents of grandparents' expectations of their roles has been underscored in work by Somary and Stricker (1998), who studied grandparents prior to and after the birth of their grandchildren. This issue has yet to be explored in custodial grandparent research, and longitudinal work might be particularly valuable.

Not unexpectedly, the present findings are limited in that they rely on a self-selected sample of both early and late adolescents, as well young adults, and therefore may not generalize to either younger or older adult grandchildren. Being self-report in nature, these findings might also benefit from confirmatory data gathered from the grandparents themselves to examine the congruence of intergenerational perceptions of the grandchild-grandparent relationship. We also encourage others to cross-validate these findings with either minority or economically disadvantaged samples of grandchildren, as well as stepgrandparents.

Despite these limitations, the data suggest an enhanced role for future cohorts of grandparents in shaping their grandchildren's lives, in contrast to a perspective that clearly delineates parental and grandparental role boundaries as influences on the well-being and life adjustment of grandchildren. In view of the increasing numbers of grandparents who are raising their grandchildren, greater attention to those factors laying a positive groundwork for grandchildren-grandparent relationships that are both realistic and mutually supportive seems warranted.

REFERENCES

Bence, S., & Blackburn, J. (1992, November). *The effect of mothers' and grandmothers' perceived responsibility for children on children's compliance.* Paper presented at the annual scientific meeting of the Gerontological Society of America. Washington, DC.

Bengtson, V. L., Rosenthal, C., & Burton, L. (1990). Families and aging: Diversity and heterogeneity. In R. Binstock & E. Shanas (Eds.), *Handbook of aging and the social sciences* (pp. 267–287). New York: Academic Press.

Cherlin, A., & Furstenberg, F. (1986). *The new American grandparent: A place in the family, a life apart.* New York: Basic Books.

Emick, M., & Hayslip, B. (1996). Custodial grandparenting: New roles for middle-aged and older adults. *International Journal of Aging and Human Development, 43,* 135–154.

Emick, M., & Hayslip, B. (1999). Custodial grandparenting: Stresses, coping skills, and relationships with grandchildren. *International Journal of Aging and Human Development, 48,* 38–61.

Greasey, G., & Kahiler, G. (1994). Differences in grandchildren's perceptions of relations with grandparents. *Journal of Adolescence, 17,* 411–426.

Hagestad, G. (1988). Demographic change and the life course: Some emerging trends in the family realm. *Family Relations, 37,* 405–410.

Hayslip, B., Shore, R. J., Henderson, C., & Lambert, P. (1998). Custodial grandparenting and the impact of grandchildren with problems on role satisfaction and role meaning. *Journal of Gerontology: Social Sciences, 53B,* 5164–5174.

Hodgson, L. (1992). Adult grandchildren and their grandparents: The enduring bond. In J. Hendricks (Ed.), *Ties in later life* (pp. 155–170). Amityville, NY: Baywood.

Hoffman, E. (1979–1980). Young adults' relations with their grandparents: An exploratory study. *International Journal of Aging and Human Development, 10,* 299–309.

Kahana, E., & Kahana, B. (1970). Grandparenthood from the point of view of the developing grandchild. *Developmental Psychology, 3,* 98–105.

Kahana, E., & Kahana, B. (1971). Theoretical and research perspectives on grandparenthood. *Aging and Human Development, 2,* 261–268.

Kennedy, G. (1990). College students' expectations of grandparent and grandchild role behaviors. *Gerontologist, 30,* 43–48.

Kennedy, G. (1992a). Quality in grandchild/grandparent relationships. *International Journal of Aging and Human Development, 35,* 83–98.

Kennedy, G. (1992b). Shared activities of grandparents and grandchildren. *Psychological Reports, 70,* 221–227.

Kivett, V. (1991). The grandparent-grandchild connection. *Marriage and Family Review, 16,* 267–290.

Kornhaber, A. (1996). *Contemporary grandparenting.* Thousand Oaks, CA: Sage.

Roberto, K., & Stroes, J. (1992). Grandchildren and grandparents: Roles, influences, and relationships. *International Journal of Aging and Human Development, 34,* 227–239.

Rosow, I. (1985). Status and role change throughout the life span. In R. Binstock & E. Shanas (Eds.), *Handbook of aging and the social sciences* (pp. 62–93). New York: Van Nostrand Reinhold.

Sanders, G., & Trystad, D. (1993). Strengths in the grandchild-grandparent relationship. *Activities, Adaptation, and Aging, 17,* 43–53.

Shore, R. J., & Hayslip, B. (1994). Custodial grandparenting: Implications for children's development. In A. Gottfried & A. Gottfried (Eds.), *Redefining families: Implications for children's development* (pp. 171–218). New York: Plenum.

Somary, K., & Stricker, G. (1998). Becoming a grandparent: A longitudinal study of expectations and early experiences as a function of sex and lineage. *Gerontologist, 38,* 53–61.

Stricker, G., & Hillman, J. (1994, November). *Attitudes toward older adults: The perceived value of grandparents as a social role.* Paper presented at the annual scientific meeting of the Gerontological Society of America, Atlanta.

Tetrick, A. N. (1990). The grandchild-grandparent bond: Its relationship to child adjustment in intact and divorced/separated family structures. *Dissertation Abstracts International, 46,* 2827A.

Uhlenberg, P., & Hammill, B. (1998). Frequency of grandparent contact with grandchild sets: Six factors that make a difference. *Gerontologist, 38,* 276–285.

Walther-Lee, D., & Stricker, G. (1998, August). *The bases of closeness between grandchildren and grandparents.* Paper presented at the annual convention of the American Psychological Association, San Francisco.

CHAPTER 4

Custodial Grandparenting of the Difficult Child: Learning from the Parenting Literature

Persephanie Silverthorn
and Sarah L. Durrant

Mental health problems affect a significant number of children, with as many as 14%–22% of children experiencing an emotional or behavioral problem during childhood or adolescence (e.g., Anderson, Williams, McGee, & Silva, 1987; Cohen et al., 1993; Costello et al., 1996; Costello, Farmer, Angold, Burns, & Erkanli, 1997; Schaffer et al., 1996; Simonoff et al., 1997). Childhood disorders are typically divided into internalizing (e.g., depression, anxiety) and externalizing disorders (e.g., attention problems, conduct problems) (Frick, 1998b; Frick & Silverthorn, in press). Although both types of disorders are problematic for children, externalizing behaviors are the most likely to cause difficulties with parents, teachers, and peers. During childhood and adolescence, between 7% and 25% of children are diagnosed with ODD (oppositional defiant disorder) or CD (conduct disorder) (Webster-Stratton & Hammond, 1997), although estimates range as high as 35%

(McDermott, 1996). These disorders are also the most common diagnoses seen by school mental health teams (Atkins, McKay, Talbott, & Arvantis, 1996) and practicing psychologists (Kazdin, Siegel, & Bass, 1990), accounting for one-third to one-half of referrals. Early intervention is important for these children, since approximately 75% of boys diagnosed with ODD retain their diagnoses or progress to CD, and approximately 50% of all boys diagnosed with CD in childhood can be expected to continue their conduct problems through adolescence and adulthood (e.g., Frick, 1998a; Lahey et al., 1995; Lahey, Loeber, Quay, Frick, Grimm, 1992; Moffitt, 1993). Girls with disruptive behavior problems are also at considerable risk, with the vast majority (up to 86%) manifesting psychological disturbances in adulthood (Silverthorn & Frick, 1999).

Grandparents may be particularly susceptible to parenting children with disruptive behavior problems. For example, children born to substance-abusing mothers are at substantial risk for developmental and behavioral problems (Pinson-Milburn, Fabian, Schlossberg, & Pyle, 1996; Zuckerman & Frank, 1992) and the increased use of crack cocaine is considered one of the primary reasons for the dramatic increase in the number of children placed in foster care since the mid-1980s (Grant, Gordon, & Cohen, 1997). Recent epidemiological data suggest that custodial grandparenting is by no means transitory or inconsequential: nearly half of grandparents (43%) become custodians for their grandchildren when the child is an infant, and an almost equal number (41%) care for their grandchildren for 5 or more years (Fuller-Thomson, Minkler, & Driver, 1997).

Research on the prevalence of behavior problems in grandchildren raised by custodial grandparents and on psychological treatments obtained for these children is limited. The prevailing belief is that increasing numbers of grandparents are seeking psychological help for their grandchildren (e.g., Emick & Hayslip, 1996), and recent data from a community-recruited sample showed that 40% of custodial grandparents had obtained therapeutic services for their grandchildren and 25% were planning to seek mental health services in the immediate future (Shore & Hayslip, 1990, 1994). Data from a large epidemiological sample indicate that children living with their custodial grandparents are at a greater risk of experiencing school problems than are children residing with two biological parents, but they share similar risks with those living with a single parent (Solomon & Marx, 1995). However, the data suggest that children residing solely with their grandparents differ from those in two-parent and one-parent families in important ways. Specifically, grand-parent-headed families are more likely to be African-American (49.5%), to be unemployed (57.8%), and to have fewer years of education (10.4%), compared to two-parent families (12%, 37.4%, and 12.9%, respectively) and one-parent families (32%, 36.4%, and 12.1%, respectively) (Solomon & Marx, 1995).

Although information about behavior problems in grandchildren living with custodial grandparents is limited, it is important for custodial grandparents to be aware of potential behavior problems in their grandchildren and to know when those behaviors warrant psychotherapeutic intervention. In addition, it is important for custodial grandparents to be aware of empirically supported treatments that may offer amelioration of these behavior problems. Although few, if any, interventions have been specifically investigated with custodial grandparents, the child behavior disorder literature currently offers several empirically supported treatments for disruptive behavior disorders, which have the potential to be generalizable to grandparents.

DISRUPTIVE BEHAVIOR DISORDERS IN CHILDREN AND ADOLESCENTS

As noted, disruptive behavior disorders are frequently found in children and adolescents, with rates estimated to be as high as 25% to 35% (McDermott, 1996; Webster-Stratton & Hammond, 1997). The current *Diagnostic and Statistical Manual of Mental Disorders* (DSM-IV) separates disruptive behavior disorders into two categories: ODD and CD (American Psychiatric Association, 1994). ODD is characterized by a pattern of negativistic, hostile, and defiant behaviors lasting at least 6 months; and CD is characterized by a persistent pattern of violation of societal norms or the rights of others, lasting at least 12 months, with at least one behavior exhibited during the previous 6 months. When symptoms warrant both diagnoses, CD supersedes the diagnosis of ODD (American Psychiatric Association, 1994; Rapoport & Ismond, 1996). Considerable debate has existed as to whether these two disorders are separate and unique or if ODD is simply a mild form of CD. Although many children with ODD do eventually meet criteria for CD, enough evidence exists to support maintaining the distinction between the two disorders (e.g., Lahey et al., 1994).

Understanding both ODD and CD are important, given that these disorders often portend long-lasting negative effects. Recent research suggests that in boys, CD is a heterogeneous disorder with at least two trajectories: a childhood-onset type and an adolescent-onset type (Hinshaw, Lahey, & Hart, 1993; Moffitt, 1993). For girls, there appears to be one trajectory to antisocial behavior: a delayed-onset type (Silverthorn & Frick, 1999). Among boys with childhood onset of CD, a full 50% continue to evidence a persistent pattern of negative behaviors, often lasting through adolescence and adulthood (Frick, 1998b; Lahey et al., 1995; Moffitt, Caspi, Dickson, Silva, & Stanton, 1996), and girls on the delayed-onset pathway tend to exhibit negative outcomes and psychological maladjustment through adulthood (Silverthorn & Frick, 1999). Thus, it is important to intervene as early as possible, with both boys and girls, to lessen the current and future negative impact of antisocial behaviors.

Children exhibiting ODD or CD typically exhibit problem behaviors severe enough to warrant attention from adults; hence the reason that those behaviors are the most frequent cause of referrals to mental health practitioners (Atkins et al., 1996; Kazdin et al., 1990). However, grandparents may avoid treatment for these children, hoping that the behaviors will improve with the passing of time as grandchildren become accustomed to their new living arrangements (e.g., de Toledo & Brown, 1995; Takas, 1995). The DSM-IV designates a category for behaviors due to a particular stressor, adjustment disorder, and requires that the disruptive behaviors appear within 3 months of a particular stressor and resolve within 6 months after the termination of the stressor (American Psychiatric Association, 1994). In addition, if the disruptive behaviors meet criteria for a specific diagnosis (e.g., ODD or CD), regardless of whether other stressors have been present, then that specific diagnosis should be made rather than a diagnosis of adjustment disorder (American Psychiatric Association, 1994; Rapoport & Ismond, 1996). Given these specific criteria and the difficulty in determining when a behavior began, it would appear prudent for custodial grandparents to obtain an assessment from a mental health professional to determine whether the disruptive behaviors are severe enough to warrant diagnosis and intervention.

EFFECTIVENESS OF TREATMENTS FOR DISRUPTIVE BEHAVIOR DISORDERS

At the same time that researchers are beginning to understand the developmental trajectories of disruptive behavior disorders, they are also focusing on the most effective intervention strategies to interrupt the course of those disorders. Due to a variety of sociopolitical forces, psychologists are under pressure to define empirically supported treatments, leading to several "special" issues of journals devoted to describing such types of interventions (e.g., Chambliss & Hollon, 1998; Lonigan, Elbert, & Bennett, 1998). Meta-analytic techniques are often used to determine the overall effectiveness of psychological interventions (e.g., Weisz & Weiss, 1993). Within the past decade, several large meta-analytic studies have been conducted for child and adolescent treatments, and the effect sizes suggest that, by the end of treatment, 76% to 81% of children and adolescents in the treatment groups made improvements when compared to control (no-treatment) children (Weisz & Hawley, 1998). Several different types of treatments have been found to be efficacious according to meta-analysis, including cognitive-behavioral (parent training, problem solving, skills training) and family therapy (Weisz & Hawley, 1998; Weisz & Weiss, 1993). Unfortunately, these positive effects typically come from laboratory-based investigations; the few treatments from "everyday clinical practice" have not yielded significant treatment effects (Weisz & Hawley, 1998; see also Weisz, Weiss, & Donenberg, 1992). In addition, research describing the effectiveness of these treatments rarely reports the family composition. Thus, it is not known what proportion of children in these studies live with custodial grandparents nor whether the effectiveness rate differs for children in nontraditional families.

As part of the movement toward defining empirically supported treatments, researchers are attempting to define "well-established treatments" and "probably efficacious treatments" (Lonigan et al., 1998). As might be expected, different treatments emerge as efficacious for children with internalizing disorders and externalizing disorders (Kazdin & Weisz, 1998). According to "29 years, 82 studies, and 5,272 kids," two treatments were designated as "well-established," both of which are parent-training models designed for young children (e.g., up to age 6 or 8 years) (Brestan & Eyberg, 1998). However, neither has been investigated for use with caretakers other than biological parents.

In addition to the two treatments designated as well established, 10 treatment programs were designated as probably efficacious (Brestan & Eyberg, 1998). Of these 10, 4 were designed for preschool children, 2 were designed for school-age children, and 4 were designed for adolescents. Also, four of these treatments are based on parent-training models and another four on cognitive-behavioral skills–training models (see also, Frick, 1998b). Kazdin and Weisz (1998) simultaneously evaluated empirically supported treatments and, similar to Brestan and Eyberg (1998), reported that the two most efficacious interventions for conduct problems and oppositional behaviors are parent-training models and cognitive-behavioral skills–training models (including problem-solving skills training; see also Frick, 1998b). Importantly, treatments based on both models have shown positive effects lasting between 1 and 3 years after treatment or longer (e.g., Kazdin, 1997; Kazdin & Weisz, 1998). Thus, researchers agree that the most effective and empirically supported treatments for oppositional behaviors and conduct problems are based on parent-training models, with cognitive-behavioral skills–training models also showing probable efficacy.

Despite the enthusiasm for these empirically supported treatments, some caveats are warranted. As noted earlier, most of the research investigating treatments have been conducted in the laboratory or university clinic; few are conducted in community-based clinics (Kazdin & Weisz, 1998). This is problematic for several reasons. First, most research studies use families specifically recruited for a clinic-based treatment study. This situation differs from community-based clinics, where the therapists typically have heavier caseloads and the clients often have more stressors and comorbid disorders (Weisz & Hawley, 1998). Second, research typically compares those who completed training with those in a no-treatment control group. However, in the "real world," between 40% and 60% of families drop out of treatment prematurely (Kazdin, 1996), which may be higher for parent-management models (Kazdin, 1997) and may differ for households headed by custodial grandparents or caretakers other than the biological parent. Premature termination can have the effect of increasing the perceived effectiveness of therapy, because only completers are included in the final analysis. In addition, most manualized treatments, including empirically supported treatments, require between 8 and 24 sessions to complete the program. However, most terminations from therapy occur prior to the eighth session (Kazdin & Hawley, 1998).

Third, research supporting the effectiveness of parent-training and cognitive-behavioral skills–training models are typically based on rather homogeneous samples; very little is known about the effectiveness of such treatments across gender and ethnicity. As Brestan and Eyberg (1998) note, the "the 'typical' conduct-disordered child in treatment studies is a 9-year-old Caucasian boy from a lower middle income background" (p. 187). Results of meta-analyses found mixed effects for gender (Weisz & Weiss, 1993), although one recent controlled study found no Gender × Treatment effects (Webster-Stratton, 1996). Nevertheless, the gender and ethnicity composition of research participants potentially differs from that of children seen at community clinics. Fourth, most manualized treatments employed in empirical investigations are designed for younger children with mild to moderate conduct problems. This often does not mirror clients at community clinics, where the children tend to be older and the behaviors tend to be more severe (Kazdin & Weisz, 1998; Weisz & Hawley, 1998). There is some evidence that research-based treatments are effective for adolescents, especially when the behaviors are not severe (see Kazdin & Weisz, 1998); however, treatments for conduct problems are most effective in children age 8 and younger (Frick, 1998b). Recent empirically supported treatments do offer multicomponent packages designed for severe, violent adolescent offenders (e.g., Henggeler & Bourdin, 1990; see also Frick, 1998b). At this stage of development, however, such treatments have yet to be replicated by research teams outside the original team that developed the program (Kazdin & Weisz, 1998).

Finally, a word of caution must be offered concerning the recent push toward empirically supported treatments. As noted, the number of special issues devoted to investigating such treatments has increased in the past several years, with task forces designed to determine which treatments are efficacious and which are not (e.g.,

Chambless & Hollon, 1998; Lonigan et al., 1998). However, in the 1990s an attempt was made to determine which treatments were effective with children and adolescents, and the two most supported treatments were parent-training models and cognitive-behavioral, skills-training models (Kazdin, 1991). Thus, despite the push in the past several years, the treatments deemed efficacious have not changed substantially. Nevertheless, the research literature offers support of effective interventions that exist for children with disruptive behaviors, with parent-training models receiving the most consistent support, generally with children of all ages (cf., Kazdin, 1997), and with cognitive-behavioral skills training a close second, particularly for children 8 years and older (e.g., Brestan & Eyberg, 1998; Kazdin & Weisz, 1998). Given that no research has investigated the effectiveness of these treatments with children living with custodial grandparents, however, it is unknown if they would be as effective in that population.

THE HOW-TO'S OF PARENT-MANAGEMENT MODELS

As noted, for oppositional, defiant behaviors and mild to moderate conduct problems, parent-management techniques are the first treatment of choice. As described by Frick (1998b), parent-management techniques and the associated components appear deceptively easy (see also, Kazdin, 1997). However, it is important to implement the techniques effectively and appropriately; otherwise, problem behaviors may become even more entrenched. Thus, it is important that parents consult a mental health professional to assist in the implementation of parent-management programs. Most parent-management programs begin with using positive control strategies before any punitive measures are employed. This is based on the notion that (a) relations between parent and child are often coercive and antagonistic prior to the implementation of therapy, and (b) children will learn what to do, rather than what not to do, if their behaviors are praised (Frick, 1998b; Kazdin, 1997). As noted above, research has not been conducted to examine the applicability and efficacy of the parent-management models with nontraditional families. However, custodial grandparents as well as other nonbiological caretakers should be able to make effective use of the basic skills taught in these programs.

Frick (1998b) summarized three of the most popular and available parent-training manuals that therapists employ in the treatment of conduct disorders: *Parent-Child Interaction Therapy* (Hembree-Kigin & McNeil, 1995), *Helping the Noncompliant Child* (Forehand & McMahon, 1981), and *Defiant Children: A Clinician's Manual for Parent Training* (Barkley, 1987). The first step for all three parent-training models is to begin with a description of the rationale for the particular program. From there the models diverge, although the focus for all three is on increasing positive behaviors and reducing negative behaviors. For parent-child interaction therapy, step 2 involves teaching behavioral play therapy skills to parents, including using special playtime for children (child-directed interactions [CDIs]). During CDIs, the parent uses strategic attention and selective attention. Step 3 includes teaching discipline skills to parents, emphasizing consistency, predictability, and follow-through; giving effective instructions; praising compliance; using time-outs effectively; developing house rules; and improving public behaviors.

In *Helping the Noncompliant Child,* step 2 involves using differential attention to shape behavior, including attending to CDIs and using attention to increase positive behaviors, ignoring misbehavior, and implementing contingency management programs for specific behaviors. Step 3 involves compliance training, which means giving effective commands, reinforcing compliance training, using time-outs, and emphasizing consistency. In *Defiant Children,* step 2 also involves using parental attention to shape behaviors. Step 3 consists of increasing the child's compliance through the use of acknowledgments, appreciation, and praise; and in step 4 independent play, that is, playing by oneself while the parent is busy, is reinforced. Step 5 involves developing effective contingency management programs, step 6 teaches time-out, and step 7 teaches how to manage noncompliance in public places. The final step teaches how to manage future problems (summarized in Frick, 1998b).

Although all three of these programs focus on the parent's interactions with a difficult child, they could be adapted for grandparent-grandchild relationships. However, because extenuating circumstances, such as parental substance abuse and parental mental illness, typically contribute to the decision for a child to live primarily with his or her grandparent (Minkler, Roe, & Price, 1992; Woodworth, 1996), it would be wise for a grandparent to seek consultation with a mental health professional to assist with the implementation of these programs. In addition, it is not uncommon for the dynamics of a grandparent-grandchild relationship to differ from the parent-child relationship, not only from the parenting relationship the child has experienced but also from the way in which the grandparent raised the grandchild's parent. For these reasons, assistance with parenting via a mental health specialist is highly recommended (de Toledo & Brown, 1995).

Although the three programs described in Frick (1998b) are designed for use by parents and therapists with preschool and school-age children, similar techniques are effective with adolescents and may be applicable for custodial grandparents. For example, *Parents and Adolescents Living Together* (Patterson & Forgatch, 1987) emphasize similar principles, with a focus on negotiating between the parents' desire for control and the adolescents' desire for autonomy. Step 1 teaches the three levels of compliance training: immediate compliance, cooperation, and following house rules. Step 2 involves teaching how to give effective commands, and step 3 involves teaching the concepts of monitoring (who, what, where, and when) combined with tracking behaviors to see if changes are actually occurring. Step 4 involves implementing effective contingency behavior plans, and using praise and encouragement, followed by introduction of a point-based system. The final step involves the implementation of punishment in three stages: (1) describing for the parent what punishment is and is not; (2) implementing small consequences, with removal of privileges as a backup punishment; and (3) implementing larger consequences that are appropriate and within reason (Patterson & Forgatch, 1987). Again, this program could be implemented by grandparents; however, the energy investment required from the parent or grandparent is considerable, and the grandparent would have to have the ability to follow through with the program. In addition, these programs are often difficult to implement with an adolescent whose behavior problems have been present for some time, which may be the case for children residing with custodial grandparents.

Each of the programs described above is based on parent-management training and is consistent with recent research identifying these techniques as an empirically supported treatment (e.g., Brestan & Eyberg, 1998; Kazdin & Weisz, 1998; see also Frick, 1998b). For children with disruptive behavior disorders, parent-management training appears to be the treatment of choice, and most therapists trained in working with children will be familiar with these types of programs. It would appear that they could be used with custodial grandparents; however, this has not been investigated and is only speculative at this time. Of note, approaches other than parent training have been used, and child cognitive-behavioral skills training also appears to be efficacious, with recent research suggesting that the combination with parent training is especially effective in ameliorating conduct problems in children (Kazdin & Weisz, 1998; Webster-Stratton & Hammond, 1997; see also Frick, 1998b).

APPLICATION OF EMPIRICALLY SUPPORTED TREATMENTS FOR CUSTODIAL GRANDPARENTS AND GRANDCHILDREN

The previous section describes empirically supported treatments for disruptive behavior disorders in children and adolescents. Of these, parent training appears to have the most robust research support, appearing particularly effective for younger children with relatively mild to moderate conduct problems. Given that nearly 88% of custodial grandparents are caring for grandchildren aged 10 or younger (Fuller-Thomson et al., 1997), there is reason to believe that parent-management strategies may be effective for custodial grandparents as well. However, little empirical evidence has investigated this possibility, and studies may at times require that children live with a biological parent as an inclusion criteria for entrance into therapy treatment studies, meaning that those families are excluded from research participation (e.g., Weisz & Hawley, 1998).

Although research has not investigated the efficacy of parent-training models for custodial grandparents, there is reason to be concerned about grandparents' ability to complete such a program. Specifically, Kazdin (1996; Kazdin, Holland, & Crowley, 1997) has been a vocal advocate of determining why children terminate from therapy prematurely and what barriers to treatment are encountered by children and their families. Several studies have found that socioeconomic disadvantage (Ambruster & Fallon, 1994; Kazdin et al., 1997; Prinz & Miller, 1994; Weisz & Weiss, 1993; Wierzbicki & Pekarik, 1993), minority group status (Ambruster & Fallon, 1994; Kazdin et al., 1997; Wierzbicki & Pekarik, 1993), living in a single-parent family (Ambruster & Fallon, 1994; Kazdin et al., 1997; Wierzbicki & Pekarik, 1993), high levels of family stress (Kazdin et al., 1997), and the presence of child antisocial behaviors (Kazdin et al., 1997) are all related to premature termination from therapy. Unfortunately, these same characteristics are found to differ significantly for custodial grandparents as compared to noncustodial grandparents (Fuller-Thomson et al., 1997). Specifically, for custodial grandparents, 46% were single parents, 38% were of a minority status, and 22.9% were living under the poverty line. These rates were significantly worse than for noncustodial grandparents, of whom only 32% were currently single, 16% belonged to an ethnic minority status, and 13.7% lived below the poverty line. In addition, custodial grandparents had a significant number of concomitant stressors compared to noncustodial grandparents, including more children in the home (3.94% vs. 3.25%), one or more coresident child(ren) (52.8% vs. 30.4%), more grandchildren (7.29% vs. 5.39%), and recently (within 5 years) losing a child by death (6.5% vs. 2.7%). Thus, although parent-training techniques have not been investigated among grandchildren living with their custodial grandparents, there is reason to suspect that dropout rate may be high. Given that between 40% and 60% of children in general will never complete therapy (Kazdin, 1996), this rate may be quite high indeed.

SUMMARY

In this chapter we have attempted to describe disruptive behavior disorders that are frequently present in children and adolescents. Given the stressors that are often present for the children prior to and during transitions in living arrangements, it is probable that many custodial grandparents may have to deal with a grandchild with ODD or CD. We have attempted to describe these disorders and delineate when they may be transitory and when they may be more severe and warrant diagnosis and treatment. We then described the research investigating the efficacy of treatments for disruptive behavior disorders, as well as describing what these interventions actually look like when implemented. Finally, we have tried to extrapolate from the existing literature whether these treatments may be applicable for custodial grandparents. Although there is no reason to suggest that these treatments would not be effective, there is some research to suggest that custodial grandparents experience many of the stressors that are associated with premature termination from therapy and thus may not be good candidates for treatment completion.

At this point, we are merely extrapolating from the parent literature and assuming that there is a chance that these interventions may be effective for custodial grandparents. However, what is needed are empirical investigations utilizing empirically supported interventions (e.g., parent-management training) with custodial grandparents. In addition, investigators must learn from the parent literature, particularly the barriers to treatment and factors associated with premature termination, and also to learn from the burgeoning literature investigating stress and role adjustment in custodial grandparents in order to offer treatments to meet the needs of custodial grandparents.

REFERENCES

American Psychiatric Association. (1994). *Diagnostic and statistical manual of mental disorders* (4th ed.). Washington, DC: Author.

Ambruster, P., & Fallon, T. (1994). Clinical, sociodemographic, and systems risk factors for attrition in a children's mental health clinic. *American Journal of Orthopsychiatry, 64,* 577–585.

Anderson, J. C., Williams, S., McGee, R., & Silva, P. (1987). DSM-III disorders in preadolescent children. *Archives of General Psychiatry, 44,* 69–76.

Atkins, M. S., McKay, M. M., Talbott, E., & Arvantis, P. (1996). DSM-IV diagnosis of conduct disorder and oppositional defiant disorder: Implications and guidelines for school mental health teams. *School Psychology Review, 25,* 274–283.

Barkley, R. A. (1987). *Defiant children: A clinician's manual for parent training.* New York: Guilford.

Brestan, E. V., & Eyberg, S. M. (1998). Effective psychosocial treatments of conduct-disordered children and adolescents: 29 years, 82 studies, and 5272 kids. *Journal of Clinical Child Psychology, 27,* 180–189.

Chambless, D. L., & Hollon, S. D. (1998). Defining empirically supported therapies. *Journal of Consulting and Clinical Psychology, 66,* 7–18.

Cohen, P., Cohen, J., Kasen, S., Velez, C. N., Hartmark, C., Johnson, J., Rojas, M., Brook, J., & Streuning, E. L. (1993). An epidemiological study of disorders in late childhood and adolescence: 1. Age- and gender-specific prevalence. *Journal of Child Psychology and Psychiatry, 34,* 851–867.

Costello, E. J., Angold, A., Burns, B. J., Stangl, D. K., Tweed, D. L., Erkanli, A., & Worthman, C. M. (1996). The Great Smoky Mountains study of youth: Goals, design, methods, and the prevalence of DSM-III-R disorders. *Archives of General Psychiatry, 53,* 1129–1136.

Costello, E. J., Farmer, E. M., Angold, A., Burns, B. J., & Erkanli, A. (1997). Psychiatric disorders among American Indian and White youth in Appalachia: The Great Smoky Mountains study. *American Journal of Public Health, 87,* 827–832.

de Toledo, S., & Brown, D. E. (1995). *Grandparents are parents: A survival guide for raising a second family.* New York: Guilford.

Emick, M. A., & Hayslip, B., Jr. (1996). Custodial grandparenting: New roles for middle-aged and older adults. *International Journal of Aging and Human Development: A Journal of Psychosocial Gerontology, 43,* 135–154.

Forehand, R., & McMahon, R. J. (1981). *Helping the noncompliant child: A clinician's guide to parent training.* New York: Guilford.

Frick, P. J. (1998a). Callous-unemotional traits and conduct problems: Applying the two-factor model of psychopathy to children. In D. J. Cooke, A. Forth, & R. Hare (Eds.), *Psychopathy: Theory, research, and implications for society* (pp. 161–188). Dordrecht, The Netherlands: Kluwer Academic Publishers.

Frick, P. J. (1998b). *Conduct disorders and severe antisocial behavior.* New York: Plenum Press.

Frick, P. J., & Silverthorn, P. (in press). Psychopathology in children and adolescents. In H. E. Adams (Ed.), *Comprehensive handbook of psychopathology* (3rd ed.). New York: Plenum Press.

Fuller-Thomson, E., Minkler, M., & Driver, D. (1997). A profile of grandparents raising grandchildren in the United States. *Gerontological Society of America, 37,* 406–411.

Grant, R., Gordon, S. G., & Cohen, S. T. (1997). An innovative school-based intergenerational model to serve grandparent caregivers. *Journal of Gerontological Social Work, 28,* 47–61.

Hembree-Kigin, T. L., & McNeil, C. B. (1995). *Parent-child interaction therapy.* New York: Plenum.

Henggeler, S. W., & Bourdin, C. M. (1990). *Family therapy and beyond: A multisystemic approach to teaching the behavior problems of children and adolescents.* Pacific Grove, CA: Brooks/Cole.

Hinshaw, S. P., Lahey, B. B., & Hart, E. L. (1993). Issues of taxonomy and comorbidity in the development of conduct disorder. *Development and Psychopathology, 5,* 31–49.

Kazdin, A. E. (1991). Effectiveness of psychotherapy with children and adolescents. *Journal of Consulting and Clinical Psychology, 59,* 785–798.

Kazdin, A. E. (1996). Dropping out of child psychotherapy: Issues for research and implications for practice. *Clinical Child Psychology and Psychiatry, 1,* 133–156.

Kazdin, A. E. (1997). Parent management training: Evidence, outcomes, and issues. *Journal of the American Academy of Child and Adolescent Psychiatry, 36,* 1349–1356.

Kazdin, A. E., Holland, L., & Crowley, M. (1997). Family experience of barriers to treatment and premature termination from child therapy. *Journal of Consulting and Clinical Psychology, 65,* 453–463.

Kazdin, A. E., Siegel, T. C., & Bass, D. (1990). Drawing on clinical practice to inform research on child and adolescent psychotherapy: Survey of practitioners. *Professional Psychology: Research and Practice, 21,* 189–198.

Kazdin, A. E., & Weisz, J. R. (1998). Identifying and developing empirically supported child and adolescent treatments. *Journal of Consulting and Clinical Psychology, 66,* 19–36.

Lahey, B. B., Applegate, B., Barkley, R. A., Garfinkel, B., McBurnett, K., Kerdyk, L., Greenhill, L., Hynd, G. W., Frick, P. J., Newcorn, J., Biederman, J., Ollendick, T., Hart, E. L., Perez, D., Waldman, I., & Shaffer, D. (1994). DSM-IV field trials for oppositional defiant disorder and conduct disorder in children and adolescents. *American Journal of Psychiatry, 151*(8), 1163–1171.

Lahey, B. B., Loeber, R., Hart, E. L., Frick, P. J., Applegate, B., Zhang, Q., Green, S. M., & Russo, M. F. (1995). Four-year longitudinal study of conduct disorders: Patterns and predictors of persistence. *Journal of Abnormal Psychology, 104,* 83–93.

Lahey, B. B., Loeber, R., Quay, H. C., Frick, P. J., & Grimm, J. (1992). Oppositional defiant disorders and conduct disorders: Issues to be resolved for DSM-IV. *Journal of the American Academy of Child and Adolescent Psychiatry, 31,* 539–546.

Lonigan, C. J., Elbert, J. C., & Bennett, J. S. (1998). Empirically supported interventions for children: An overview. *Journal of Clinical Child Psychology, 27,* 138–145.

McDermott, P. A. (1996). A nationwide study of developmental and gender prevalence for psychopathology in childhood and adolescence. *Journal of Abnormal Child Psychology, 24,* 53–66.

Minkler, M., Roe, K. M., & Price, M. (1992). The physical and emotional health of grandmothers raising grandchildren in the crack cocaine epidemic. *Gerontologist, 32,* 752–761.

Moffitt, T. E. (1993). Adolescence-limited and life-course-persistent antisocial behavior: A developmental taxonomy. *Psychological Review, 100,* 674–701.

Moffitt, T. E., Caspi, A., Dickson, N., Silva, P., & Stanton, W. (1996). Childhood-onset versus adolescent-onset antisocial conduct problems in males: Natural history from ages 3 to 18 years. *Development and Psychopathology, 8,* 399–424.

Patterson, G. R., & Forgatch, M. (1987). *Parents and adolescents living together: Part 1. The basics.* Eugene, OR: Castalia.

Pinson-Milburn, N. M., Fabian, E. S., Schlossberg, N. K., & Pyle, M. (1996). Grandparents raising grandchildren. *Journal of Counseling and Development, 74,* 548–554.

Prinz, R. J., & Miller, G. E. (1994). Family-based treatment for childhood antisocial behavior: Experimental influences on drop-out and engagement. *Journal of Consulting and Clinical Psychology, 3,* 645–650.

Rapoport, J. L., & Ismond, D. R. (1996). *DSM-IV training guide for diagnosis of childhood disorders.* New York: Brunner/Mazel.

Schaffer, D., Fisher, P., Dulcan, M. K., Davies, M., Piacentini, J., Schwab-Stone, M. E., Lahey, B. B., Bourdon, K., Jensen, P. S., Bird, H. R., Canino, G., & Regier, D. A. (1996). The NIMH Diagnostic Interview Schedule for Children version 2.3 (DISC-2.3): Description, acceptability, prevalence rates, and performance in the MECA study. *Journal of the American Academy of Child and Adolescent Psychiatry, 35,* 865–877.

Shore, R. J., & Hayslip, B., Jr. (1990, November). *Comparisons of custodial and noncustodial grandparents.* Paper presented at the annual scientific meeting of the Gerontological Society, Boston.

Shore, R. J., & Hayslip, B., Jr. (1994). Custodial grandparenting: Implications for children's development. In A. D. Gottfried & A. W. Gottfried's (Eds.), *Redefining families: Implications for children's development.* New York: Plenum Press.

Silverthorn, P., & Frick, P. J. (1999). Developmental pathways to antisocial behavior: The delayed-onset pathways in girls. *Development and Psychopathology, 11,* 101–126.

Simonoff, E., Pickles, A., Meyer, J. M., Silberg, J. L., Maes, H. H., Loeber, R., Rutter, M., Hewitt, J. K., & Eaves, L. J. (1997). The Virginia twin study of adolescent behavioral development: Influences of age, sex, and impairment of rates of disorders. *Archives of General Psychiatry, 54,* 801–808.

Solomon, J. C., & Marx, J. (1995). "To grandmother's house we go": Health and school adjustment of children raised solely by grandparents. *Gerontological Society of America, 35,* 386–394.

Takas, M. (1995). *Grandparents raising grandchildren: A guide to finding help and hope.* Crystal Lake, IL: Brookdale Foundation Group.

Webster-Stratton, C. (1996). Early-onset conduct problems: Does gender make a difference? *Journal of Consulting and Clinical Psychology, 64,* 540–551.

Webster-Stratton, C., & Hammond, M. (1997). Treating children with early-onset conduct problems: A comparison of child and parent training interventions. *Journal of Consulting and Clinical Psychology, 65,* 93–109.

Weisz, J. R., & Hawley, K. M. (1998). Finding, evaluating, refining, and applying empirically supported treatments for children and adolescents. *Journal of Clinical Child Psychology, 27,* 206–216.

Weisz, J. R., & Weiss, B. (1993). *Effects of psychotherapy with children and adolescents.* Newbury Park, CA: Sage Publications.

Weisz, J. R., Weiss, B., & Donenberg, G. R. (1992). The lab versus the clinic: Effects of child and adolescent psychotherapy. *American Psychologist, 47,* 1578–1585.

Wierzbicki, M., & Pekarik, G. (1993). A meta-analysis of psychotherapy dropout. *Professional Psychology: Research and Practice, 2,* 190–195.

Woodworth, R. S. (1996). You're not alone . . . you're one in a million. *Child Welfare, 5,* 619–635.

Zuckerman, B., & Frank, D. A. (1992). Prenatal cocaine and marijuana exposure: Research and clinical implications. In I. S. Zagon & T. A. Slotkin (Eds.), *Maternal substance abuse and the developing nervous system.* San Diego, CA: Academic Press.

CHAPTER 5

Intergenerational Continuity: Transmission of Beliefs and Culture

Karen Kopera-Frye and Richard Wiscott

Because people are living longer today than in any other point in history (Hooyman & Kiyak, 1999), there are new opportunities for individuals to experience roles such as grandparenthood for longer periods of time and in ways that are different than in the past. Previously, grandparents could expect to be involved in traditional pursuits such as indulging grandchildren, serving a companion function, and being keeper of family customs, beliefs, and values (Gratton & Haber, 1996). However, with current societal changes in family composition, more grandparents are finding themselves in a custodial role, often as primary caregivers of their grandchildren (e.g., Downey, 1995; Minkler, Driver, Roe, & Bedian, 1993). How changes in role responsibilities affect traditional intergenerational relationships is currently unknown.

When perceptions of grandparent influences on grandchild behaviors are examined (e.g., King & Elder, 1998), much variability is evident. However, except for a few early studies (e.g., Strom & Strom,

1992) examining the perceptions and quality of cross-generational linkages, little has been done to examine the impact on these relationships of specific beliefs that grandchildren hold about grandparents. As more grandparents now are involved in greater amounts of caregiving, coupled with a traditional role of culture keeper, a fruitful line of inquiry is how grandparents share cultural beliefs and how they affect grandchild ideologies. This chapter is one of the first to examine this premise by employing a comprehensive framework to investigate grandchildren's perceptions of grandparent influence on cultural beliefs.

HISTORICAL CONCEPTUALIZATIONS OF GRANDPARENT ROLES

Utilizing case study approaches, early research centered on the symbolic meaning the grandparent held in the psyche of the grandchild, especially in regard to the development of psychopathology (e.g., LaBarre, Jessner, & Ussery, 1960; Rappaport, 1958). In the 1960s, Neugarten and Weinstein (1964), utilizing a psychoanalytic and sociological foundation, investigated three dimensions of grandparenthood: degree of comfort, significance of role, and the ways in which the role was enacted. In their interviews with 70 middle-class, primarily Caucasian grandmother-grandfather pairs, they found that only 60% viewed the role as pleasant, and a surprising 36% were experiencing difficulty, disappointment, or lack of positive reward. Data from this study generated a typology of grandparenting styles: Formal, Fun-Seeking, Surrogate Parent, Reservoir of Family Wisdom, and Distant Figure. Of grandparents under the age of 65, the vast majority fell into two categories: 37% were classified as Fun-Seeking (informal and playful), and for 32% of the sample the Distant Figure role style was prominent (infrequent contact, usually only at holidays or special occasions). However, among grandparents over the age of 65, the Formal role predominated. Approximately 59% followed a prescribed role for grandparents, characterized by a clear disdain for offering advice on parenting but including a great interest in the grandchildren and, commonly, indulgence with gifts. The role of Surrogate Parent (caretaking responsibility) and Reservoir of Family

Wisdom (dispenser of special skills or resources) were rarely endorsed by any of the respondents.

Kahana and Kahana (1970) were among the first to consider the meaning of grandparenthood from the perspective of the grandchild. In a sample of 85 Caucasian grandchildren aged 4 to 12 years, they found that perceptions of grandparents changed as a function of the child's stage of cognitive development. For example, the youngest children viewed grandparents in concrete terms (e.g., grandma is nice), whereas older children were able to describe grandparents in more abstract ways. On the basis of their findings, Kahana and Kahana suggested that perceptions of grandparents by grandchildren vary both developmentally and characteristically as a function of grandchild age.

Kivnick (1983) posited a typology that incorporates the dualistic nature of both grandparent function and impact of that function on the grandchild. Using data from 286 Caucasian grandparents, she found that grandparent meaning could be classified along five dimensions: Centrality (how central the role is to the person), Valued Elder (passing on traditions), Immortality Through Clan (identification with grandchildren), Reinvolvement with Past (reliving earlier life experiences through grandchildren), and Indulgence (attitudes of leniency). Each dimension provided a conceptual framework on which researchers could base findings and better understand how intergenerational relationships could have reciprocal effects. Additionally, Kivnick (1986, 1988) stressed the importance of life review to older adults, suggesting that her five dimensions of grandparent meaning could be examined in an Eriksonian framework to further understand the functions and effects of this role. For example, the dimension of Valued Elder could be used to understand how the older adult fulfilled the need to give back to younger generations (i.e., generativity)—in this case, the giving of family traditions.

CUSTODIAL GRANDPARENTING

As in the past, roles that grandparents fulfill continue to evolve. As a result of increased longevity, divorce, and remarriage rates, coupled with greater geographic mobility (Giarrusso, Silverstein, & Bengston, 1996), a different pattern of grandparenting is emerging: custodial grandparenting. With this increasing trend, researchers have begun to focus on the consequences of this role to grandparents. Presumably, positive or negative affective states and/or efficacy of role performance should affect the grandparent-grandchild relationship.

Burton (1992) found that despite custodial grandparents finding emotional satisfaction in their role, a number of contextual (e.g., neighborhood crime), familial (e.g., caregiving for other family members while raising prenatally exposed crack cocaine children), and individual factors (e.g., role strain, no time for self) contributed to severe negative economic, health-related, and psychological costs to them (e.g., depression). Similarly, Shore and Hayslip (1994) found lower grandparent satisfaction to be related to more negative well-being among a group of 203 primarily Caucasian custodial grandparents and a greater likelihood of seeking professional help for their grandchildren rather than for themselves, even though reporting poorer well-being, greater social isolation, and more disruptive relationships with their grandchildren. Surveying 71 African American caregiving grandmothers, Minkler, Roe, and Price (1992) found that 65% of the grandmothers were concerned about their own health, with a third indicating worse health since assuming caretaking. Fuller-Thomson and colleagues (Fuller-Thomson, Minkler, & Driver, 1997) found that custodial demands led to increased physical, emotional, and economic vulnerability, with caregiving grandparents twice as likely as noncaregiving grandparents to experience depression.

Although existing data suggest that custodial grandparents may experience a myriad of negative consequences as a result of assuming this role, many report that the emotional reward of caring for a grandchild offsets the extensive role demands. Burton and deVries (1992) found 15 African American grandmothers who cited a very important reward of their custodial role, that of parenting again with the goal of being more effective this time. Dressel and Barnhill (1994) found that grandparents caring for children of incarcerated mothers expressed satisfaction derived from their grandchildren's accomplishments, growth, and overall presence in their lives. The existing research paints a picture of mixed rewards and stresses among this newly emergent grandparent function. How can we reconcile this seemingly paradoxical situation?

A particularly insightful framework first was discussed in 1971 by Bengston and Kuypers in examining data from their longitudinal study of generations. Representing 300 three-generation family lineages over a 20-year span, this research targeted how intergenerational relationships change as well as exhibit continuity across time. Two constructs examined then are still of particular importance to today's changing roles of grandparenting: intergenerational solidarity (characterizing dimensions of interaction, cohesion, sentiment, and support between successive generations) and intergenerational conflict (negative, conflicting, and nonaffirming dimensions). Using the 1991 wave of data, they found that both intergenerational solidarity and conflict were common, suggesting that a life course theoretical framework has merit. Others have found additional support for this contemporary perspective (Bengtson & Allen, 1993; Elder, 1994; Holladay et al., 1998; Mangen, Bengtson, & Landry, 1988; Strom & Strom, 1992), which provides a useful framework from which to view the reciprocity of grandparent-grandchild interactions, particularly with respect to understanding the transmission of cultural beliefs.

CULTURAL SHARING WITHIN AN INTERGENERATIONAL PERSPECTIVE

Today, one of the most primary roles of the grandparent function is that of keeper of family heritage. As a working definition, *culture* is the set of attitudes, beliefs, values, and behaviors shared by a group of people and communicated from one generation to the next (Matsumoto, 1996). These shared behaviors are often observable either as rituals or as common, automatic behavior patterns that result from shared cultural values and norms. If we apply the intergenerational life course framework to this notion, we can see how grandparents can indeed be valuable transmitters of culture or conduits of cultural transmission.

Although few in number, studies examining the role of grandparents as conduits in ethnic families have employed an intergenerational framework. For example, Schmidt and Padilla (1983) interviewed 31 Mexican American grandchildren and grandparents about their interaction patterns. They found a high degree of involvement with grandchildren by most grandparents. Although there were no significant differences between grandmothers and grandfathers in the degree to which each was involved in the socialization of their grandchildren, grandmothers did report speaking Spanish (one measure of cultural transmission) more often to granddaughters.

The role of grandparents as keepers of culture also has been studied in various Native American tribes. Herring (1989) examined three types of Native American families with respect to preservation of traditional values: (a) a traditional group (overtly adheres to traditional practices as defining their lifestyle), (b) a nontraditional group (a bicultural group that seems to have adopted aspects other than those of Native American groups), and (c) a pan-traditional group that struggles to redefine and reaffirm previously lost cultural ways. The very essence of the conflict often felt within Native Americans in their struggle to create or preserve ethnicity and assure the connection of future children with their heritage is inherent in this simplified typology. Bahr (1994) and Bahr and Bahr (1995) reported that Apache grandmothers were instrumental in preserving customs, beliefs, and traditions from the past. Using an in-depth case study approach ($N = 13$), they found that these grandmothers universally enjoyed a high status position as agents of socialization for their grandchildren (Bahr, 1994). However, it also was noted that the media (i.e., television, radio) worked to undermine this important role; time once spent teaching Native American traditions to younger generations now was spent watching favorite television shows (Bahr & Bahr, 1995). Strauss (1995), in a reflective examination of his life and the sharing of culture within his family, suggested that the tribal community, extended family, and immediate physical environment all provide the opportunity for each Native American member to interact daily in spiritual ways, resulting in a shaping of one's personality, identity, notion of power, and understanding of one's place in the world. The importance of relational bonding provided by relatives to cultural identity development in youth is critical to preservation of Native American ways in various tribes (Shoemaker, 1989; Weibel-Orlando, 1990).

Considerably more research has been conducted with African American grandparenting (both custodial and noncustodial) in regard to roles and cultural beliefs. Cherlin and Furstenberg (1986) found that African American grandparents were significantly more involved in day-to-day aspects of their grandchildren's lives relative to Caucasian groups. These grandparents reported routinely engaging in cultural practices (sharing particular family songs, rituals, and foods) that were conducive to increased family interactions. Kivett (1991) found that the role of grandparent was reported to be more salient (i.e., meaningful and important) to African American grandfathers and centered on higher expectations, greater assistance given, and more interpersonal closeness with their grandchildren relative to the Caucasian grandfathers. Further, these men more often emphasized future goals as compared to past ethnic practices.

Strom, Collingsworth, Strom, and Griswold (1993) interviewed 204 African American grandparents and 175 Caucasian and 295 African American grandchildren. Results indicated that both African American grandparents' self-reports and reports by grandchildren portrayed the grandparents as more active teachers, more influential in providing a sense of direction through utilizing lessons of respecting others' feelings, placing greater worth on religion, using good manners, giving advice, reinforcing right and wrong, and teaching the importance of learning as a lifelong pursuit. Caucasian grandchildren were more apt to see their grandparents as better able to cope with difficult situations, more effective managers of frustration, and excellent sources of information. Timberlake and Stukes-Chipungu (1992) examined the symbolic meanings or values of grandparenting in 100 African American grandmothers and 100 of their grandchildren. For 85% of the grandmothers, their grandchildren represented an expansion of themselves and were an important link to carrying on the family line and traditions. Pearson, Hunter, Ensminger, and Kellam (1990), in their study of the influence of 130 African American grandmothers on their grandchildren, reported that parenting involvement was substantial and characterized by two types of activity patterns: control and punishment and support and punishment. Greater parenting involvement of grandmothers was found in mother-absent homes. Increased centrality and involvement of grandparents in their grandchildren's lives is more readily apparent among studies of African American families in which custodial responsibilities were undertaken because of parental substance abuse (Burton, 1992; Burton & deVries, 1992; Minkler et al., 1993; Minkler, Roe, & Robertson-Beckley, 1994).

Whereas research on cultural sharing in both custodial and non-custodial grandparents often has focused on diverse ethnicities, studies examining cultural practices and transmission among Caucasian grandparents are almost nonexistent. Occasionally beliefs, practices, or behaviors of Caucasian grandparents are examined but typically in a comparative fashion, with a different ethnic group as the targeted focus of study. Quite possibly this state of affairs stems from our fascination with studying that which is perceptually different or from our erroneous equating of culture with ethnicity. Matsumoto (1996) cautions that culture does not necessarily conform to nationality, race, or geographic region. Whatever the operating bias, there clearly is a need for research investigating cultural sharing among varied heritages found in Caucasian individuals.

GRANDCHILD PERCEPTIONS OF GRANDPARENT INFLUENCE

Much of the literature to date has focused on grandparent perceptions of their satisfaction, roles, and influence on grandchildren's beliefs. Despite the consistent finding of a "culture keeper" function prevalent in grandparenthood, little research has examined how grandparents share or transmit cultural ways to their grandchildren. If most grandparents are currently spending increased time with grandchildren relative to the past, this becomes an important area of inquiry. Moreover, we are aware of no study to date that examined the sharing of culture as viewed from the grandchildren's perspective. That is, although studies (e.g., Kennedy, 1992) have assessed reports of the types of activities shared with grandchildren, none has examined what the grandchildren report that they have learned from grandparents in terms of culture.

To more fully explore how cultural sharing between generations occurs, we conducted a study to assess grandchildren's perceptions of the influence of grandparents on their lives. Specifically, participants were queried on issues related to belief and value formation, relationship quality, and the intergenerational sharing of culture. Of particular interest to us was how our newly created instruments of intergenerational sharing of culture would relate to established grandparenting measures (e.g., shared activities [Kennedy, 1992]). Overall, we expected that the sharing of culture would be a predominant theme in respondents' protocols because of the historical role of grandparents as keepers of culture.

METHOD

Procedure and Participants

Participants (N= 246) from various undergraduate psychology classes were instructed to think of one particular grandparent they felt especially close to while answering the questions. If no grandparents were living, respondents were instructed to remember past experiences with a close grandparent while answering the survey. The sample was 78% Caucasian, 16% African American, and 6% other or mixed racial heritage. Ages ranged from 18 to 54 years (M = 22.5 years, SD = 5.5), and 67% of the sample was female. Average education level was 13.4 years, and student monthly income levels ranged from $0 to $8,000 per month ($M$ = $786, SD = $1086). Approximately 29% of the respondents were Catholic, 13% Baptist, 8% Methodist, and 30% other; 16% of the sample reported no religious affiliation. The majority of the participants (83%) were single. Approximately 10% of the sample reported no living grandparents; 19%, one living grandparent; 33%, two living grandparents; and 36%, three or more living grandparents.

Established Measures

Perceived frequency of grandparent and grandchild–shared activities was measured by the Grandparenting Shared Activities Scale (Kennedy, 1992). Responses were summed, with a higher sum indicating a greater degree of shared activities. A modified version of the Belief Development Scale (Roberto & Stroes, 1992) assessed the degree to which grandchildren felt that grandparents have influenced them in eight domains—religion, sexual, political, family, educational, work, moral, and personal identity—in addition to an overall estimation of influence. Response categories ranged from 1 (none) to 4 (a great deal), with a higher total score indicating an overall greater effect of the grandparent on the grandchild's beliefs. Relationship quality was assessed by using questions from the Bengtson Positive Affect Scale (cf., Roberto & Stroes, 1992), which measured the degree to which participants understood and felt close to their nominated grandparents. Participants responded to four items (e.g., how much do you feel you understand your grandparent?), with a higher overall score indicating a stronger relationship between grandchild and grandparent.

Newly Created Measures

Three new measures were created for this project (Wiscott & Kopera-Frye, in press). The Shared Cultural Activities Scale is an 11-item scale that measured how frequently grandparents and grandchildren engaged in activities relating to cultural heritage. Examples of these items included how often grandchildren and grandparents discussed cultural heritage and attended events spotlighting their cultural background. Using a 5-point Likert scale (ranging from not at all to very typical), responses were summed, with a higher total score indicating a greater degree of shared cultural activities. This scale performed well in the current sample; Cronbach's alpha = .90. The Attitudes About Grandparenting Scale is a 12-item measure that tapped possible stereotypical attitudes held about older adults and grandparents. Sample items included "I am embarrassed by the way my grandparent dresses" and "I think my grandparents act a lot younger than their age." Negative items were reverse-coded so that a total higher score indicated more positive attitudes about grandparents and showed moderately strong internal consistency reliability in this sample (Cronbach's alpha = .74). Finally, the Cultural Sentence Completion Test (CSCT) was devised, using a projective type of response style, where participants completed sentence stems focusing on cultural transmission such as "The things I like most about our culture are . . . " Responses were analyzed in terms of whether the completed stem reflected positive, neutral, or negative affective tone. Protocols were quantified by total number completed and proportions of positive, negative, neutral, or uncodeable responses. Interrater agreement on a randomly selected subsample of 237 sentence stems was excellent (96%).

RESULTS

Existing Grandparenting Scales

Results indicated that grandchildren perceived that it was somewhat typical to engage in shared activities with grandparents ($M = 82.22$ for the Shared Activities Scale; $SD = 26.51$, range, 29 to 145), that grandparents exerted a moderate influence on the grandchild's beliefs ($M = 27.98$ for the Shared Beliefs Scale; $SD = 6.50$; range, 10 to 40), and that most grandchildren felt that the relationships with their grandparents were moderately strong ($M = 2.65$ for the Relationship Quality measure; $SD = .36$; range, 1.17 to 3.83). Additionally, the Grandparenting Shared Activities Scale was positively correlated with the Shared Beliefs Scale ($r = .68$, $p < .001$) and the Relationship Quality measure ($r = .15$, $p < .05$). The Shared Beliefs Scale and the Relationship Quality measure were also positively related ($r = .27$, $p < .05$).

Cultural Sharing and Relationship Indices

The four most frequently endorsed items of the new Shared Cultural Activities Scale included sharing of cultural customs, listening to stories from grandparent's childhood, looking at family photo albums together, and teaching of traditions and customs by grandparents. Most grandchildren in the sample reported that these cultural sharing activities were at least somewhat typical of the grandparenting relationship ($M = 3.20$). Additionally, the sample reported moderately positive attitudes about their grandparents as evidenced by scores on the Attitudes About Grandparenting Scale ($M = 43.75$; $SD = 6.74$; range, 27 to 60). Respondents completed an average of 9 items on the Cultural Sentence Completion Test ($SD = 3.34$; range, 0 to 12). Coding for affective tone of the individual responses to each completed stem resulted in an average of 80.2% ($SD = 25$) positive, 13.3% ($SD = 19.9$) negative, and 3.1% ($SD = 8.5$) neutral responses.

The Shared Cultural Activities Scale was positively correlated with the Attitudes About Grandparenting Scale ($r = .14$, $p < .05$) and the proportion of positive responses to the Cultural Sentence Completion Test stems ($r = .41$, $p < .001$); whereas it was negatively correlated with the proportion of negative responses to the Cultural Sentence Completion Test stems ($r = -.40$, $p < .001$). The Attitudes About Grandparenting Scale was positively related to the proportion of positive responses to the Cultural Sentence Completion Test stems ($r = .21$, $p = .001$) and negatively correlated with the proportion of negative responses to the Cultural Sentence Completion Test stems ($r = -.20$, $p < .01$).

We also tested the relationship between our newly created culture measures and established measures of intergenerational relationships. Increased frequency of cultural sharing was significantly related to greater sharing of nonculturally specific activities ($r = .68$, $p < .001$), and greater perceived influence of grandparents on beliefs ($r = .58$, $p < .001$); quality of relationship was unrelated. More favorable attitudes toward grandparents was significantly associated with greater shared activities ($r = .27$), greater perceived influence on beliefs ($r = .27$), and better quality of relationship ($r = .29$), all p's $< .001$. Overall, the pattern of correlations suggests a moderately positive relationship between existing and newly created instruments.

Together, these results suggest that the newly created measures of intergenerational sharing of culture were significantly related to each other and to existing measures of grandparent-grandchild relationships. Because of the large sample size, several of these correlations are small in terms of the amount of variance they capture. We are currently cross-validating these results in a larger study to examine whether these reported relationships continue to hold.

Demographic Correlates of Relational Sharing

Pearson and point biserial correlation coefficient analyses were undertaken to examine the relationship among key study variables. Table 5.1 provides a summary of the obtained results. Although significant, it was surprising that the obtained correlation coefficients were not stronger. As expected, African American grandchildren were more likely to share culture with their grandparents. Race was significantly and positively related to shared everyday activities, shared cultural activities, and the proportion of completed cultural

TABLE 5.1 Relationship Among Variables in the Study

	1	2	3	4	5	6	7	8	9	10	11	12
1. Gender	—											
2. Race	.05	—										
3. Marital	.05	-.01	—									
4. Educ.	-.04	.03	.22***	—								
5. Share	.22***	.15*	-.04	-.13*	—							
6. Beliefs	.17**	.09	.07	-.03	.68***	—						
7. Relat.	-.03	.07	.14*	.05	.15*	.27***	—					
8. Culture Share	.17**	.26***	.04	-.02	.68***	.58***	.05	—				
9. #CSCT	-.01	.07	-.01	.06	.09	.05	.02	.23***	—			
10. Pro-Pos CSCT	.06	.16*	.11	.09	.28***	.31***	.12	.41***	.30***	—		
11. Pro-Neg CSCT	-.14*	-.11	-.06	-.04	-.26***	.27***	-.08	-.40***	.01	-.72***	—	
12. Attitud.	-.04	.07	.07	-.01	.27***	.27***	.29***	.14*	-.04	.21**	-.20**	—

*p < .05.
**p < .01.
***p < .001.

77

sentence stems reflecting positive affective tone. Surprisingly though, race was not related to any of the measures tapping relationship quality between grandchildren and grandparents.

Granddaughters engaged in more activities with their grandparents (both everyday and culture-related) and were more likely to say that their grandparents influenced the development of their beliefs. Additionally, granddaughters were less likely than grandsons to have completed culture sentence stems reflecting negative affect. Interestingly, education was negatively related to the number of shared culture activities but had no effects on other variables in the study. Similarly, marital status also was a rather weak correlate. Being married was related only to more positive relationship quality between grandchildren and grandparents.

Implications of Current Findings for Custodial Grandparents

The present study expanded on prior research by examining the role of cultural sharing from the grandchild's perspective, a construct not previously examined in studies of grandparent-grandchild relationships. Although prior research has investigated scale indices of relationship quality (Kennedy, 1992; Roberto & Stroes, 1992; Hayslip, Shore, Henderson, & Lambert, 1998), this study suggests the importance of new measures that tap a critical component of this reciprocal relationship, that of sharing of cultural ways. As our findings suggest, the majority of grandchildren (regardless of ethnicity or cultural background) reported some vestiges of familial traditions to be an important part of their lives. Although this work focused primarily on grandchild perceptions, without regard to whether they were a product of custodial grandparenting, the strength of the grandchildren's beliefs and attitudes regarding heritage clearly occupied a central theme in their identity formation. Thus, if we think about the intense amounts of time custodial grandparents invest in their grandchildren and their reported perceptions of viewing the grandchildren as extensions of themselves and the family line, this caregiving context becomes an invaluable, natural opportunity to preserve heritage in the successive generations.

Especially interesting were the relationships between gender, race, and intergenerational sharing. Overall, minority and female participants were more likely to engage in both more general and more culturally related activities. Additionally, on the projective sentence stems, minority grandchildren were more likely to report a greater proportion of positive responses, with granddaughters overall noting a lower proportion of negative reactions. This differential pattern of intergenerational shared activities found among minorities in this study is even more relevant to the custodial context in light of figures showing that minority grandchildren are more likely to be cared for by grandparents than are nonminority grandchildren (Minkler & Roe, 1993; Strom et al., 1993). Further research that includes larger numbers of minority grandchildren should focus on the extent to which shared culture affects grandchildren's beliefs and behaviors.

An important finding was the extent to which grandparents influenced grandchildren's belief formation. The majority of our grandchildren reported that their grandparents had moderate to great influence on their beliefs in six of eight domains: religion (strongest), family, education, work, moral, and personal identity; minimal influence was reported on sexual and political beliefs. These results are in accord with prior data by Bengtson (1996), Kennedy (1992), and Roberto and Stroes (1992), who reported that grandchildren are greatly influenced by grandparents in formation of identity, values, and life beliefs. Thus, grandchildren appear to report that this influence is real and perceived as an important role accorded to grandparents. Although the custodial grandparenting relationship was not the focus of these prior studies, intergenerational caregiving provides a unique opportunity for grandparents to have a profound impact on young adult grandchildren's identity formation and belief system.

Because we know that custodial grandparenting is increasing today due to a myriad of societal changes (e.g., parental substance abuse patterns), the results from our study suggest that custodial grandparents may have sizable influence on grandchildren's beliefs while additionally serving as a positive role model for grandchildren relative to parental models. Studies by Minkler et al. (1993) and Burton (1992) highlight the importance of grandparents' perceptions that revolve around the goal of "doing a better job this time." Many were dissatisfied with their own child-rearing outcomes for a host of reasons and see this new responsibility of caregiving as a chance to rectify wrongdoings of the past in order to excel with the current surrogate child.

Our newly created measures offer a promising approach to our understanding of dynamic interrelationships within a life course framework (Bengston & Kuypers, 1971). Data obtained from the established measures in this study provide support for our new instruments. General activity sharing and greater influence on grandchild beliefs, but not overall relationship quality, were strongly related to cultural sharing. Overall, the construct of cultural sharing appears to be a valid line of inquiry.

FUTURE DIRECTIONS FOR RESEARCH ON CULTURAL SHARING

Most research has focused on understanding characteristics of traditional grandparenting contexts, but far less is known about custodial grandparenting. With the handful of noteworthy efforts undertaken by researchers such as Hayslip and colleagues (Emick & Hayslip, 1996; Hayslip et al., 1998; Shore & Hayslip, 1994), Burton and colleagues (1992), and Minkler and colleagues (1993), both the rewards and costs of this new grandparenting form are beginning to emerge. However, much more work remains to be done. Piecemeal and often sparse support for these grandparents, coupled with ambiguous legal issues (e.g., custody), precipitates role confusion among grandparents. What parameters define their role as full-time custodial grandparents? Given their huge investment in nurturing and overseeing the welfare of their grandchildren, how might this role ambiguity play itself out in grandchildren's belief formation and identity development? With the demands of parental responsibility, how are traditional grandparenting functions, such as the transmission of cultural heritage and values, accomplished?

A promising line of inquiry is how these contextual stressors and supports experienced by grandparents may trickle down, if at all, to affect belief formation in successive generations. Further, with the exception of our study, no other work has examined grandchildren's perceptions of cultural sharing and the value of this sharing in their lives. Understanding how the transmission of culture may be different (e.g., patterns, extent) in custodial grandparenting contexts is an area yet to be explored. Additionally, other types of special custodial or noncustodial situations (e.g., stepgrandparents, great-grandparents) must be investigated. Overall, whereas research over the past 25 years has provided valuable insight on grandparents and intergenerational relations, our understanding of these issues is still in the infancy stage.

ACKNOWLEDGMENTS

We would like to thank Krys Gesen, Lisa Cognata, Dean Blevins, and Thomas Yerkey for their assistance in data entry and coding and especially Marybeth Mersky for her editorial assistance. Requests for reprints should be sent to Karen Kopera-Frye, PhD.

REFERENCES

Bahr, K. S. (1994). The strength of Apache grandmothers: Observations on commitment, culture and caretaking. *Journal of Comparative Family Studies, 25,* 233–248.

Bahr, K. S., & Bahr, H. M. (1995). Autonomy, community, and the mediation of value: Comments on Apachean grandmothering, cultural change, and the media. In C. K. Jacobson (Ed.), *American families: Issues in race and ethnicity* (pp. 229–260). New York: Garland.

Bengtson, V. L. (1996). Continuities and discontinuities in intergenerational relationships over time. In V. L. Bengtson (Ed.), *Adulthood and aging: Research on continuities and discontinuities* (pp. 271–303). New York: Springer Publishing Co.

Bengtson, V. L., & Allen, K. R. (1993). The life course perspective applied to families over time. In P. Boss, W. Doherty, R. LaRossa, W. Schumm, & S. Steinmetz (Eds.), *Sourcebook of family theories and methods: A contextual approach* (pp. 469–498). New York: Plenum.

Bengtson, V. L., & Kuypers, J. A. (1971). Generational differences and the "developmental stake." *Aging and Human Development, 2,* 249–260.

Brussoni, M. J., & Boon, S. D. (1998). Grandparental impact in young adults' relationships with their closest grandparents: The role of relationship strength and emotional closeness. *International Journal of Aging and Human Development, 46,* 267–286.

Burton, L. M. (1992). Black grandparents rearing children of drug-addicted parents: Stressors, outcomes, and social service needs. *Gerontologist, 32,* 744–751.

Burton, L., & deVries, C. (1992). African American grandparents as surrogate parents. *Generations, 16,* 51–54.

Cherlin, A. J., & Furstenberg, F. F. (1986). *The new American grandparent: A place in the family, a life apart.* New York: Basic.

Downey, T. (1995, March). Untitled presentation to mini-White House Conference on Grandparents Raising Grandchildren, College Park, MD.

Dressel, P. L., & Barnhill, S. K. (1994). Reframing gerontological thought and practice: The case of grandmothers with daughters in prison. *Gerontologist, 34,* 685–691.

Elder, G. H., Jr. (1994). Adult lives in a changing society. In K. Cook, G. Fine, & J. S. House (Eds.), *Sociological perspectives on social psychology* (pp. 231–244). Boston: Allyn and Bacon.

Emick, M. A., & Hayslip, B. (1996). Custodial grandparenting: New roles for middle-aged and older adults. *International Journal of Aging and Human Development, 43,* 135–154.

Fuller-Thomson, E., Minkler, M., & Driver, D. (1997). A profile of grandparents raising grandchildren in the United States. *Gerontologist, 37,* 406–411.

Giarrusso, R., Silverstein, M., & Bengtson, V. L. (1996). Family complexity and the grandparent role. *Generations, 20,* 17–23.

Gratton, B., & Haber, C. (1996). Three phases in the history of American grandparents: Authority, burden, companion. *Generations, 20,* 7–12.

Hayslip, B., Jr., Shore, J., Henderson, C. E., & Lambert, P. L. (1998). Custodial grandparenting and the impact of grandchildren with problems on role satisfaction and role meaning. *Journal of Gerontology: Social Sciences, 53B,* S164–S173.

Herring, R. D. (1989). The American Native family: Dissolution by coercion. *Journal of Multicultural Counseling and Development, 17,* 4–13.

Holladay, S., Lackovich, R., Lee, M., Coleman, M., Harding, D., & Denten, D. (1998). (Re)constructing relationships with grandparents: A turning point analysis of granddaughters' relational development with maternal grandmothers. *International Journal of Aging and Human Development, 46,* 287–303.

Hollingshead, A. B. (1975). *Four factor index of social status.* Unpublished manuscript, Yale University.

Hooyman, N., & Kiyak, H. A. (1999). *Social gerontology.* Boston: Allyn and Bacon.

Jackson, J. J. (1986). Black grandparents: Who needs them? In R. Staples (Ed.), *The black family: Essays and studies.* Belmont, CA: Wadsworth.

Kahana, B., & Kahana, E. (1970). Grandparenthood from the perspective of the developing grandchildren. *Developmental Psychology, 3,* 98–105.

Kennedy, G. E. (1992). Quality in grandparent/grandchild relationships. *International Journal of Aging and Human Development, 35,* 83–98.

King, V., & Elder, G. H., Jr. (1998). Perceived self-efficacy and grandparenting. *Journal of Gerontology: Social Sciences, B53,* S249–S257.

Kivett, V. R. (1991). Centrality of the grandfather role among older rural Black and White men. *Journal of Gerontology: Social Sciences, 46,* S250–258.

Kivnick, H. Q. (1983). Dimensions of grandparenthood meaning: Deductive conceptualization and empirical derivation. *Journal of Personality and Social Psychology, 44,* 1056–1068.

Kivnick, H. Q. (1986). Grandparenthood and a life cycle. *Journal of Geriatric Psychiatry, 19,* 39–55.

Kivnick, H. Q. (1988). Grandparenthood, life review, and psychosocial development. *Journal of Gerontological Social Work, 12,* 63–81.

LaBarre, M. B., Jessner, L., & Ussery, L. (1960). The significance of grandmothers in the psychopathology of children. *American Journal of Orthopsychiatry, 30,* 175–185.

Mangen, D. J., Bengtson, V. L., & Landry, P.H., Jr. (Eds.). (1988). *The measurement of intergenerational relations.* Beverly Hills, CA: Sage.

Matsumoto, D. (1996). *Culture and psychology.* Pacific Grove, CA: Brooks/ Cole.

Minkler, M., Driver, D., Roe, K. M., & Bedeian, K. (1993). Community interventions to support grandparent caregivers. *Gerontologist, 33,* 807–811.

Minkler, M., & Roe, K. (1993). *Grandmothers as caregivers: Raising children of the crack cocaine epidemic.* Newbury Park, CA: Sage Publications.

Minkler, M., Roe, K. M., & Price, M. (1992). The physical and emotional health of grandmothers raising grandchildren in the crack cocaine epidemic. *Gerontologist, 32,* 752–761.

Minkler, M., Roe, K. M., & Robertson-Beckley, R. (1994). Raising grandchildren from crack-cocaine households: Effects on family and friendship ties of African-American women. *American Journal of Orthopsychiatry, 64,* 20–29.

Neugarten, B. L., & Weinstein, K. K. (1964). The changing American grandparent. *Journal of Marriage and the Family, 11,* 199–205.

Pearson, J. L., Hunter, A. G., Ensminger, M. E., & Kellam, S. G. (1990). Black grandmothers in multigenerational households: Diversity in family structure and parenting involvement in the Woodlawn community. *Child Development, 61,* 434–442.

Rappaport, E. (1958). The grandparent syndrome. *Psychoanalytic Quarterly, 27,* 518–537.

Roberto, K. A., & Stroes, J. (1992). Grandchildren and grandparents: Roles, influences, and relationships. *Journal of International Aging and Human Development, 34,* 227–239.

Schmidt, A., & Padilla, A. M. (1983). Grandparent-grandchild interaction in a Mexican-American group. *Hispanic Journal of Behavioral Sciences, 5,* 181–198.

Shoemaker, D. J. (1989). Transfer of children and the importance of grand-mothers among the Navajo Indians. *Journal of Cross-Cultural Gerontology, 4,* 1–18.

Shore, R. J., & Hayslip, B. (1994). Custodial grandparenting: Implications for children's development. In A. E. Gottfried & A. W. Gottfried (Eds.), *Redefining families: Implications for children's development* (pp. 171–218). New York: Plenum Press.

Strauss, J. H. (1995). Reframing and refocusing American Indian family strengths. In C. K. Jacobson (Ed.), *American families: Issues in race and ethnicity* (pp. 105–118). New York: Garland.

Strom, R., Collingsworth, P., Strom, S., & Griswold, D. (1993). Strengths and needs of Black grandparents. *International Journal of Aging and Human Development, 36,* 255–268.

Strom, R., & Strom, S. (1992). Grandparents and intergenerational relation-ships. *Educational Gerontology, 18,* 607–624.

Timberlake, E. M., & Stukes-Chipungu, S. (1992). Grandmotherhood: Con-temporary meaning among African American middle-class grandmoth-ers. *Social Work, 37,* 216–222.

Weibel-Orlando, J. (1990). Grandparenting styles: Native American per-spectives. In J. Sokolovsky (Ed.), *The cultural context of aging: Worldwide perspectives* (pp. 109–125). New York: Bergo and Gravely.

Wiscott, R., & Kopera-Frye, K. (in press). Sharing of culture: Adult grand-childrens' perceptions of intergenerational relationships. *International Journal of Aging and Human Development.*

Variations in Surrogate Parenting in Middle and Late Life

Emotional Well-Being Among Grandparents Raising Children Affected and Orphaned by HIV Disease

Daphne Joslin

B y the early 1990's, HIV disease had "come to rival or surpass other important causes of death in taking the lives of mothers of young children" (Michaels & Levine, 1992). Although the use of combination antiretroviral therapies has reduced AIDS mortality and extended the time between HIV infection and major disease symptoms, the number of grandparents raising HIV-affected and orphaned children will increase over the coming decade. Female infection incidence continues to increase, especially among African American and Latino women (CDC, 1994, 1995). AIDS continues to be a leading cause of death among women between the ages of 25 and 44 (CDC, 1997). The decline in AIDS mortality rates due to earlier and more effective treatments has been much less dramatic among women; African American and Latino women's death rates have declined even less markedly (CDC, 1997). With the proportion of American women who are HIV-infected increasing (Ickovics & Rodin, 1992; CDC, 1995), growing numbers of third- and even fourth-generation relatives (i.e., great-grandmothers) will assume parental responsibility for thousands of affected children.

Yet despite this and the projected 82,000 to 125,000 minor children orphaned by AIDS in the year 2000, grandparents raising HIV-affected and orphaned grandchildren have received scant attention in recent gerontological research on grandparents as parents, nor have service programs and policy initiatives addressed the special concerns of grandparents raising grandchildren in the wake of HIV/AIDS. This chapter focuses on the prevalence of grandparents raising children orphaned and affected by parental HIV disease and death, the uniqueness of these circumstances, findings from recent descriptive research, and relevant research, program, and policy issues. It also emphasizes the psychosocial needs of caregivers, the unique circumstances of grandparents raising children orphaned and affected by parental HIV infection and disease, findings from recent descriptive research, and relevant program and policy issues.

PREVALENCE OF GRANDPARENTS RAISING CHILDREN ORPHANED AND AFFECTED BY HIV DISEASE

Documentation of custodial responsibility for HIV-affected children has found that grandmothers are the surrogate parent in nearly two thirds of these circumstances (Cohen & Nehring, 1994; Draimin, 1995; Schable et al., 1995). If this proportion is used, an estimated 54,100 to 82,500 AIDS-orphaned children and adolescents will be raised by grandmothers as we enter the next century. A recent study found that AIDS-affected grandmothers were raising, on average, two children (Joslin, Mevi-Triano, & Berman, 1997). This would place the number of grandmothers in the United States who will be raising AIDS-orphaned children at between 27,060 and 41,250 by the year 2001. These projections do not include the thousands who will be intermittent or permanent parental surrogates, where the children's primary parent, usually a mother, is living with HIV disease but is too incapacitated to assume full responsibility. No estimates exist on the number of grandparents caring for children of infected mothers.

EMOTIONAL WELL-BEING AND CAREGIVING: RELEVANT LITERATURE

Despite satisfaction in providing help to a relative, deleterious psychological effects are well documented among caregivers to impaired elderly (Montgomery, Gonyea, & Hooyman, 1985; Zarit, Reever, & Bach-Peterson, 1980). With the exception of one study (Szinovacz, Deviney, & Atkinson, 1997) custodial grandparents face greater risk of psychological distress, especially depression. Grandparents raising children were more likely to report depression, especially if female, older, and in poorer health (Minkler, Fuller-Thompson, Miller, & Driver, 1997). Increased psychological distress was found among White, middle-class grandparents and was found to be associated with social isolation and loss of important life roles, such as "traditional" (noncustodial) grandparenting, leisure pursuits, and free time (Kelly, 1993). Among an ethnically diverse sample, high stress and low self-esteem were associated with caregiver poor health, perception of low social support, and grandchildren's poorer health (Dowdell, 1995).

Family members, partners, and friends caring for persons with HIV disease also experience high emotional distress (Pearlin, Semple, & Turner, 1988; Raveis & Siegel, 1991), given the unpredictable roller-coaster course of HIV infection and disease (Raveis & Siegel, 1990), the infected person's housekeeping, personal care and emotional needs, caregiver anticipatory bereavement, and contamination risk (Clipp, Adinolfi, Forrest, & Bennett, 1995). Helping the infected person manage disease symptoms and medication side effects produced feelings of helplessness and depleted emotional and physical strength (Clipp et al., 1995), as well as measurable depressive symptoms (LeBlanc, Aneshensel, & Wight, 1995). AIDS stigma compounds emotional stress as caregivers feel "guilty by association" with a stigmatized illness and its transmission modes—homosexuality, intravenous drug use, and promiscuous sex (Powell-Cope & Brown, 1992; Cannon & Linsk, 1999; Dew, Gagni, & Nimorwicz, 1991). Pearlin, Anenshensel, and LeBlanc (1997) find that AIDS caregivers are "exposed to difficulties and challenges over and above the ordinary burdens of providing assistance to those unable to care for themselves," given the stigma associated with HIV and the death of younger persons which "violates normative life-course expectations."

Multiple deaths within a family or social network, fear of contagion, and the uncertain course of HIV disease are also uniquely associated with HIV/AIDS (Brown & Powell-Cope, 1991).

UNIQUE STRAINS ASSOCIATED WITH RAISING HIV-AFFECTED AND ORPHANED CHILDREN

As suggested by a review of the literature, grandparents raising HIV-affected and orphaned children face unique emotional stress. In addition to the common issues shared with other custodial grandparents, such as financial needs, loss of personal time, and lack of child care, HIV-affected grandparents confront distinct challenges that undermine emotional well-being: providing direct care to an infected adult or child, HIV disclosure, AIDS stigma, death and bereavement. In families of infected mothers, the grandmother's caregiving role includes not only parental surrogacy but also emotional and social support, personal care, housekeeping, and financial assistance to her infected adult daughter or daughter-in-law. More than 80% of young children's infected mothers reported their own mother as part of their support network (Williams, Shahryarinejad, Andrews, & Alcabes, 1997). Only 3 of 20 older surrogate parents in a convenience sample of HIV-affected grandparents had not been the primary caregiver of the dying mother (Joslin, Mevi-Triano, & Berman, 1997). Grandparents must learn the special nutritional and feeding needs of infected adults and children (Marder & Linsk, 1995; Shevlov, 1994), become adept at reducing the risk of viral transmission, and monitor even minor children's illnesses, such as ear infections and colds, because of compromised immunity. As new treatments lengthen the time between HIV diagnosis and terminal illness, grandparents are likely to provide assistance to the infected adult for a longer period (Theis, Cohen, Forrest, & Zelewsky, 1997).

Grandmothers also must negotiate the complicated issue of HIV diagnosis and disclosure within the family. The children's mother or parents may resist disclosure and prohibit the grandparents from telling the grandchildren about their parent's status and even their own viral infection. Grandparents may become messengers who tell the child the cause of their parent's death and even the child's own infected status. Then, because the child has not had the opportunity to express fear, rage, or grief to her or to his parent, the grandparent becomes the target of the child's profound distress.

Fear, anger, denial, anguish, despair, confusion, and uncertainty confront caregivers and persons with HIV disease (Macklin, 1989). Shame and stigma associated with HIV infection exacerbate the emotional time bomb (Roth, Siegel, & Black, 1994) for both infected and affected family members. Grandparents and infected and uninfected children face disgrace, hostility, and rejection from family members, friends, neighbors, and even professionals (Christ & Wiender, 1994; Fair, Spencer, & Winer, 1995; Herek & Capitanio, 1993; Land & Haragody, 1990; Lesar, Gerber, & Semmel, 1995/6; Macks, 1990; Maj, 1991; McGinn, 1996; Poindexter & Linsk, 1999; Roth et al., 1994). Others isolate themselves, in fear and anticipation of stigma and rejection.

Dying, death, and bereavement are a central part of the HIV-affected grandparent's stress. Because HIV is a terminal disease, when their child or grandchild dies, a grandparent outlives the younger generation, a disordering of the normal phases of the life cycle. Among African American and Latino women of child-bearing years (i.e., 25 to 44 years), AIDS is the leading cause of death in the United States (CDC, 1997). Nationwide, AIDS is the seventh leading cause of death among children ages 1–4 in New York, and in New Jersey it is the second leading cause of death for children in this age group (Chu, Beuhler, Oxtoby, & Kilbourne, 1991). Families of infected women, more likely to be poor, often experience multiple deaths within a short period of time (Bunting, 1996; Honey, 1988; Lesar, Gerber, & Semmel, 1995/6), thus prolonging and intensifying the bereavement process. Two grandmothers in the study reported in this chapter each buried a daughter and a grandchild within the same year.

Grief over the loss of a daughter, a potential caregiver to that parent, may be heightened by powerful guilt about having failed to keep her from deadly life choices (Tiblier, Walker, & Rolland, 1989). As grandparents help grandchildren through the grieving process, they may suspend their own bereavement in order to attend to the grandchildren's emotional needs. With the loss of an adult child, the older parent faces intense, prolonged, and incomparable grief (Levine-Perkell, 1996). Disenfranchised grief, associated with a stigmatized disease or relationship, interferes with the grieving process by isolating the bereaved from potential sources of support (Doka, 1989). Grandparents may not be able to disclose AIDS as the cause of death out of fear of social rejection. A conspiracy of silence may envelop both grandparents and grandchildren (Dane, 1993), disturbing the children's mourning process and contributing to even greater psychosocial and interpersonal distress to which grandparents must respond.

PURPOSE OF THE STUDY

Current research strongly points to compromised physical and psychological well-being of grandparents raising HIV-affected and orphaned children. An exploratory study was conducted to gather information about physical and emotional health and to identify factors associated with poorer self-reported physical and psychological well-being.

METHODS

A convenience sample of 20 older caregivers was recruited from HIV/AIDS service programs in Passaic and Bergen counties in northern New Jersey, including home care agencies, case management programs, and pediatric and adult HIV outpatient programs. Criteria for participant selection included being at least 45 years of age and a third or fourth generation relative of a child whose primary parent has died from or is living with HIV disease. African American, Euro-American, and Latino caregivers were chosen through representative sampling. Face-to-face interviews were conducted during 1996; all but two occurred in the caregivers' homes. Five interviews were conducted in Spanish and 15 in English. Study participants received $25 per interview. Participant responses were written on the questionnaire and quantitative data entered on SPSS 7.0.

Because study participants were recruited through the HIV/AIDS service network, it was possible to identify characteristics of those who met sample criteria yet declined to participate. These characteristics suggest that those participating in the study faced relatively less stressful circumstances or felt less shame attached to the HIV diagnosis within their family. Caregivers who declined to participate were those who had lost an adult child or grandchild to AIDS within the prior month; were experiencing a family crisis related to substance abuse or incarceration; were experiencing severe emotional distress; were unwilling to discuss family issues outside the family or beyond an established relationship with a nurse or social worker. These characteristics suggest that study participants may have faced less stressful circumstances.

The research instrument was modified from a questionnaire used in a study of custodial Latino grandparents living in New York City (Burnette, 1997), which integrated questions from a study of grandmothers raising children affected by the crack cocaine epidemic (Minkler & Roe, 1993). Participants described reported emotional health at the present time as "excellent," "good," "fair," or "poor," and as either "better," "the same," or "worse" than 1 year ago. Self-reported demographic information included caregiver age, race/ ethnicity, marital status, education, household income, and occupation. Caregivers were asked whether they were currently using psychotropic medications and how often in the past 6 months they had felt burdened by surrogate parenting. Selected items from the Brief Symptoms Inventory (BSI) (Derogatis & Spencer, 1982), a measure of psychological distress, included "Tell me how much . . . feeling depressed or very sad, . . . feeling hopeless about the future, . . . feeling lonely . . . has been a problem for you in the past seven days?"

Sample size and lack of random selection precluded more than tentative bivariate analysis. Descriptive findings present patterns of poorer emotional health in relationship to six variables: raising an infected child, being the sole caregiver, raising more than one child, being 60 years of age or older, having a household income below the study median of $19,500, and the HIV-related death of an adult child within the past year.

FINDINGS

Although 21 interviews were completed, 1 was excluded because the grandmother could not identify her daughter's death from sudden pneumonia as AIDS-related. An adult child, grandchild, or other immediate relative of each caregiver had been or was a client of an HIV/AIDS medical or social service program.

Selected sociodemographic characteristics are presented in Table 6.1. The sample's age profile is similar to other studies of older relative caregivers in which mean ages were 53 (Minkler & Roe, 1993), 63 (Burnette, 1997), and 55 (Joslin & Brouard, 1995). Although the sample was primarily low-income, with more than one

TABLE 6.1   Demographic Characteristics of Sample

	No.	%
Age		
47–49	2	10%
50–54	2	10%
55–59	7	35%
60–64	5	25%
65–69	1	5%
70–75	3	15%
Mean 59.6, *SD* 7.21		
Race/Ethnicity		
African American	9	45%
Hispanic	5	25%
Euro-American	6	30%
Asian	—	0%
Native American	—	0%
Marital Status		
Never married	3	15%
Divorced, separated	6	30%
Widowed	5	25%
Married	6	30%
Education		
No formal education	1	5%
5th–8th grade	3	15%
Some high school	5	25%
High school grad.	8	40%
Some college/grad.	3	15%
Household Income		
Under $7,499	1	5%
$7,500–13,499	3	15%
$13,500–19,499	7	35%
$19,500–24,499	3	15%
$25,000+	6	30%

half reporting household incomes of less than $19,500 per year, there was some heterogeneity of education and occupation. Forty-two percent were employed at the time of the interview, primarily in semiskilled, service, or industrial jobs. Two caregivers held administrative or professional positions.

Table 6.2 presents children's characteristics and the circumstances of child rearing. All caregivers were grandparents except one that was a great aunt. Participants were raising at least one child under the age of 18 whose primary parent had died or was too ill from HIV disease to be the primary caregiver. Custodial responsibility of 45% of the sample was due to parent's drug use ($n = 4$), child abuse or neglect ($n = 2$), or parent's incarceration ($n = 1$). Similar to findings from the studies cited earlier (Minkler & Roe, 1993; Joslin &

TABLE 6.2   Characteristics of Children and Child-Rearing Responsibility

Characteristic	No.	Percent
Primary caregiver	17	85%
Sole caregiver	8	40%
Number of children being raised		
1	12	60%
2	2	10%
3	2	10%
5	2	10%
6	1	5%
7	1	5%
Mean: 2.25, *SD:* 1.94		
HIV-positive children	13	65%
Relationship to child		
Grandmother	18	90%
Grandfather	1	5%
Great aunt	1	5%
Primary reason for caregiving		
HIV illness of mother	30% (6)	
HIV death of mother	30% (6)	
HIV death/other	5% (1)	
Drug use	20% (4)	
Incarceration	5% (1)	
Abuse/neglect	5% (1)	
Other	5% (1)	

Brouard, 1995; Burnette, 1997), the number of children being raised ranged from one to seven, with a mean of two. Children's ages ranged from 3 months to 17 years. Three grandparents were caring for an adult child with HIV disease. Six others had lost a child to AIDS within the past year. One grandmother had buried a daughter and infant grandson and was caring for an infected 3-year-old granddaughter. Only three participants had not directly cared for an HIV-infected person, although one grandmother was trying to decide whether to have her granddaughter tested for HIV infection.

SELF-REPORTED EMOTIONAL HEALTH

Global self-assessed health was rated positively as either "excellent" ($n = 3$) or "good ($n = 6$) by nearly one half of the participants and as either "fair" ($n = 7$) or "poor" ($n = 4$) by 55% of the sample. As Table 6.3 shows, those whose adult child had died from AIDS within the past year, who were raising an infected child, or who had lower incomes were more likely to rate emotional health more negatively.

Only 10% ($n = 2$) said emotional well-being improved; 40% (n = 8) said it was "about the same"; and 45% (n = 9) said it was "worse" than the prior year. A grandfather rated his emotional health as "good" and said he did not know if it had changed over the past year but that he felt "more alert" and added, "A lot of stresses isn't necessarily negative." As Table 6.4 shows, poorer grandparents and those whose adult child or grandchild died from AIDS within the year were more likely to report deterioration of emotional health.

PERCEIVED BURDEN

Grandparent responses to being asked, "Overall, how often in the past six months have you felt burdened from raising your grandchildren?" clustered at the middle, with 35% ($n = 7$) reporting "sometimes," and at the extremes, with one quarter each ($n = 5$) reporting "never" or "nearly always." Fifteen percent reported "rarely" or "quite frequently." To obtain a profile of those reporting greater feelings of burden, a new variable, "great burden," was constructed, in which "nearly always" and "quite frequently" were grouped together, and

TABLE 6.3 Current Self-Reported Emotional Well-being

	All	Sole caregiver		Infected Grandchild		Death in Year	
		Yes	No	Yes	No	Yes	No
Positive well-being	9 (45%)	4 (50%)	5 (42%)	5 (39%)	4 (57%)	1 (17%)	8 (57%)
Negative well-being	11 (55%)	4 (50%)	7 (58%)	8 (61%)	3 (43%)	5 (83%)	6 (43%)
Total	20 (100%)	8 (100%)	12 (100%)	13 (100%)	7 (100%)	6 (100%)	14 (100%)

	No. of Children		Household Income		Caregiver Age	
	1	2 or more	Below $19,499	$19,500+	<59 yr.	>59 yr.
Positive well-being	5 (42%)	4 (50%)	4 (36%)	5 (55%)	5 (45%)	4 (44%)
Negative well-being	7 (58%)	4 (50%)	7 (64%)	4 (45%)	6 (55%)	5 (56%)
Total	12 (100%)	8 (100%)	11 (100%)	9 (100%)	11 (100%)	9 (100%)

"sometimes," "rarely," and "never" were grouped as one category. In this scheme, 35% of the sample reported feelings of greater burden. As Table 6.5 shows, these caregivers tended to be raising an infected child and had lost an adult child to AIDS within the past year. The data suggest that those with higher incomes, those who are not sole caregivers, and those who are older also may perceive a greater burden of custodial parenting.

Feelings of hopelessness and depression over the past 7 days were reported by 45% of the sample, with 50% saying they had felt lonely during the past week. Those more likely to report feelings of depression were grandparents whose adult child died of AIDS (83% vs. 17%) and those who were not the sole caregivers (66% vs. 12%). Older grandparents (56% vs. 36%) and those who were not poor (56% vs. 36%) were more likely to report feeling depressed. Among

TABLE 6.4   Emotional Health Compared with 1 Year Ago

		Sole caregiver		Infected Grandchild		Death in Year	
	All	Yes	No	Yes	No	Yes	No
Same/better[a]	11 (55%)	5 (63%)	5 (42%)	6 (46%)	4 (57%)	1 (17%)	8 (57%)
Worse	9 (45%)	3 (37%)	7 (58%)	7 (54%)	3 (43%)	5 (83%)	6 (43%)
Total	20 (100%)	8 (100%)	12 (100%)	13 (100%)	7 (100%)	6 (100%)	14 (100%)

	No. of Children		Household Income		Caregiver Age	
	One	Two or more	Below $19,499	$19,500+	<59 yr.	>59 yr.
Same/better[a]	5 (42%)	4 (50%)	4 (36%)	6 (66%)	5 (45%)	5 (55%)
Worse	7 (58%)	4 (50%)	7 (64%)	3 (33%)	6 (55%)	4 (45%)
Total	12 (100%)	8 (100%)	11 (100%)	9 (100%)	11 (100%)	9 (100%)

[a]"Don't know" grouped with same/better.

the 45% reporting feelings of hopelessness, recently bereaved parents (83% vs. 29%), those with lower incomes (64% vs. 22%), and younger caregivers (53% vs. 33%) had greater levels of reported distress. Greater feelings of loneliness were reported by bereaved parents (100% vs. 29%), those raising only one child (67% vs. 25%), and those who were not sole caregivers (67% vs. 25%).

Psychotropic medication use also indicated emotional distress. The five participants (25%) who reported taking medications "for nerves" were either raising an infected grandchild and/or had lost an adult child within the past year.

Caregivers' elaboration on their experience gives insight into additional dimensions of emotional well-being. Social isolation was a theme in many interviews. A 62-year-old Euro-American widow living in a working-class suburb and caring for her infected daughter and granddaughter, both ill with HIV disease, said poignantly, "I don't go out much any more. I'm only relating to doctors, nurses and family so I don't see other people. I don't have the money to go out and I don't have many people I can trust." An African American grandmother living in a city housing project echoed these feelings

TABLE 6.5   Perceptions of Greater Burden

	Total	Sole Caregiver		Infected Grandchild		Death in Year	
		Yes	No	Yes	No	Yes	No
Low burden	13 (65%)	6 (75%)		6 (46%)	6 (100%)	2 (33%)	11 (79%)
High burden	7 (35%)	2 (25%)		7 (54%)	0	4 (67%)	3 (21%)
	20 (100%)	8 (100%)		13 (100%)	6 (100%)	6 (100%)	14 (100%)

	No. of Children		Household Income		Age	
	1	2 or more	Below $19,499	$19,5000+	<59 yr.	>59 yr.
Low burden	8 (67%)	5 (63%)	8 (73%)	5 (56%)	8 (73%)	5 (56%)
High burden	4 (33%)	3 (37%)	3 (27%)	4 (44%)	3 (27%)	4 (44%)
	12 (100%)	8 (100%)	11 (100%)	9 (100%)	11 (100%)	9 (100%)

of isolation as she described not being able to tell friends at church that her daughter and grandson both died of AIDS. Another African American grandmother in the same housing project tearfully described helping her three grandsons, ages 11, 15, and 17, cope with their mother's HIV disease and anticipated death and the taunts of other children who teased them about their mother having AIDS. "They'd throw it up in their faces. My grandsons wanted to move."

A 60-year-old Puerto Rican grandmother whose son and daughter-in-law both died of AIDS within the past year describes her struggle in raising an infected 15-year-old grandson whose rage spills over into the interview itself as he screams at her, "I hate you. You're not my mother. I want to die. I don't want to live this life anymore."

DISCUSSION

Given the circumstances of parental surrogacy, it is surprising that the self-assessed emotional health of these caregivers is as positive as it is, with nearly one half assessing it as "excellent" or "good." Study findings underscore the emotional resiliency of older relatives who assume parental surrogacy under conditions of great emotional distress and pain. As observed with regard to the physical health of older surrogate parents (Minkler, Roe, & Price, 1992; Joslin & Harrison, 1998), custodial grandparents may be a self-selected group whose hardiness enables them to assume this responsibility. This hardiness may extend to their emotional health, particularly their resiliency and capacity to endure loss, grief, HIV stigma, and the anxiety associated with HIV disease. However, signs of emotional distress, such as depression, hopelessness, and anxiety, suggest a vulnerability masked by their determination to care for their grandchildren.

In their study of grandmothers in the crack cocaine epidemic, Minkler and Roe (1993) found that more than one half of their sample reported "excellent" or "good" emotional health. A slightly smaller proportion (45%) of HIV-affected grandparents gave such assessment. However, 45% of the HIV-affected caregivers reported their emotional health as worse than 1 year ago, compared with 30% of the crack cocaine–affected grandmothers.

Minkler and Roe (1993) found subgroups with greater risk of emotional strain: those also caring for an elder family member and those employed in caregiving jobs. In the study of HIV-affected grandparents reported here, poorer emotional well-being was found among the recently bereaved, those caring for an infected grandchild, and those with lower incomes. Although no age differences were found in self-reported emotional health, older grandparents expressed a greater sense of child-rearing burden as well as concern about their capacity to continue in this role.

Poorer self-assessed emotional health was also greater among those with lower incomes. Yet the imperative of parental surrogacy in a context of daily economic survival (Joslin & Harrison, 1998) may mean that one's own emotional needs, like one's physical health, must be ignored because of the immediacy of greater priorities. Ironically, a smaller proportion of poorer grandmothers reported feeling burdened by child rearing. As a poor Latina grandmother stated, "I have other people to worry about before myself." Persistently poorer emotional well-being was found among those who had lost a child or grandchild to AIDS within the past year. Although this is not surprising, the particular vulnerability of these caregivers must be underscored, given that child rearing may preempt the caregiver's mourning. Moreover, greater risk of isolation in bereavement must also be anticipated, because of AIDS stigma and the demands of child care, which may mean that the grandparents are less likely to self-identify as needing supportive services and less likely to be able to use services that are available.

The stigma of HIV continues to be a psychological toxin for grandparents raising HIV-affected and orphaned children and a stigma encountered even within the aging network (Joslin, 1999; Joslin & DeGraw, 1998; Lloyd, 1989). Professionals in aging and other human services often lack the necessary sensitivity and respect, and this treatment becomes another social strain that isolates and shames. Given that some grandparents blame themselves for how their adult child became infected, the added burden of a stigmatized disease further diminishes self-esteem.

Several areas call for closer research attention. First, as others have noted (Joslin & Brouard, 1996; Minkler & Roe, 1993), longitudinal studies are needed to investigate changes in emotional and physical health over time. Because the experiences of HIV-affected grandparents are determined by the course of HIV infection, illness, and dying, often in multiple events within the same family, a cross-sectional approach is insufficient to capture grandparent well-being over time. Research on effective coping strategies and supports is also essential to develop effective and appropriate interventions.

How the new combination antiviral therapies are transforming HIV caregiving and parental grandparenting has not been examined. It is likely that the new treatments will mean protracted care of the infected over a longer period of time and greater likelihood that the grandparent generation will be helping to manage the disease in both their adult children and grandchildren at the same time. Another issue concerns those grandparents who are raising pre- or perinatally infected children who survive to adolescence and then cope with the new developmental issues that puberty and peer culture brings, such as lack of medication adherence, risk of depression (especially among females), and defiant behavior (J. Grosz, personal communications, 1998).

The multigenerational impact and implications of HIV disease have not been integrated by recent research on grandparents as parents, nor have they been given sufficient focus in program initiatives. This group's invisibility within grandparenting and HIV literature is juxtaposed to the epidemic's continued imposition of parental surrogacy on large numbers of grandparents, typically grandmothers. As we enter the 21st century the numbers of grandparents and other relatives raising HIV-affected children will continue to rise in the United States and around the globe, particularly in Southeast Asia, sub-Saharan Africa, and Latin America. Women, especially the poor and those of color, are in the pandemic's direct course, with fewer public, community, and interpersonal resources to prevent infection, to reduce maternal transmission, and to improve treatment outcomes. Grandparents in families affected by HIV disease will continue to absorb the emotional costs of caregiving.

REFERENCES

Brown, M. A., & Powell-Cope, G. M. (1991). AIDS family caregiving: Transitions through uncertainty. *Nursing Research, 40,* 338–345.

Bunting, S. M. (1996). Persons with AIDS and the family care givers: Negotiating the journey. *Journal of Family Nursing, 2,* 399–417.

Burnette, D. (1997). Grandmother caregivers in inner city Latino families: A descriptive profile and informal supports. *Journal of Multicultural Social Work, 5,* 121–138.

Cannon-Poindexter, C., & Linsk, N. (1999). HIV-related stigma in a sample of HIV affected older female African American caregivers. *Social Work, 44,* 46–61.

Centers for Disease Control and Prevention. (1997, July). HIV/AIDS and women in the United States. *CDC Update.*

Chu, S., Buehler, J., Oxtoby, M. J., & Kilbourne, B. W. (1991). Impact of the human immunodeficiency virus epidemic on mortality in children, United States. *Pediatrics, 87,* 806–810.

Clipp, E. C., Adinolfi, A. J., Forrest, L., & Bennett, C. L. (1995). Informal caregivers of persons with AIDS. *Journal of Palliative Care, 11,* 10–18.

Cohen, F. L., & Nehring, W. L. (1994). Foster care of HIV positive children in the United States. *Public Health Reports, 109,* 60–67.

Derogatis, L., & Spencer, P. (1982). *Administration and Procedures: BSI manual.* Baltimore, MD: Johns Hopkins Press.

Doka, K. (1989). *Disenfranchised grief.* New York: Lexington.

Dowdell, E. N. (1995). Caregiver burden: Grandmothers raising their high risk grandchildren. *Journal of Psychosocial Nursing, 33,* 27–30.

Draimin, B. (1995). A second family? Placement and custody decisions. In S. Geballe, J. Gruendel, & W. Andiman (Eds.), *Forgotten children of the AIDS epidemic* (pp. 125–139). New Haven: Yale University Press.

Gaynor, S. E. (1990). The long haul: The effect of home care on caregivers. *Image: Journal of Nursing Scholarship, 22,* 208–212.

Honey, E. (1988). AIDS and the inner city. *Social Casework, 37,* 365–370.

Ickovics, J., & Rodin, J. (1992). Women and AIDS in the United States: Epidemiology, natural history and mediation mechanisms. *Health Psychology, 11,* 1–16.

Joslin, D. (1999). Grandparents raising children orphaned and affected by HIV/AIDS. In C. Cox (Ed.), *To grandmother's house we go* (pp. 167–183). New York: Springer Publishing Co.

Joslin, D., & Brouard, A. (1995). The prevalence of grandmothers as primary caregivers in a poor pediatric population. *Journal of Community Health, 20,* 383–401.

Joslin, D., & DeGraw, C. (1998). *OASIS final report.* Paterson, NJ: Coalition on AIDS in Passaic County.

Joslin, D., & Harrison, R. (1998). The "hidden patient": Older relatives raising children orphaned by AIDS. *Journal of the American Medical Women's Association, 53,* 65–71.

Joslin, D., Mevi-Triano, C., & Berman, J. (1997, November). *Grandparents raising children orphaned by HIV/AIDS: Health risks and service needs.* Paper presented at the 50th annual scientific meeting of the Gerontological Society of America. Cincinnati, OH.

Kelly, S. J. (1993). Caregiver stress in grandparents raising grandchildren. *Image: Journal of Nursing Scholarship, 25,* 331–336.

LeBlanc, A. J., Aneshensel, C. S., & Wight, R. G. (1995). Psychotherapy use and depression among AIDS caregivers. *Journal of Community Psychology, 23,* 127–142.

Lesar, S. M., Gerber, M., & Semmel, M. I. (1995/6). HIV infection in children: Family stress, social support and adaptation. *Exceptional Children, 62,* 224–236.

Levine-Perkell, J. (1996). Caregiving issues. In K. Nokes (Ed.), *HIV/AIDS and the older adult* (pp. 20–41). Washington, DC: Taylor & Francis.

Lloyd, G. (1989). AIDS and elders: Advocacy, activism and coalitions. *Generations, XIII*(4), 32–35.

Macklin, E. D. (1989). Introduction. In E. D. Macklin (Ed.), *AIDS and families.* New York: Harrington Park Press.

Marder, R., & Linsk, N. L. (1995). Addressing AIDS long-term care issues through education and advocacy. *Health and Social Work, 20,* 75–80.

Michaels, D., & Levine, C. (1992). Estimates of the number of motherless youth orphaned by AIDS in the United States. *Journal of the American Medical Association, 268,* 3456–3461.

Minkler, M., Fuller-Thompson, E., Miller, D., & Driver, D. (1997). Depression in grandparents raising grandchildren: Results of a national longitudinal study. *Archives of Family Medicine, 6,* 445–452.

Minkler, M., & Roe, K. (1993). *Grandmothers as caregivers: Raising children of the crack cocaine epidemic.* Thousand Oaks, CA: Sage Publications.

Minkler, M., & Roe, K. (1996). Grandparents as surrogate parents. *Generations, 20*(1), 34–38.

Minkler, M., Roe, K., & Price, M. (1992). The physical and emotional health of grandmothers raising grandchildren in the crack cocaine epidemic. *The Gerontologist, 32,* 752–761.

Montgomery, J. F. V, Gonyea, J. G., & Hooyman, N. R. (1985). Caregiving and the experience of subjective and objective burden. *Family Relations, 34,* 19–26.

Pearlin, L. I., Anenshensel, C. S., & LeBlanc, A. J. (1997). The forms and mechanisms of stress proliferation: The case of AIDS caregivers. *Journal of Health and Social Behavior, 39,* 337–356.

Pearlin, L. I., Semple, S., & Turner, H. (1988). Stress of AIDS caregiving: A preliminary overview of the issues. *Death Studies, 12,* 501–517.

Poindexter, C. C., & Linsk, N. (1998). HIV-related stigma in the lives of a sample of HIV-affected older female African American caregivers. *Social Work, 44,* 46–61.

Powell-Cope, G. M., & Brown, M. A. (1992). Going public as an AIDS family caregiver. *Social Science and Medicine, 34,* 571–580.

Raveis, V. H., & Siegal, K. (1991). The impact of caregiving on informal and familial caregivers. *AIDS Patient Care, 5,* 39–43.

Roth, J., Siegal, R., & Black, S. (1994). Identifying the mental health needs of children living in families with AIDS or HIV infection. *Community Mental Health Journal, 30,* 581–592.

Schable, B., Diaz, T., Chu, S., Caldwell, M. B., & Conti, L. (1995). Who are the primary caregivers of children born to HIV infected mothers? Results from a multi state surveillance project. *Pediatrics, 95,* 511–515.

Shevlov, S. P. (1994). The children's agenda for the 1990s and beyond [Editorial]. *American, Journal of Public Health, 84,* 1066–1067.

Szinovacz, M., DeViney, S., & Atkinson, M. (1997, November). *Effects of surrogate parenting on grandparents' depression and self-esteem: A panel analysis.* Paper presented at the 50th annual scientific meeting of the Gerontological Society of America, Cincinnati, OH.

Theis, S. L., Cohen, F. L., Forrest, J., & Zelewsky, M. (1997). Needs assessment of caregivers of people with HIV/AIDS. *Journal of the Association of Nurses in AIDS Care, 8,* 76–84.

Tiblier, K. B., Walker, G., & Rolland, J. (1989). Therapeutic issues when working with families of persons with AIDS. In E. D. Macklin (Ed.), *AIDS and families* (pp. 33–58). New York: Harrington Park Press.

Williams, A. B., Shahryarinejad, A., Andrews, S., & Alcaebes, P. (1997). Social support of HIV infected mothers: Relationship to HIV care seeking. *Journal of the Association of Nurses in AIDS Care, 8*, 91–98.

Zarit, S. H., Reever, K. E., & Bach-Peterson, J. (1980). Relatives of the impaired elderly: Correlates of feelings of burden. *Gerontologist, 20*, 649–655.

CHAPTER 7

Cross-Cultural Differences in Custodial Grandparenting

J. Rafael Toledo, Bert Hayslip Jr., Michelle A. Emick, Cecilia Toledo, and Craig E. Henderson

That individual differences in the experience of aging are substantial is now well established (Nelson & Dannefer, 1992). Consequently, given the potential for variability across persons, it should not be surprising to find that as individuals grow older they experience life transitions and adapt to age-grade roles in unique ways; this is true, for example, for phenomena such as retirement (Braithwaite, Gibson, & Bosly-Craft, 1986), caregiving (Aneshensel, Pearlin, Mullan, Zarit, & Whitlatch, 1995), and adjustment to nursing home life (O'Connor & Vallerand, 1994). Variations in adjustment to grandparenting have been explored in terms of the meaning of grandparenthood (Kivnick, 1982) and grandparental styles (Cherlin & Furstenberg, 1986), but there is comparatively little work on variations in custodial grandparenting. What research does exist has focused on the difficulties African American grandparents face in caring for a grandchild (Burton & deVries, 1993; Minkler &

Roe, 1993; Minkler, Roe, & Price, 1992; Minkler, Roe, & Robertson-Beckley, 1994) and on interventions to aid such grandparents (Minkler, Driver, Roe, & Bedeian, 1993), as well as on those African Americans not raising their grandchildren (Strom, Collinsworth, Strom, & Griswold, 1992).

Given that there appear to be both subcultural and/or ethnic differences in the experiences of custodial grandparents, it would not be surprising to observe cross-cultural differences in custodial grandparenting, though no such published work exists in this regard. Such differences, if they indeed do exist, may be mediated by either socioeconomic, health-related, family compositional, or role-expectation influences. Cultural differences in custodial grandparenting also may influence the mental health, role satisfaction, and role meaning of grandparents raising grandchildren who are experiencing behavioral or emotional difficulties, either arising from the divorce of or abuse by their parents or related to difficulties in adjusting to their grandparents, who now must raise them (Emick & Hayslip, 1999; Hayslip, Shore, Henderson, & Lambert, 1998).

Little work exists regarding grandparenting in other cultures. Regarding Mexican grandparents, Schmidt (1982) reported a high degree of involvement based on gender preferences. However, grandparents and grandchildren did not live in the same household; thus, the study did not focus on grandparents' ongoing interactions with their grandchildren.

Despite the paucity of grandparent research in Mexican culture, the family unit is central in the worldview of Mexicans, and grandparents play a very meaningful role in this society. Culbertson and Margaona (1981) reported that whereas most U.S. students considered elderly relatives who choose to live with their children as burdens, 26% of Mexican students had aged relatives living in their homes, and 77% indicated that they helped their families in some way and were perceived as a source of comfort by the majority of their older family members. Selby, Murphy, and Lorenzen (1990) concluded that the nuclear family was definitely the most important context of experience for every Mexican and that poverty and adverse living conditions have not destroyed the Mexican family, as it "seems to have in the U.S. American underclass" (p. 53).

In Mexico even nuclear families establish frequent contact with their relatives, to the extent that they could be considered as functioning in fact as extended families. There is a marked tendency for parents to encourage their children to remain in the parental home until they marry or to remain close to them after their marriage, sometimes living in the same household with the grandchildren. The extended family gathers on weekends regularly, and intergenerational interactions are quite dynamic. To say that grandparents have a great deal of visibility in Mexican families is an understatement. They play a very important role in modern urban Latin America, where Adler-Lomnitz and Perez-Lizar (1987) suggest that the "grand family" is the most significant family unit.

Selby et al. (1990) further describe the family as an ideological construction based on the notions of *respeto*, an agreement of respect toward the elders; *macho*, the ideal male figure; *abnegation*, the most important maternal quality of selflessness; and *confianza*, a contract of trust as part of being a family member. Children are generally obedient and definitely represent a very important economic asset given the precarious conditions experienced by a large segment of the population that includes children in the "locus of Mexican production." A child who consistently refuses to help in a household is considered to be of "inferior quality" and "seriously defective."

Despite the centrality of the family in Mexico, Selby et al. (1990) point out that the "ideal" family does not always reflect the reality of family life, which may be full of contradictions. Poverty further separates the real from the ideal household in Mexico, leading to alcoholism, violence, cynicism, and psychological pathology (Lewis, 1959). Gramajo and Norah (1988) report that 40%–80% of the families in Guadalajara donate their children to the grandparents. Some of these families may be migrants from small villages; among members of the upper class the arrangement may be temporary.

This orientation toward the primacy of the family in Mexico, as is true of African American families (see Bengtson, Rosenthal, & Burton, 1990), may mitigate the stresses of raising one's grandchild, especially if this child is problematic in nature (see above). In this light, the purpose of the present study is to explore cultural (United States vs. Mexico) differences in custodial grandparenting as they interact with the differences noted above between grandparents not raising their grandchildren, those raising apparently normal grandchildren, and those raising problem grandchildren (e.g., Emick & Hayslip, 1999).

METHOD

Participants

U.S. Sample

Seventy-eight middle-aged and older adults participated in this study (see Emick & Hayslip, 1999). Grandparents were recruited through newspaper, radio, and television advertisements, as well as through presentations to local retirement communities, senior centers, grandparents' clubs, and mental health agencies. Additionally, school principals, medical and dental practitioners, and legal professionals were approached to solicit grandparent volunteers.

Selection criteria specified that grandparents report on a grandchild 18 years or younger (a) who may or may not have been in their legal custody but for whom they exclusively provided parental supervision and care and with whom they coresided or (b) for whom primary responsibility of care lay with parents, whom respondents saw the most frequently of all their grandchildren, and for whom they provided only minimal or nominal care. Criteria (a) defined the parental, or custodial, grandparental groups; criteria (b) defined the traditional grandparental group.

The extent to which the grandchildren in the Emick and Hayslip (1999) study were experiencing physical, behavioral, school-related, emotional, or neurological difficulties, as perceived by grandparents, was assessed in several ways. First, in an initial interview with each grandparent, individuals were asked an open-ended question regarding whether the grandchild had experienced problems of the above varieties and were asked to describe these problems in as much detail as possible. Second, individuals were asked, as a part of a questionnaire each completed, to indicate the extent to which the grandchild about whom they were reporting was experiencing a variety of difficulties. On the basis of these open-ended data, individuals were defined as belonging to one of two custodial groups of grandparents.

These objective problem-rating data suggest substantial agreement between the open-ended and objective measures of the difficulties grandchildren were experiencing as perceived by their grandparents. Indeed, the difference across groups in perceived grandchildren's difficulties was statistically significant, multivariate $F(20, 122) = 2.75$, $p < .01$; particular to resisting authority, $F(2, 71) = 10.97$, $p < .01$; hyperactivity, $F(2, 71) = 10.71$, $p < .01$; learning difficulties, $F(2, 71) = 4.54$, $p < .01$; depression, $F(2, 71) = 10.45$, $p < .01$; and, to a lesser extent, other miscellaneous problems, $F(2, 71) = 2.98$, $p < .06$. For total perceived difficulties, grandparent group differences were substantial as well, $F(2, 71) = 16.80$, $p < .01$ (see Emick & Hayslip, 1999). Overall, these data suggest that both traditional and custodial grandparents raising grandchildren whom they perceived to be experiencing few problems indeed reported that their grandchildren were experiencing few difficulties relative to those custodial grandparents who reported their grandchildren to be having a variety of problems.

The traditional group of grandparents consisted of 23 participants, 5 males and 18 females, all of whom were Caucasian. Respondents ranged in age from 40 to 77 years ($M = 60.22$, $SD = 10.14$). Seventeen participants were married, two were divorced, and four were widowed. Years of education completed ranged from 12 to 20 ($M = 15.96$, $SD = 2.88$). Annual income ranged from less than \$10,000 to greater than \$60,000, with most participants falling within the \$40,000 to \$60,000 range. Self-rated health ranged from 3 (fair) to 5 (very good) ($M = 4.39$, $SD = .78$). The age of the grandchild about whom the participants completed the survey ranged from less than 1 year of age to 18 ($M = 7.22$, $SD = 6.53$). Eight of the grandchildren were male, and 15 were female. No persons in this group reported full-time responsibility for a grandchild's care.

The custodial group of grandparents raising grandchildren who were not demonstrating problems consisted of 24 participants, 8 males and 16 females. Twenty-three were Caucasian, and one was African American. Respondents ranged in age from 47 to 70 years ($M = 56.75$, $SD = 6.60$). Twenty-one participants were married, two were divorced, and one was widowed. Years of education completed ranged from 11 to 20 ($M = 14.08$, $SD = 2.19$). Annual income ranged from less than \$10,000 to greater than \$60,000, with most participants falling within the \$30,000 to \$40,000 range. Self-rated health ranged from 3 (fair) to 5 (very good) ($M = 4.37$, $SD = .77$). The age of the grandchild about whom the respondents completed the survey ranged from less than 1 year of age to 17 ($M = 7.04$, $SD = 5.76$). Eleven of the grandchildren were male, and 13 were female. Ten participants had legal custody of their grandchildren, and 13 did not. One participant failed to answer the question pertaining to custody.

The custodial group of grandparents raising grandchildren manifesting problems consisted of 28 participants, 4 males and 24 females. Twenty-four of the participants were Caucasian, and four were Hispanic. Respondents ranged in age from 44 to 71 years ($M = 56.07$, $SD = 7.43$). Twenty-four participants were married, three were divorced, and one was separated. Years of education completed ranged from 5 to 18 ($M = 12.43$, $SD = 2.52$). Annual income ranged from less than \$10,000 to greater than \$60,000, with most participants falling within the \$20,000 to \$40,000 range. Self-rated health ranged from 3 (fair) to 5 (very good) ($M = 3.79$, $SD = .74$). The age of the grandchild about whom the respondents completed the survey ranged from less than 1 year of age to 18 ($M = 8.46$, $SD = 4.69$). Nineteen of the grandchildren were male, and nine were female. Eighteen participants had legal custody of their grandchildren, and 10 did not. Grandchildren being raised by these grandparents were receiving treatment for oppositional behavior, drug use, attention deficit/hyperactivity disorder, learning disabilities, and depression. Other problems perceived by the grandparents for which the grandchildren were to varying degrees being treated included alcohol use, mental retardation, sexual identity disturbance, and legal problems (i.e., breaking the law).

The circumstances under which grandparents assumed responsibility for their grandchildren included divorce; incarceration; mental, emotional, or physical impairment of the parent; death of the parent; child abuse; and parents' drug abuse, with divorce, child abuse, and the parents' drug abuse being most common.

Mexican Sample

Volunteers in Mexico were selected from the town of Ciudad Guzman, in the state of Jalisco. Both male and female grandparents served as participants. Criteria (primarily based on interview data, supplemented by problem ratings due to missing data for 18 grandparents) defining each grandparent group were identical to those utilized in the American sample.

The traditional group of grandparents consisted of 4 males and 12 females (M age = 45, range = 36–75). Ten were married, and the remainder were either divorced or widowed. Self-rated health ranged from very poor (1) to very good (5) ($M = 2.9$). Years of education ranged from less than 1 year to 12 years, and all reported earning less than $10,000 annually. The age of the grandchild about whom respondents reported ranged from less than 1 year to 18 years ($M = 5.1$ years); 10 were male, and 4 were female (missing data = 2). No persons in this group reported full-time responsibility for a grandchild's care.

The custodial group of grandparents raising children experiencing few problems consisted of 5 men and 11 women (M age = 46.8). Thirteen were married, and the remainder were divorced or widowed. Level of education ranged from less than 1 year to 12 years, and all earned less than $10,000 annually. Self-rated health ranged from very poor (1) to very good (5) ($M = 2.95$). The age of the grandchild whom the grandparents were raising ranged from less than 1 year to 17 years ($M = 7.8$ years); 8 were female, and 8 were male. Only one grandparent had legal custody of the grandchild (s)he was raising (missing data = 3). Only drug abuse ($n = 2$), oppositional behavior ($n = 1$), mental retardation ($n = 1$), hyperactivity ($n = 3$), sexual identity ($n = 2$), learning difficulties ($n = 1$), depression ($n = 2$), and other miscellaneous difficulties ($n = 1$) were mentioned by grandparents in this group as moderate or serious problems in their grandchildren.

The custodial group of grandparents raising problem grandchildren consisted of 3 men and 14 women (M age = 61.1, range = 42–79). Ten were married, and the remainder were either separated or widowed. Level of education ranged from less than 1 year to 6 years (missing data = 3); all reported earning less than $10,000 annually. Self-reported health ranged from very poor (1) to very good (5) ($M = 2.8$). The age of the grandchild being raised ranged from less than 1 year to 18 years (M age = 9.1); 9 were male, and 5 were female. Only two grandparents reported having custody of the grandchildren they were raising. Problems reportedly experienced by these grandchildren were related to drug or alcohol use ($n = 2$), oppositional behavior ($n = 2$), mental retardation ($n = 2$), hyperactivity ($n = 4$), learning difficulties ($n = 3$), depression ($n = 3$), and other miscellaneous behavioral, emotional, and neurological difficulties ($n = 1$). Most Mexican grandparents assumed responsibility for their grandchildren because of cognitive or emotional impairment in their children, parental child abuse, parental abuse of drugs or alcohol, or death of the parent.

Questionnaires

For the U.S. sample, initial interviews were conducted in volunteers' homes, after which individuals were asked to complete a self-report questionnaire, the initial section of which focused on demographic information such as age, gender, level of education, health status, work history (previous occupations, current work status), marital status, and income.

The first step in the gathering of data from the Mexican sample involved the translation of the questionnaire utilized with the U.S. sample into Spanish. The items on the questionnaire matched those from the one utilized for the U.S. sample (Emick & Hayslip, 1999) and was translated by a bilingual/bicultural individual; we chose not only a bilingual person but one who was bicultural as well to prevent the loss of the actual meaning of each question. Next, the typist and translator, in addition to two other bilingual/bicultural people, proofread each question to further ensure its validity with Mexican individuals.

Once this questionnaire was ready for use, volunteers were gathered from the Mexican university Centro Universitario del Sur, located in Ciudad Guzman, for assistance in administering the questionnaires on a one-to-one basis. In addition, a bilingual/bicultural psychology student (the fourth author) volunteered assistance in this task. Once this group was formed, three practice sessions were held, consisting of understanding the meaning behind each question, and explanations of each scale were undertaken, with much detail to ensure proper comprehension of each question's meaning. Moreover, various scenarios were role-played to present "live" cases to each participant. At the end of the second session, each volunteer was issued a practice questionnaire and was asked to bring this questionnaire, as complete as possible, to the third session, which consisted of discussing any difficulties experienced by the volunteers and did not end until every question was answered. These training sessions were held under the supervision of the first author, a bilingual/bicultural psychology professor.

For the Mexican sample, all interviews were held in the participating grandparent's home or in a private room in the local senior citizen center. The completion of each questionnaire was at the participant's time and place of choosing so as to provide as relaxed an atmosphere as possible for interviewing. All volunteers were thoroughly counseled regarding their rights, risks, and benefits associated with participation, as per Human Subjects Research guidelines. Approximate time for the completion of this questionnaire was anywhere from 2 to 25 hours (spread out over a weeklong period).

Measures

For each person, a formal measure of social support (Sarason, Shearin, Pierce, & Sarason, 1987) was administered, indexed by the total number of persons listed who provided both physical and psychosocial support perceived as effective or beneficial in nature. Respondents were asked to report on salient features of their relationship with only one grandchild, age 18 or younger, according to the procedure of Thomas (1988). This procedure was used because different grandchildren affect grandparent feelings and perceptions in different ways (Cherlin & Furstenberg, 1986). Satisfaction with grandparenting was assessed with 15 Likert-type questions—for example, "Life has more meaning for me because of my grandchild," "Sometimes it is hard to say I love my grandchild" (alpha = .79)—used in the Thomas work. The meaning of grandparenthood was evaluated with Likert-type items from the Thomas questionnaire, for example, "I value the fact that my grandchild confides in me," "I value being able to teach things to my grandchild." These items reflected five dimensions of meaning pertaining to grandparenthood (i.e., Centrality, Valued Elder, Immortality through Clan, Reinvolvement with Past, and Indulgence), where scores for each meaning dimension were used here (Kivnick, 1982). Coefficient alphas range from .68 (Indulgence) to .90 (Centrality) (Kivnick, 1982).

Grandparents' perceptions of their relationships with a grandchild were measured by the Positive Affect Index and Negative Affect Index (Bence & Thomas, 1988). Two single questions each asked the respondent to rate the quality of the relationship with the grandchild (Very Negative to Very Positive) and the satisfaction with this relationship (Very Unsatisfied to Very Satisfied). Psychological distress was assessed with the Center for Epidemiologic Studies Depression Scale (CES-D) (Radloff, 1977). The scale exhibits high internal consistency (alpha = .85), adequate test-retest stability (correlations range from .45 to .70) (see Radloff, 1977). Psychological well-being was evaluated using Liang's (1985) 15-item self-report scale, which is designed to measure respondents' feelings about their lives. The scale integrates items from the Bradburn Affect Balance Scale (Bradburn, 1969) and the Life Satisfaction Index A (Neugarten, Havighurst, & Tobin, 1961). The Structure of Coping Scale (Pearlin & Schooler, 1978) was used to identify potential strains in participants' roles as marriage partners, economic managers, parents, and workers, as well as to identify emotional stress experienced by participants connected to these roles. Only those questions relating to role stress and role strain as economic managers and parents were used here, as not all participants were employed or married.

RESULTS

Data were analyzed via a 2 (culture—U.S. vs. Mexico) × 3 (grandparent group) MANOVA, utilizing the above measures of satisfaction with grandparenting, grandparental meaning, positive and negative affect, relationship quality and relationship satisfaction, role (parental, financial) stress, depression, well-being, social support, and attitudes toward mental health care as dependent variables. At the multivariate level of analysis, both cultural, $F(16, 91) = 8.18, p < .01$, and grandparent group, $F(32, 180) = 2.21, p < .01$, differences were substantial for the linear combination of measures, and the Culture × Group interaction was not statistically different from zero. At the univariate level of analysis, cultural differences were specific to four of five dimensions of grandparent meaning (indulgent, centrality, reinvolvement with past, immortality through clan), satisfaction with grandparenting, financial and parental stress, positive affect, relationship quality, and depression [all $Fs(1, 92) > 6.09, p < .01$]. Although means for the above dimensions of grandparent meaning favored Mexican grandparents, such persons also had higher depression scores, experienced more parental and financial stress, reported less satisfying relationships with their grandchildren, less mutual understanding and trust in such relationships (positive affect), and reported less satisfaction with grandparenting (see Table 7.1).

Regarding the univariate findings for grandparent group effects (see Table 7.1), differences were obtained for perceptions of the grandchild's behavior as irritating (negative affect) and parental and financial stress, all $Fs(2, 106) > 4.62$, $p < .01$. In each case, grandparents raising problem grandchildren scored highest, followed by those raising grandchildren with few problems, and traditional grandparents.

The above grandparent group and cultural effects were then examined via statistically controlling (using MANCOVA) for the effects of grandparent age, grandchild age, grandparent health, grandparent level of education, grandparent income, and number of grandchildren. A two-way (Culture × Grandparent group) MANOVA had indicated that grandparent groups differed ($p < .01$) in terms of grandchild age, education, health, and number of grandchildren. Moreover, cultural differences existed ($p < .01$) for income, education, health, and number of grandchildren, with Mexican grandparents being in poorer health, earning less money, being less highly educated, and having more grandchildren. This additional analysis suggested that, whereas the grandparent Group × Culture interaction remained nonsignificant, the multivariate grandparent group effect remained substantial ($p < .01$), and particular to parental and financial stress. However, the multivariate effect of culture was no longer statistically different from zero ($p < .10$). Post hoc examination of cultural differences at the univariate level revealed them nevertheless to be statistically reliable ($p < .01$) and particular to indulgent and immortality through clan grandparental meaning (still favoring Mexican grandparents), depression, self-esteem, and social support (where the U.S. sample was less depressed, had higher self-esteem, and more social support).

DISCUSSION

These data suggest that there are cultural differences in the experience of grandparenting and that the personal and role-related difficulties associated with raising a grandchild, especially a problematic grandchild, relative to being a traditional grandparent, are universal

TABLE 7.1 Grandparent Group by Cultural Differences in Custodial Grandparenting

| | United States | | | | | | Mexico | | | | | |
| | T (n = 21) | | C-LP (n = 19) | | C-PC (n = 26) | | T (n = 16) | | C-LP (n = 16) | | C-PC (n = 14) | |
	M	SD	M	SD	M	SD	M	SD	M	SD	M	SD
GP satisfaction	61.66	5.83	58.84	7.36	55.00	9.33	55.89	10.15	53.68	7.46	55.28	10.35
Valued Elder	29.04	3.18	29.47	3.64	28.03	4.94	28.68	4.46	28.62	4.82	29.38	6.02
Centrality	27.19	4.92	27.26	5.24	28.50	4.22	30.61	4.90	31.46	5.49	32.15	6.74
Immortality	19.71	4.64	21.26	3.91	18.65	4.69	23.35	4.54	24.75	4.56	24.38	5.03
Reinvolvement	11.09	3.88	9.31	4.34	10.84	4.77	14.43	3.24	14.28	3.94	13.46	4.08
Indulgence	12.33	4.05	10.42	3.46	9.73	2.92	14.06	2.86	14.68	3.04	14.23	4.30
Pos. affect[a]	41.31	11.06	39.41	12.18	41.00	9.61	38.73	6.28	40.31	6.94	41.50	6.67
Neg. affect[b]	38.81	6.43	36.29	6.19	32.21	5.70	32.28	6.31	35.37	5.52	34.28	5.69
Relationship quality	4.77	.68	4.88	.48	4.53	.83	4.25	.68	4.37	.72	4.14	1.23
Relationship satisfaction	4.68	.78	4.54	.98	4.21	1.13	4.25	.85	4.31	.79	3.92	1.32
Parental Stress[c]	31.36	6.39	38.25	7.90	48.71	11.13	40.40	16.99	53.31	18.28	55.21	17.59
Financial Stress[c]	26.22	8.47	27.95	5.12	32.78	7.10	31.33	8.64	39.18	7.69	35.07	5.92
Depression	29.90	11.85	29.16	9.30	33.92	13.28	40.00	12.10	43.66	11.38	43.35	9.47
Self-esteem	52.50	16.78	50.95	12.77	46.89	11.89	48.31	12.66	48.66	8.60	46.00	11.08
Social support	22.00	14.40	21.37	12.37	13.71	11.48	15.31	8.45	16.31	8.60	15.07	11.90

T = Traditional.

C-LP = custodial, low problem.

C-PC = Custodial, problem child.

GP = Grandparent.

[a]Grandchild's behavior, positive.

[b]Grandchild's behavior, negative.

[c]Structure of Coping Scale (Pearlin & Schooler, 1978).

across U.S. and Mexican samples of grandparents. These grandparental group differences that generalized across cultures remained, for the most part, when controlling for the effects of a variety of sociodemographic variables differentiating samples both within and across each culture.

Importantly, Mexican grandparents reported enhanced grandparental meaning relative to those in the United States, despite experiencing less role satisfaction and more role stress compared to their U.S. counterparts. It is important to note, however, that although we found significant cultural differences in the experience of grandparenting, these differences may be slowly lessening, due mostly to factors such as heavy migratory and trade patterns between Mexico and the United States, as well as the impact that U.S. television and movies have in the Mexican population (Selby et al. 1990). In this respect, Hondagneu-Sotelo (1992) studied the behavior of migrating Mexican husbands and found that lengthy separations diminished their patriarchal authoritary upon return, thus providing some evidence of the U.S. influence on Mexican traditions. In a significant proportion of impoverished families, the common law type of marriage is very frequent. Lewis (1959) found this to be the case in 46% of the families he studied. Yet the incidence of separation and divorce have risen considerably in Mexico City (Pick & Butler, 1997).

That Mexican grandparents in this sample experienced enhanced role meaning despite the greater financial and parental stress, as well as diminished grandparental role satisfaction, is noteworthy. This is similar to what we have observed with male grandparents, who derive personal meaning from their roles as grandparents despite the stresses of raising their grandchildren (Hayslip et al., 1998). This, in fact, may be the source of much psychological distress in Mexican society and may at least in part explain the high scores on grandparental depression we found in our sample. This apparent discrepancy between role meaning and role satisfaction also may reflect the perception of the family in Mexico, wherein individuals' needs are subjugated to those of the family unit, and the family in reality functions in an extended manner. As individuals' egos, privacy, and power are viewed as secondary to the integrity of the family, this may permit grandparents to retain meaning in their role as family caretakers (most Mexican grandparents in this sample were women), enabling them to tolerate disagreements with both children and grandchildren, to sustain themselves in face of having to make ends meet financially, and to permit them to deal with the demands of raising their grandchildren. The Mexican grandparent sample's higher scores on immortality, centrality, and reinvolvement may therefore be a reflection of the importance they attribute to their family as an extension of themselves. Their indulgence scores may indicate a compensation for the strictness and authoritarianism typical of Mexican parents. Grandparenting, therefore, provides a second opportunity for parental benevolence.

The perception of the family as one and the same with the individual may explain the fact that Mexican grandparents reported less formal social support than did U.S. grandparents, due to their rejection of others outside the family as resources on which to draw to deal with the difficulties of raising a grandchild. As role-specific designations are less clear among Mexican families, asking for help from others in the family with the expectation of receiving it may be easier, underscored by the lower SES (i.e., income) of Mexican grandparents in this sample. It also may reflect the greater likelihood of both the husband and wife sharing caregiving responsibilities, permitting them to persist in the face of role demands, in contrast to American grandparents, where women have assumed primary responsibility for raising the grandchildren (Burton, 1992; Minkler, Roe, & Price, 1992). This orientation toward formal help sources is similar to that of African-American families in caring for their elderly family members (see Bengtson et al., 1990).

In concert with higher grandparental meaning scores, Mexican grandparents reported less role satisfaction than did U.S. grandparents. It may be that Mexican grandparents' parenting responsibilities are, comparatively speaking, prolonged into an age in which economic resources usually shrink, when they have increasing health problems of their own, and when there are no professional or institutional agencies available for them. Dietz (1995) found that only 31% of older Mexican Americans received significant help from their relatives. This also could be true of the families in this sample: they did belong to the lower socioeconomic class wherein their social circle is burdened by the demands of their own survival, permitting them little time to help their aged relatives. This also could account for lower scores in self-esteem and coping and higher depression scores among Mexican grandparents. Raymond, Rhoads, and Raymond (1980) compared Anglos, Blacks, and Chicanos and found that, for Chicanos, family satisfaction was more predictive of overall well-being and positive affect than was social satisfaction, suggesting that the Chicano family may function primarily to provide a positive environment for its members, rather than mitigating the stressful effects of a negative environment.

Though this study is quite exploratory and is in need of replication, it nevertheless helps us realize how much more we need to learn about the impact of grandparental roles on the economic and psychological well-being of Mexican grandparents. Consequently, this study raises more questions than it answers. Indeed, although we know that grandparenting and parenting together can be a source of distress and that the demands of raising grandchildren are, to a certain extent, universal, these cross-cultural findings do shed some light on the coping mechanisms some grandparents have developed to help them deal with the demands of raising their grandchildren. Indeed, these cross-cultural data suggest that some grandparents are able to carry on in the face of poorer health, lower incomes, and a lack of formal support from others by drawing on the family and by maximizing the family's protective, sustaining function in caring for its young. Thus, they can derive meaning from their roles as caretakers and as grandparents who are symbols of the family's persistence in face of role change and economic hardship.

REFERENCES

Adler-Lomnitz, L., & Perez-Lizaur, M. (1987). *A Mexican elite family, 1820–1980: Kinship, class, and culture.* Princeton, NJ: Princeton University Press.

Aneshensel, C. S., Pearlin, L. I., Mullan, J. T., Zarit, S. H., & Whitlatch, C. J. (1995). *Profiles in caregiving: The unexpected career.* New York: Academic Press.

Bence, S. L., & Thomas, J. L. (1988, November). *Grandparent-parent relationships as predictors of grandparent-grandchild relationships.* Paper presented at the annual scientific meeting of the Gerontological Society of America. San Francisco.

Bengtson, V. L., Rosenthal, C., & Burton, L. (1990). Families and aging: Diversity and heterogeneity. In R. H. Binstock & L. K. George (Eds.),

Handbook of aging and the social sciences (3rd ed., pp. 263–287). New York: Academic Press.

Bradburn, N. M. (1969). *The structure of psychological well-being.* Chicago: Aldine.

Braithwaite, V. A., Gibson, D. M., & Bosly-Craft, R. (1986). An exploratory study of poor adjustment styles among retirees. *Social Science and Medicine, 23,* 493–499.

Burton, L. M. (1992). Black grandparents rearing children of drug-addicted parents: Stressors, outcomes, and social service needs. *Gerontologist, 32,* 744–751.

Burton, L. M., & deVries, C. (1993). Challenges and rewards: African American grandparents as surrogate parents. In L. Burton (Ed.), *Families and aging* (pp. 101–108). Amityville, NY: Baywood Publishers.

Cherlin, A. J., & Furstenberg, F. F. (1986). *The new American grandparent: A place in the family, a life apart.* New York: Basic Books.

Culbertson, F. M., & Margaona, E. A. (1981). A study of attitudes and values toward the aged, cross-cultural comparisons. *International Journal of Group Tensions, 11,* 34–46.

Dietz, T. L. (1995). Patterns of integenerational assistance within the Mexican-American family: Is the family taking care of the older generation's needs? *Journal of Family Issues, 16,* 344–356.

Emick, M. A., & Hayslip, B. (1999). Custodial grandparenting: Stresses, coping skills, and relationships with grandchildren. *International Journal on Aging and Human Development, 48,* 35–61.

Gramajo, G., & Norah, N. (1988). La familia tapatia: "Los hijos regalados" [The family in Guadalajara: "Donated children"]. *Revista de Psicoanalisis, 45,* 187–204.

Hayslip, B., Shore, R. J., Henderson, C., & Lambert, P. (1998). Custodial grandparenting and grandchildren with problems: Impact on role satisfaction and role meaning. *Journal of Gerontology: Social Sciences, 53B,* S164–S174.

Hondagneu-Sotelo, P. (1992). Overcoming patriarchal constraints: The reconstruction of gender relations among Mexican immigrant women and men. *Gender and Society, 6,* 393–415.

Kivnick, H. G. (1982). Grandparenthood: An overview of meaning and mental health. *Gerontologist, 22,* 59–66.

Lewis, O. (1959). *Five families: Mexican case studies in the culture of poverty.* New York: Basic Books.

Liang, J. (1985). A structural integration of the Affect Balance Scale and the Life Satisfaction Index A. *Journal of Gerontology, 40,* 552–561.

Minkler, M., Driver, D., Roe, K., & Bedeian, K. (1993). Community interventions to support grandparent caregivers. *Gerontologist, 33,* 807–811.

Minkler, M., & Roe, K. M. (1993). *Grandmothers as caregivers: Raising children of the crack cocaine epidemic.* Newbury Park, CA: Sage Publications.

Minkler, M., Roe, K. M., & Price, M. (1992). The physical and emotional health of grandmothers raising grandchildren in the crack cocaine epidemic. *Gerontologist, 32,* 752–761.

Minkler, M., Roe, K. M., & Robertson-Beckley, R. J. (1994). Raising grandchildren from crack-cocaine households: Effects on family and friendship ties of African American women. *American Journal of Orthopsychiatry, 64,* 20–29.

Nelson, E., & Dannefer, D. (1992). Aged heterogeneity: Fact or fiction? The fate of diversity in gerontological research. *Gerontologist, 32,* 17–23.

Neugarten, B. L., Havinghurst, R. J., & Tobin, S. (1961). The measurement of life satisfaction. *Journal of Gerontology, 16,* 134–143.

O'Connor, B. P., & Vallerand, R. J. (1994). Motivation, self-determination, and person-environment fit as predictors of psychological adjustment among nursing home residents. *Psychology and Aging, 9,* 189–194.

Pearlin, L. I., & Schooler, C. (1978). The structure of coping. *Journal of Health and Social Behavior, 19,* 2–21.

Pick, J. B., & Butler, E. W. (1997). *Mexico megacity.* New York: Westview Press.

Radloff, L. S. (1977). The CES-D Scale: A self-report depression scale for research in the general population. *Applied Psychological Measurement, 1,* 385–401.

Raymond, J. S., Rhoads, D. L., & Raymond, R. I. (1980). The relative impact of family and social involvement on Chicano mental health. *American Journal of Community Psychology, 8,* 557–569.

Sarason, B., Shearin, E., Pierce, G., & Sarason, H. (1987). Interrelations of social support measures: Theoretical and practical applications. *Journal of Personality and Social Psychology, 52,* 813–832.

Schmidt, A. (1982). *Grandparent-grandchild interaction in a Mexican American group.* Spanish Speaking Mental Health Research Center: Occasional Papers (no. 16, p. 22). Mexico City, Mexico.

Selby, H. A., Murphy, A. D., & Lorenzen, S. A. (1990). *The Mexican urban household: Organizing for self-defense.* Austin: University of Texas Press.

Strom, R., Collinsworth, P., Strom, S., & Griswold, D. (1992). Grandparent education for Black families. *Journal of Negro Education, 61,* 554–569.

Thomas, J. L. (1988, November). *Relationships with grandchildren as predictors of grandparents' psychological well-being.* Paper presented at the annual scientific meeting of the Gerontological Society of America. San Francisco.

CHAPTER 8

Custodial Grandparenting Among African Americans: A Focus Group Perspective

Annabel Baird, Robert John, and Bert Hayslip Jr.

A lthough the increase in the number of children being raised by grandparents, with or without a parent present, encompasses all ethnic and socioeconomic groups, the African American community has been hit particularly hard. In 1998, 12.1% of African American children under the age of 18 were being raised in grandparent-headed households, compared to 6.5% and 4.3% for their Hispanic and White counterparts, respectively (U.S. Bureau of the Census, 1999). Of further concern is the proportion of African American children who live in grandparent-headed households where neither parent is present. Of the 1.4 million who lived in the home of a grandparent or great-grandparent in 1998, 570,000, or 41.5%, were in split- or skipped-generation households, in which the parents and sometimes the grandparents were absent, again in comparison with 30.4% of Hispanic and 33.1% of non-Hispanic White children who lived in the same circumstances (U.S. Bureau of the Census, 1999). These households have been shown to be the most impoverished and undereducated of all grandparent-headed households (Chalfie, 1994).

Difficulties in defining the African American grandparent who serves as a surrogate parent for one or more grandchildren originate, as with the grandparent as surrogate parent population as a whole, from a lack of relevant data. The number of African American children under the age of 18 living in grandparent-headed households is easily obtainable from census data, but the reasons for the assumption of parental responsibility by the grandparent are unknown, as are other concurrent responsibilities of the grandparent, such as employment or caring for other children or elders. Studies have been conducted of African American grandparents who assumed the role of parent as a result of the drug epidemic, especially that of crack cocaine (Burton, 1992; Minkler & Roe, 1993), as well as of African Americans as grandparents in general (Strom, Collinsworth, Strom, & Griswold, 1993). Other studies, which included grandparents who took on parental responsibility for their grandchildren for a wide variety of reasons, have yielded data concerning the environment and needs of custodial grandparents but were, by circumstance, not design, conducted on predominately non-Hispanic White custodial grandparents (e.g. Hayslip, Shore, Henderson, & Lambert, 1998; Jendrek, 1994).

Therefore, a study was undertaken of African American grandparents who were currently or had been parenting one or more grandchildren, without regard to the reason for the assumption of parental responsibility, to more broadly define the demographics of African American grandparent-headed households. This study utilized two focus groups drawn from the African American community of grandparents raising grandchildren in two southwestern cities, providing a regional focus not yet explored, and endeavored to determine the challenges faced, the services needed, and the rewards gained by these grandparents.

METHOD

In order to investigate custodial grandparenting issues, two focus group discussions were organized and held with African American grandparents from Dallas and Fort Worth, Texas. Focus groups are a qualitative methodology that involves unstructured small-group discussions designed to elicit participants' opinions on a specific topic (Stewart & Shamdasani, 1990). Focus group discussion is a dynamic, interactive communicative process (Albrecht, Johnson, & Walther, 1993) that facilitates the identification of diverse viewpoints by recording the opinions, attitudes, values, feelings, and subjective perceptions of the participants. The interactive nature of this research technique allows the investigator to pursue clarification or elaboration of responses, facilitate and expand discussion on specific areas of interest (Barduhn, Furman, Kinney, & Malritz, 1991; Fuller, Edwards, Vorakitphokatorn, & Sermsri, 1993; Jarrett, 1993), and gain understanding of the *natural vocabulary*, or colloquial expressions, of research participants (Fuller et al., 1993; O'Brien, 1993; Stewart & Shamdasani, 1990).

Focus group participants were recruited by using a personalized recruitment strategy (Jarrett, 1993) with the assistance of service providers at two senior centers. To be selected to participate in the focus group discussion, the person had to be providing a substantial amount of care to a grandchild. Focus group participants were compensated at $20 for the session.

Twenty-one African American grandparents participated in the focus group discussions. Participants reported demographic information for themselves as well as for the grandchild(ren) in their care. Five of the participants were men, and 16 were women. There was one married couple in attendance, as well as a father and his adult daughter, each of whom was caring for at least one grandchild.

In all, these grandparents were providing care to 46 children (37 grandchildren and 9 great-grandchildren). Ten of the children had a physical or emotional problem, such as asthma, birth defect, sexual abuse, or gang involvement, that the grandparent viewed as a special difficulty. Five of the children had been adopted by the grandparent, and at the time of the focus group discussions, 25 children were living with the grandparent, with or without a parent present, and 16 children were receiving some form of supplemental care.

Each of the focus group discussions lasted approximately 90 minutes and were tape-recorded with the consent of the participants. To open the discussion, participants were asked to describe their experiences as surrogate parents, including the most significant types of problems they encountered in caring for a grandchild. To put the participants at ease, they were told that there were no right or wrong answers to the questions and that the issues might or might not be relevant to their experience. Both focus group discussions were transcribed. The resulting material was analyzed by the constant comparative method (Strauss & Corbin, 1990) to identify salient themes, conceptual categories, and associations among the categories that emerge from the data. The constant comparative method involves the systematic examination and reexamination of the text to define and code units of meaning (Knodel, 1993; Strauss & Corbin, 1990).

The focus group findings are presented below in terms of the qualitative themes that describe the framework within which African American grandparents discussed grandparenting issues. Because these grandparents frequently, if not always, insisted on identifying the broader context or cultural framework and the interrelationships among the issues that represented their sense of meaning, their responses to the specific questions are discussed within the broad context of this framework rather than being treated as independent and discrete issues.

RESULTS

Scope of Responsibility

Placing each participant in a "grandparent type" proved difficult because of the fluidity of the arrangements. These family units demonstrated remarkable adaptability and flexibility as children, grandchildren, and great grandchildren came and went as needs dictated. In addition, some grandparents had differing degrees of involvement with various grandchildren.

The most common form of arrangement involved the grandchild living with the grandparent, with or without any form of legal custody and with or without a parent present. Parents often came and went, and it was difficult at times to distinguish whether a parent in residence was the child of the grandparent who headed the household.

Five of the children had been formally adopted, one by a great-grandmother in an effort to obtain needed financial and medical services.

A substantial number of group participants were providing what could be termed supplemental care for grandchildren, in an effort to assist parents whose work and school schedules left little time for the needs of their children. Providing transportation to and from school, medical appointments, and other activities was the most often mentioned form of assistance rendered. Only one grandparent mentioned providing day care, probably attributable to the age of the grandchild, leading to the possibility that the supplemental role is, for many, an extension of a previous grandparental responsibility.

Reasons for Assumption of Responsibility

Although previous research focused primarily on drug abuse, particularly crack cocaine, as the reason for the assumption of parental responsibility among African American grandparent caregivers (Burton, 1992; Minkler, Roe, & Price, 1992), the participants in these focus groups described a variety of circumstances that led to their assumption of the responsibility for grandchildren or great-grandchildren. The death of a parent, child abuse (physical or sexual, or severe neglect), inability to parent, marital disruption, and incarceration of a parent were all represented. Many of the grandparents were providing care because both parents were in the workforce or in school and time constraints were such that they could not care adequately for the grandchildren.

Whereas previous research has demonstrated a high number of difficult and perhaps emotionally disturbed children placed in the care of grandparents (Emick & Hayslip, 1999; Hayslip et al., 1998), there was a surprising number of physically handicapped children represented in these groups. Three children were severely asthmatic, one with severe hearing loss that had required corrective surgery; several suffered from mild to moderate asthma; one had been born prematurely with multiple complications; one had a clubfoot; and one had a hole in his heart. Grandparents made it clear that the parents lacked either the time or emotional or financial capacity to cope with these special-needs children. A grandmother who cared for her granddaughter reflected the feelings of those similarly involved:

> She was also born premature. She was in [name of service organization] from 2 weeks old until she was 2 years old. And, so, therefore, it . . . brought me into being a person to take her to these appointments and to reinforce the therapy that they were giving her. As a matter of fact, I have been told over and over, she would have never made the strides she made had she not had one-on-one therapy . . . somebody [who] didn't have others to attend to other than her. Her mother and her father worked. And you can't be at home working too. . . . I think it's been invaluable, the fact that she had me.

Benefits/Rewards

The most pronounced finding from the two focus groups was the complete devotion of the participants to the grandchildren (and great-grandchildren) they were raising, coupled with a sense of confidence in their ability to do a good job. Most expressed extensive gratification in fulfilling their role as supplemental or surrogate parent in spite of almost universal frustration with the service network, and in only a few cases, to be discussed later, were any personal sacrifices or difficulties mentioned. Although all had assumed some, if not total, parental responsibility and the term "my child" was used frequently when referring to the grandchild for whom they cared, the sense of being a grandparent remained, as had been found in previous studies of predominately non-Hispanic White samples (Emick & Hayslip, 1999; Shore & Hayslip, 1994).

Companionship, combined with a sense of purpose, appeared to be the most prevalent reward voiced by the grandparents. One grandmother, who had assumed custody of three grandchildren upon the death of her daughter, put it this way:

> Well, it has helped me a lot because I was by myself, you know, for awhile. And then after they, after my daughter passed away, they gave me custody of the children. . . . So they give me custody of 'em. And I'm really enjoying them. Because I would be by myself, you know. And everything is just, we just going along together real nicely. And I'm enjoyin' them.

And a grandfather who was responsible for a 3-year-old grandson went so far as to credit his grandson with saving his life: "This little boy has really helped me, I tell ya. Once, you know, I felt like I might just go on and die. But he gave me life. Gave me something to live for."

Another frequently mentioned benefit was that of keeping "up with the times" when raising grandchildren: "So I think that they keep you in touch with the changing world. And even the part that you don't like, it allows you to *deal* with it. From, with them, from *their* perspective."

Echoing a theme reported by Burton (1992), several of the participants voiced satisfaction at being able to do what they considered to be a better job raising their grandchildren than they were able to do with their children. One great-grandmother, who was raising the son of a granddaughter whom she had also raised, said: "I enjoy him because I can always uh . . . when my children were growing up I was working and I didn't have a lot of chances to do things for them. But now I can take him fishing, I can do all kinds of things with him. And he's really a good kid."

Finally, there was a sense that the needs of the grandchild were being met when he or she was with the grandparent. Although these grandparents were older and were caring for few grandchildren under school age, participants agreed that they would rather the child be with them than in day care or with a babysitter. After discussing her difficulties adjusting to her new lifestyle as well as the financial strains placed on her by the assumption of responsibility for a 5-year-old grandson, one grandmother said:

> . . . rather [for him] to be with me than be with some babysitters . . . so I rather know that he's there with grandmother. If, if we don't have nothing to eat I give you some bread and water, where if you out there with somebody [else], they may not even give you that. And that's worrisome.

However, despite expressing pleasure, if not joy, at parenting their grandchildren, all but one participant said that they had not expected to have to take responsibility for a grandchild when they thought about their future.

Adjustments

New Parenting Skills

Chief among the series of adjustments encountered when assuming responsibility for a grandchild was the need to learn how to parent this generation. Although Strom, Collinsworth, Strom, and Griswold (1993) had found Black grandparents lacking in the ability to treat each grandchild as a individual, these grandparents evidenced a willingness to listen to a grandchild in order to understand him as a unique person, as well as having a clear awareness of the need to change their previous parenting styles and techniques.

> . . . So like I say, the things that I done with C, R, and A, I can't do with M, J, and C, because it's a *whole* different generation. And that's uh, I catches myself a lot a times, I really do, you know, and then my baby girl, who's C, says, "Mama, I told you, you cannot raise these kids the way you did us."

and

> But I know it changed me 'cause each generation as they come along, you *have* to learn to listen, they need a lookout. I think the problem with most of us is that we don't look and listen to anything and we have developed one way of thinking and that's the way it goes. I have changed *so* many ways . . . raising children . . . until I never have to, never, very seldom have to, after they're five, six years old, seven years old, I never have to touch em. I learned how to punish *without* my hands.

There was not unanimous agreement, however, that the change in parenting was a positive development, only that it was necessary if only to avoid the involvement of child protective services.

Loss of Personal Time

The majority of the focus group participants were caring for grandchildren of school age; therefore, little mention was made of the loss of time for friends and activities. Some expressed relief at no longer having to deliver the constant care required when the grandchildren were younger, and one grandmother recalled the difficulties she experienced when having to deliver grandchildren at three different schools each morning. Another grandmother lamented: "A lot of times, you know, *I* would like to go out, . . . and my friends want to go somewhere. . . . And looks like I'm the one what has to stay here. . . . And sometimes we just have to give up what *we* need." However, the most general agreement was that their routines had changed in order to accommodate the grandchildren as well as their own activities:

> . . . it's just been a change of schedule, I'll put it like that. Because before my grandchild came into my life to live, everything was, I could do just about whatever I wanted to do. I had a time to get myself ready to go to community service to work or volunteer or whatever. I had time to get myself leisurely dressed for church. I had time to do whatever I wanted to do. But then when he came into my life, that changed. I had to fix time where I could work him in there, too, and keep him happy. So now, like this morning, we were comin' over here and I'm goin' to work, too. Now if I hadn't a had him, I could have just got up, took a bath, got dressed, waited for my ride. But as it was this morning, I had to get up, get his breakfast, get him dressed, take him to school, *then* come back and get myself ready for them to pick me up. When we leave here, I'm goin' to work. *So* havin' my grandbaby with me is a joy, I wouldn't change it, *but* the most thing that it changed for me is that it just made my *whole* life take on a different new time pattern.

Loss of Community

The members of the focus groups clearly felt the loss of community in the parenting of their grandchildren. Detailed accounts were related of their own growing-up years, as well as those of their children, during which neighbors, church members, school personnel, and other parents would work together to reenforce morals and values taught at home. One grandmother who was herself raised by an aunt, said: "Not only did they raise me, but the neighborhood raised me. Whatever I did, if I did a durn thing wrong, it was reported before I got back. . . . " And a great-grandmother talked about her childhood experience of getting in trouble at school and subsequently being stopped on her walk home by neighbors who had somehow heard of her misdeed, and she was reprimanded at house after house before finally reaching home, where she found her mother waiting on the front porch.

More troublesome than the loss of community for these grandparents, however, were the experiences of having their authority as parents to their grandchildren subverted by others.

> These days when a parent or somebody sees you doing, sees a child going wrong in the street, they may call [him] in, but it's not to chastise [him]. They'll add to whatever it is they see, the wrong that they see [him] doing. And that will let the child know, "that if I get in trouble, I can go over here and stay." And where that parent or that person in the house that sees the person doing wrong, instead of chastising them, or telling the parent about it, they just cover it up and just keep letting that child keep doing wrong, instead of straightening up. Now I found that to be very true.

It had also been made clear to anyone who attempted to admonish a young person that they had no right to interfere in the lives of others, and, in one case, a grandparent had witnessed the killing of a person who had stepped in to stop a disturbance in which he was not personally involved.

Not only were the previously utilized community resources unavailable, focus group participants perceived that they received little or no support when they accessed the legal or school systems as well. While counseling was sought for a variety of reasons and appeared readily available when requested, although some questioned its effectiveness, no other recourse presented itself when a grandchild defied authority. In their opinion, the removal of prayer from the schools was the definitive antecedent to the loss of discipline, and when coupled with the elimination of corporal punishment, they felt teachers had been rendered impotent, and no one was left with authority over the students. In addition, those grandparents with "problem" grandchildren had found the legal authorities unwilling or unable to take action until actual crimes had been committed, leaving them with a sense of helplessness in the face of gang- and drug-related occurrences. As one particularly distraught great grandmother who had repeatedly sought help for her gang-involved sixteen-year-old great-grandson put it, "Just can't get no help. We've been, been for the last month trying to get help. Ain't got none yet . . . and when they get through talking, they say he hasn't done no crime, ain't nothing against him, they got nothing on him. He either got to be killed or kill."

Great-Grandmothers

A portion of the generational effects of teen pregnancy and childbearing was evident in the relatively high number of participants with parental responsibility for one or more *great*-grandchild. In three of the five cases of custodial great grandparents, the great-grandmother had also raised the grandchild who was the parent of the great-grandchild. With an exceptionally high number of African American girls, many of whom were themselves born to teenage mothers, giving birth to children while they are still teenagers (Burton & Dilworth-Anderson, 1991; Ladner, 1988), the young mother is often deemed incapable of raising the child. Because the grandmother is often still actively involved in the workforce, as well as with her own childbearing and rearing, the care for the newborn is often passed up the generational structure to the great grandmother. In such cases, it is not unusual for her to be responsible for one or more grandchildren as well (Burton & Dilworth-Anderson, 1991).

> . . . I stepped in because my granddaughter had nobody but me. So that just left me with J [great grandson]. So that's why I did it.
> *Moderator:* So you say she didn't know much about being a parent?
> . . . Nothing about being a parent. She was only sixteen.

Of particular interest was Speaker C, a great-grandmother who told of raising 5 children, 14 grandchildren, and 4 great-grandchildren. Epitomizing the Black grandmother of history (Burton, 1992; Jones, 1973; Minkler, 1997; Minkler et al., 1992; Wilson, 1986) and legend, this participant had not only taken responsibility for her own grandchildren and great-grandchildren but also for two children who were not related directly to her. In each case, the child was the half sibling of one of her grandchildren or great-grandchildren, and she would not allow them to be separated.

... She's not one of my granddaughters. But I went through court a whole year for this child. And they decided to put her with her daddy's mother. And my granddaughter with me. And when it got right up to the date we went to court to do that, the day before, her daddy's mother packed her clothes, set her on the porch, and called an' told 'em to come get her because she didn't want her ... I'm here. This is my granddaughter's sister. And I am crazy about her family. And I refuse to let her to go to [children's home].

Each half sibling had formidable problems, one suffering from severe neglect and the other from sexual abuse. This custodial great-grandmother went to great lengths to assure that each child received appropriate treatment, including surgery for the first and extensive counseling for the second, despite reporting astonishing difficulties in obtaining services for them. What is remarkable about Speaker C is not that she approximates the commonly held conception of the African American matriarch but that she was the only member of the focus groups to do so.

Problems Experienced

Related to the Grandchildren

In addition to the physical disabilities, these grandparents found themselves dealing with a variety of other problems in the parenting of their grandchildren. Although these problems often did not differ significantly from those found in the general population, when coupled with the one and sometimes two generational skips between the children and the parental figures, they posed substantial difficulties for the group participants. Academic problems, materialism, negative peer influence, and the certain belief that children were growing up too fast were all related as problematic. One set of grandparents had experienced the kidnaping and subsequent return of a granddaughter, two others were experiencing difficulties resulting from the sexual abuse of their granddaughters, and the grandson of another had expressed suicidal ideation.

Although drug abuse was not specifically mentioned as a concern for these participants, gang membership was clearly affecting several of the families represented, as told by one distraught grandfather:

. . . them leaders in them gangs got more influence on him than their parents have. They can tell them what to do and they'll do that despite what you do for them, what you tell them. And I can't reach him and so, therefore, I done lost him. . . . I didn't think I could give up on him, but. . . . He's a pain. Now, he's about spoiled the whole family by joining a gang.

In virtually every instance, the grandparents evidenced a clear willingness to seek help for their grandchildren, although as previously mentioned, the results were mixed. However, when asked about counseling or support for themselves, there was unanimous agreement that none was necessary, echoing findings from previous research (Emick & Hayslip, 1996) that custodial grandparents will readily seek help for their grandchildren but not for themselves.

Financial Strains

With the one exception of the grandmother who was parenting the three children of a daughter who had died and whose work-related benefits had transferred to the children, there was unanimous agreement that the assumption of the care of their grandchildren had placed them in substantial financial difficulty. Extensive discussions revolved around the obstacles encountered when attempting to obtain financial services for their grandchildren, almost exclusively Aid to Families with Dependent Children (AFDC) and Medicaid. (Note: These focus groups were conducted before the implementation of PWROA in 1996 and AFDC was replaced with Temporary Aid for Needy Families.) Raising the issue of obtaining financial assistance led to the following spontaneous exchange:

Speaker G: Let me ask you something. When you go for help like this and you have multiple children, do you not have to give some reason as to why you have inherited this in the first place? To get back to the responsibility of the person. I was always taught . . . you're a parent and there's no alternative to parenting. You are a parent. Your options are gone when they cut the cord. You're a *parent.* So, based upon that, I'm just wondering, when you *go,* do you not have to substantiate or say *how you got this problem* of grandchildren, 'cause there's somebody in between you and the grandchildren? You're not their biological reason they're here; there's somebody else.

Speaker C: Sweetheart, let me tell you this. When you, when I go, I carries a birth certificate. I carries the medical problems. I carries *how* I got 'em. Works and books and papers from the judge. I have briefcases with this. They sit up and read 'em . . . papers from the jurors, . . . paper from their mother, and all this.

Speaker G: But are they sensitive to you? With these problems?

Speaker E: They give you a hassle, even on AFDC, Medicaid and food stamps and all. You've got to have the history and the life of three grandkids, and they feel like you done went out on the street to get these grandkids just to get the little bit a month.

Physical

There was little discussion of physical consequences of caring for grandchildren, perhaps because there were few persons with grand-children under school age, and the care provided was less labor-intensive. There was, however, one grandmother who had suffered a heart attack she believed to be related to stress incurred while caring for her son's three children. It is worthy of note that this particular grandmother was the only participant who openly expressed her displeasure at having to take parental responsibility.

DISCUSSION

In an effort to facilitate a more accurate understanding of the range of the needs of and problems faced by African American grandparent-headed households, no criteria other than the provision of some level of instrumental support for at least one grandchild or great grandchild were required for participation in these focus groups. The reasons for the assumption of parental responsibility paralleled those found in other studies of primarily non-Hispanic white participants (Burnette, 1997; Emick & Hayslip, 1999; Fuller-Thomson, Minkler, & Driver, 1997; Generations United, 1997; Jendrek, 1994; Minkler 1997; Pinson-Milburn, Fabian, Schlossberg, & Pyle, 1996). Teen pregnancy, child abuse, unemployment, parental incarceration, marital disruption, and death of a parent were all cited. More pronounced in these African American grandparent-headed households, however, was the overwhelming need for financial assistance, whether in the form of supplemental income (Aid to Families with

Dependent Children at the time of this study) or Medicaid. Also evidenced was the sense of being discounted by providers *because* of their position as grandparents, perhaps an extension of a reluctance of welfare workers to place children within their family in the belief that it was the family dysfunction that contributed to the need for placement in the first place (Davidson, 1997; Kornhaber, 1996; Minkler, 1997).

The number of grandchildren cared for because they had physical disabilities is noteworthy. Again, as a result of the financial need of these African American households, in some instances both parents were working one or more jobs and did not have time available to see to the special needs of their children. Grandparents stepped in to provide the necessary instrumental assistance.

An extremely troublesome finding was the consistent struggle experienced by these custodial grandparents when trying to obtain services, some having so much difficulty that they gave up altogether and simply tried to make do or searched for additional employment. Story after story emerged of interminable waits and the need to prove over and over again to service providers that they indeed were responsible for their grandchildren, that the services were necessary, and/or that they were entitled to the benefits.

The theme of isolation so often found in custodial grandparents (Emick & Hayslip, 1996; Hayslip et al., 1998; Pinson-Milburn et al., 1996; Shore & Hayslip, 1994) was also prevalent in both focus groups, with mention made of the inability to meet with friends or pursue other commitments, as well as the general lack of support from other family members. With the exception of the grandmother whose daughter had died, all participants either described the absence of any support from other children, siblings, etc., or actual discord and strife among members about the parenting of the grandchildren. In one group, a father and his adult daughter, each of whom was parenting grandchildren, began arguing about the manner in which the daughter was raising those in her care. Concern over altered relationships with grandchildren not resident with the grandparents was voiced as well as over unfulfilled expectations and perceived resentments of the nonresident grandchild.

The greatest sense of isolation for these custodial grandparents, however, surfaced in discussions about the loss of the community. Unfortunately, for these custodial grandparents, the neighborhood had become a hostile environment in which they felt unsupported and that their authority as parent was subverted. Like their cohorts who assumed responsibility for grandchildren as a result of the parental drug abuse (Burton, 1992; Minkler et al., 1992), these custodial grandparents felt unsafe in their neighborhoods, the most often mentioned cause for alarm being the presence of gangs. Having looked to the schools and, in some cases, the police for support, they expressed dismay at the inability or unwillingness of these entities to provide tangible assistance in addressing any problems associated with their grandchildren and felt they had been left with few, if any, allies.

Most of the participants were deeply steeped in their religion and clearly felt a lack of spiritual foundation to be a root cause of societal difficulties today. Each drew heavily on their personal faith for consolation and strength. However, no indication was given that they looked to their church as able to solve their problems, even though children and grandchildren were taken to church on a regular basis.

Implications for Service Providers

Service providers must be educated about the value of the African American grandparent in the rescue of at-risk children if timely and accessible services are to be provided. In addition, a sense of community must be fostered to ease their sense of isolation and abandonment. Of interest are the favorable results obtained in a school-based intervention for custodial grandparents (Grant, Gordon, & Cohen, 1997), where delays and difficulties in accessing the health care system were minimized, if not eliminated. For custodial grandparents with school-age grandchildren, a school-based intervention could serve as an entry to both the medical and social service systems, as well as provide a forum for support and the re-establishment of a sense of community.

Study Limitations

Both the number and the age of the focus group participants served as limiting factors. However, these limitations were seen as necessary to deepen the understanding of the African American grandparent-headed household. Small focus groups, while perhaps restricting the number of circumstances presented, allow the participants to develop a level of comfort and afford them the opportunity to explore issues and difficulties in more depth than would be conceivable in larger groups. Each group took on its own focus, one more concerned with the problems associated with gang involvement and the other with the loss of moral and ethical teaching of the young. This might have occurred as one member "piggybacked" off the issue of another, but more likely was a representation of the concerns of the community from which each group was recruited.

The participants were older than the average grandparent who assumes parental responsibility for a grandchild, although some had clearly stepped into that role at a much younger age. However, with the "verticalization" of the African American family combined with the extended active life expectancy of its members (Szinovacz, 1998), older African Americans are at increasing risk of parenting great and even great-great-grandchildren. An understanding of the special needs of the elder black grandparent is essential in order to anticipate and/or meet their needs.

More study utilizing small focus groups is necessary to fully understand the needs and circumstances of younger African American custodial grandparents. It is in this group that the most labor-intensive, time consuming care will probably be found, and perhaps a greater occurrence of health and job related problems. In addition, the younger African American custodial grandparent will be more likely to be involved in the workforce as well as the active parenting of other children still residing in the home, circumstances which lend themselves to higher levels of stress related to role conflicts.

A Final Note

The African American custodial grandparents in these two focus groups were managing quite well in spite of substantial obstacles. All expressed great satisfaction in their roles and were confident in their ability to do a good job. Even when discussing problematic behavior or situations, most expressed a sense of pride both in their grandchildren and in their own parenting. The love that they held for their grandchildren was obvious.

ACKNOWLEDGMENTS

Partial support for this research was provided by the Louisiana Board of Regents Support Fund through the University of Louisiana at Monroe.

REFERENCES

Albrecht, T. L., Johnson, G. M., & Walther, J. B. (1993). Understanding communication processes in focus groups. In D. L. Morgan (Ed.), *Successful focus groups: Advancing the state of the art* (pp. 51–64). Newbury Park, CA: Sage Publications.

Barduhn, M. S., Furman, L. J., Kinney, M. B., & Malvitz, D. M. (1991). Using focus groups in gerontological research. *Gerontology and Geriatrics Education, 12*(2), 69–78.

Burnette, D. (1997, September-October). Grandparents raising grandchildren in the inner city. *Families in Society: The Journal of Contemporary Human Services, 78,* 489–499.

Burton, L. (1992). Black grandparents raising children of drug-addicted parents: Stressors, outcomes, and social service needs. *Gerontologist, 32,* 744–751.

Burton, L., & Dilworth-Anderson, P. (1991). The intergenerational roles of aged Black Americans. *Marriage and Family Review, 16,* 311–330.

Chalfie, D. (1994). *Going it alone: A closer look at grandparents parenting grandchildren.* Washington, DC: American Association of Retired Persons, Women's Initiative.

Davidson, B. (1997). Service needs of relative caregivers: A qualitative analysis. *Families in Society: The Journal of Contemporary Human Services, 78,* 502–510.

Emick, M., & Hayslip, B. (1996). Custodial grandparenting: New roles for middle-aged and older adults. *International Journal of Aging and Human Development, 43,* 135–154.

Emick, M., & Hayslip, B. (1999). Custodial grandparenting: Stresses, coping skills, and relationships with grandchildren. *International Journal of Aging and Human Development, 48,* 35–61.

Fuller, T. D., Edwards, J. N., Vorakitphokatorn, S., & Sermsri, S. (1993). Using focus groups to adapt survey instruments to new populations: Experience from a developing country. In D. L. Morgan (Ed.), *Successful focus groups: Advancing the state of the art* (pp. 89–104). Newbury Park, CA: Sage Publications.

Fuller-Thomson, E., Minkler, M., & Driver, D. (1997). A profile of grandparents raising grandchildren in the United States. *Gerontologist, 37*, 406–411.

Generations United. (1997, October). *Grandparents and other relatives raising children: An intergenerational action agenda.* Washington, DC: Author.

Grant, R., Gordon, S., & Cohen, T. (1997). An innovative school-based original model to serve grandparent caregivers. *Journal of Gerontological Social Work, 28*(1/2), 47–61.

Hayslip, B., Shore, R. J., Henderson, C., & Lambert, P. (1998). Custodial grandparenting and the impact of grandchildren with problems on role satisfaction and role meaning. *Journal of Gerontology: Social Sciences, 53B*, S164–S173.

Jarrett, R. L. (1993). Focus group interviewing with low-income minority populations. In D. L. Morgan (Ed.), *Successful focus groups: Advancing the state of the art* (pp. 184–201). Newbury Park, CA: Sage Publications.

Jendrek, M. (1994). Grandparents who parent their grandchildren: Circumstances and decisions. *Gerontologist, 34*, 206–216.

Jones, F. (1973). The lofty role of the Black grandmother. *Crisis, 80*(1), 19–21.

Knodel, J. (1993). The design and analysis of focus group studies: A practical approach. In D. L. Morgan (Ed.), *Successful focus groups: Advancing the state of the art* (pp. 35–50). Newbury Park, CA: Sage Publications.

Kornhaber, R. (1996). *Contemporary grandparenting.* Thousand Oaks, CA: Sage Publications.

Ladner, J. (1988). The impact of teenage pregnancy on the Black family. In H. P. McAdoo (Ed.), *Black families* (2nd ed., pp. 296–305). Thousand Oaks, CA: Sage.

Minkler, M. (1997, October). Intergenerational households headed by grandparents: Demographic and social contexts. In *Grandparents and other relatives raising children: Background papers from Generations United's expert symposium (pp. 3–18). Washington, DC: Generations United.*

Minkler, M., Fuller-Thomson, E., Miller, D., & Driver, D. (1997, September-October). Depression in grandparents raising grandchildren. Archives of Family Medicine, 6, 445–452.*

Minkler, M., & Roe, K. (1993). *Grandmothers as caregivers: Raising children of the crack cocaine epidemic. Newbury Park, CA: Sage Publications.*

Minkler, M., Roe, K. M., & Price, M. (1992). The physical and emotional health of grandmothers raising grandchildren in the crack cocaine epidemic. *Gerontologist, 32,* 5752–5761.

O'Brien, K. (1993). Improving survey questionnaires through focus groups. In D. L. Morgan (Ed.), *Successful focus groups: Advancing the state of the art* (pp. 105–117). Newbury Park, CA: Sage Publications.

Pinson-Millburn, M., Fabian, E., Schlossberg, N., & Pyle, M. (1996). Grandparents raising grandchildren. *Journal of Counseling and Development, 74,* 548–554.

Shore, R., & Hayslip, B. J. (1994). Custodial grandparenting: Implications for children's development. In A. Gottfied & A. Gottfied (Eds.), *Redefining families: Implications for children's development* (pp. 171–218). New York: Plenum Press.

Stewart, D. W., & Shamdasani, P. N. (1990). *Focus groups: Theory and practice.* Applied Social Research Methods Series, vol. 20. Newbury Park, CA: Sage Publications.

Strauss, A., & Corbin, J. (1990). *Basics of qualitative research: Grounded theory procedures and techniques.* Beverly Hills, CA: Sage.

Strom, R., Collinsworth, P., Strom, S., & Griswold, D. (1993). Strengths and needs of Black grandparents. *International Journal of Aging and Human Development, 36*(4), 255–268.

Szinovacz, M. (1998). Grandparents today: A demographic profile. *Gerontologist, 38,* 37–52.

U.S. Bureau of the Census. (1999). *Living arrangements of children under 18 years: March 1998.* Washington, DC: U.S. Government Printing Office.

Wilson, M. (1986). The Black extended family: An analytical consideration. *Developmental Psychology, 22,* 246–258.

CHAPTER 9

Custodial Grandparenting and ADHD

David B. Baker

C ustodial grandparenting presents unique challenges to older adults who have already raised a generation of children. These challenges become even greater when grandparents are responsible for the care of a grandchild with behavioral problems (Hayslip, Shore, Henderson, & Lambert, 1998). This chapter will examine and discuss issues of custodial grandparenting of children with one of the most widely recognized behavior disorders in clinical practice, attention-deficit/hyperactivity disorder (ADHD).

DEFINING AND ASSESSING ADHD

ADHD is listed in the *Diagnostic and Statistical Manual of Mental Disorders*, fourth edition (DSM-IV) (American Psychiatric Association, 1994) under the heading of "Disorders Usually First Diagnosed in Infancy, Childhood, or Adolescence." Developmentally inappropriate levels of inattention, impulsivity, and overactivity characterize ADHD. Inattention is manifested in such ways as not paying attention, daydreaming, and forgetting. Impulsivity can be observed in such things as blurting out answers to questions, starting activities while ignoring directions, engaging in dangerous acts and not waiting to take turns in group activities. Overactivity, often referred to as "hyperactivity," involves excessive motor activity, such as difficulty sitting still, fidgeting, restlessness, and a need to always be "on the go" (American Psychiatric Association, 1994). According to the DSM-IV, ADHD can be of three types depending on the severity of the three cardinal features. For those whose presentation mostly involves inattentive symptoms the diagnosis of ADHD, predominantly inattentive type, would be appropriate; when hyperactive/impulsive symptoms predominate, ADHD, predominantly hyperactive-impulsive type, is diagnosed; and when there is a combination of inattention, impulsivity, and hyperactivity, ADHD, combined type, is diagnosed. One of the most commonly diagnosed of all childhood disorders, ADHD affects approximately 3%–5% of school-age children, with male-to-female ratios ranging from 4:1 to 9:1 (American Psychiatric Association, 1994).

The effects of ADHD are rather pervasive, affecting children behaviorally (difficulty in sitting still), cognitively (difficulty in focusing), academically (lowered performance), socially (difficulty in playing cooperatively) and emotionally (low frustration tolerance). Children with ADHD often have poor self-concepts and are more likely to experience learning disabilities (Pisecco, Baker, Silva, & Brooke, 1996). The impact that the disorder has on family functioning, particularly on parental stress, can be significant (Baker & McCal, 1995).

The proper assessment of ADHD involves a multimethod approach that requires that information be collected from multiple informants across various settings. Clinicians rely not only on clinical observation but also include data gathered from the child, parent, and teacher. It is crucial that the diagnosis be made by a clinician familiar with ADHD because elements of the cardinal features of ADHD (inattention, impulsivity, and overactivity) are shared with other disorders, such as depression and anxiety. A psychologist or physician commonly diagnoses ADHD, and although assessment practices vary, it is incumbent that the assessment of ADHD include multiple informants and be conducted by a professional with expertise in the assessment of ADHD in children.

ETIOLOGY

The work of Russell Barkley has stimulated research and debate over the nature of ADHD. In the 1980s Barkley proposed that deficits in rule-governed behavior were a central feature of ADHD. By the 1990s his conceptualization had grown to encompass the concept of behavioral inhibition (Barkley, 1997). Behavioral inhibition is analogous to self-control; it includes such things as delaying gratification and being able to stop and think before responding. In Barkley's view, behavioral disinhibition characterizes ADHD and leads to deficits in executive functions, which include (1) prolongation/working memory; (2) self-regulation of affect, motivation, arousal; (3) internalization of speech; and (4) reconstitution (for a detailed discussion, see Barkley, 1997). These deficits result in, among other things, an inability to learn from past experience and an inability to plan, direct and maintain behavior toward future goals or plans.

With improvements in brain imaging technologies there is a growing body of evidence that points to a neurobiological basis for ADHD (for a review, see Barkley, 1997). ADHD also has been shown to have a strong familial association in that it is more common in first-degree biological relatives of children with the disorder.

DEVELOPMENTAL CONSIDERATIONS

Increasingly, researchers and clinicians are recognizing that the symptoms of ADHD often persist beyond childhood and can contribute to a host of difficulties in adolescence and adulthood (Weiss & Hechtman, 1993). Follow-up studies of individuals diagnosed with ADHD in childhood, for instance, show that as many as 60% to 80% continue to exhibit symptoms of the disorder into adulthood (Hechtman, 1991; Weiss, Hechtman, Milroy, & Perlman, 1985).

The diagnosis of ADHD in adulthood is frequently overlooked in individuals presenting with emotional and behavioral problems. This oversight stems partly from the fact that the assessment of ADHD in adults is still rather new and that attentional problems are common to a number of psychiatric disorders, such as schizophrenia, bipolar disorder, unipolar depression, and borderline personality disorder (Ward, Wender, & Reimherr, 1993).

Childhood symptoms of overactivity, impulsivity, and distractibility are required for the diagnosis of ADHD in adulthood and can be observed in a variety of ways. Overactivity, or hyperactivity, is less overt and is often experienced as feelings of restlessness. Impulsivity can be seen in difficulties in coping with frustration and anger and engaging in risk-taking behaviors; distractibility is often associated with poor organizational skills. It is not uncommon for adults with a history of childhood ADHD to show significant underachievement in academic and employment settings, have frequent changes in residence and employment, have difficulty in managing finances, experience emotional problems, and have difficulty in managing aggressive behavior (Weiss & Hechtman, 1993).

Of particular concern is the association of childhood ADHD with the development of antisocial behaviors (Baker, Knight, & Simpson, 1995; Glenn & Parsons, 1991; Shekim, Asarnow, Hess, Zaucha, & Wheeler, 1990). In an 8-year prospective study, Fischer, Barkley, Fletcher, and Smallish (1993) found that ADHD children continued to show significantly higher rates of emotional and behavioral disturbance in adolescence, compared to a matched control group. Aggressive, delinquent, and antisocial behaviors were found to show the greatest continuity over time.

In examining factors that predicted adult outcome of childhood ADHD, Weiss and Hechtman (1993) found that an interaction of variables related to personality, social, and family characteristics predicted such outcomes as emotional adjustment, school performance, work history, police involvement, car accidents, and nonmedical drug use. In particular, socioeconomic status, mental health of family members, IQ, aggressive behavior, emotional instability, and low frustration tolerance were found to be the strongest predictors of these measures.

TREATMENT

Treatment modalities can be divided into two major types: physiologically based (medication, diet, biofeedback, etc.) and psychologically based (behavior modification, cognitive behavior therapy, family therapy, etc.). With the vast amount of research and editorializing regarding ADHD and its management, it is no wonder that clinicians and consumers alike are often confused and bewildered by the array of opinions offered. There is general consensus that the combination of pharmacological agents (stimulant medications such as Ritalin) and behavioral interventions (parent training, behavior modification, etc.) is the most efficacious form of treatment (for a current and comprehensive review, see Pelham, Wheeler, & Chronis, 1998).

PSYCHOSOCIAL CONSIDERATIONS

Child Characteristics

Children with ADHD often present with a host of challenging behaviors. In addition to the primary symptoms of inattention, impulsivity, and overactivity, the DSM-IV also refers to associated features such as low frustration tolerance, temper outbursts, bossiness, stubbornness, demands for immediate gratification, mood lability, demoralization, dysphoria, rejection by peers, and poor self-esteem. Add poor academic achievement, and it is inevitable that conflicts with peers, parents, siblings, and teachers will occur. In their interactions, children with ADHD have a difficult time working cooperatively (Cunningham & Segal, 1987) and often receive negative evaluations from their fellow classmates (Johnston, Pelham, & Murphy, 1985). In the school setting the cognitive and behavioral manifestations of ADHD can make compliance with classroom demands an issue (Margalit, 1989).

Parenting Characteristics

Dealing with ADHD in the context of the family unit, particularly helping parents cope with and respond to the manifestations of ADHD in their children, has received increased attention in both clinical practice and research (Baker & Pisecco, 1998). Studies have consistently demonstrated that parents of children with ADHD report levels of parenting stress that are among the highest of any special-needs population of children (Abidin, 1995; Baker, 1994). By far the greatest source of parenting stress in families of children with ADHD is the behavior of the child with ADHD (Baker & McAl,

1995). The day-in and day-out experience of struggling with noncompliance, forgetfulness, moodiness, and peer conflicts often leaves parents feeling angry, isolated, and incompetent in their parenting role. A survey of parents of children with ADHD (Kottman, Baker, & Roberts, 1995) found most parents working hard to sort through the ever-growing thicket of information on ADHD. Parents frequently reported having to do a balancing act between the needs of their child and the larger environment outside the home. It was not uncommon for parents to report having to endure well-meaning family and friends who give unsolicited advice, school personnel who demand behavioral change, and professionals who often present conflicting recommendations. Finally, parents all seemed to agree that what they most wanted was education/information, behavior management strategies, and social support.

ISSUES IN CUSTODIAL GRANDPARENTING OF CHILDREN WITH ADHD

There is little to suggest that the experiences of parenting a child with ADHD would be any different for custodial grandparents than for natural parents. In fact, based on the discussion to follow, it is fair to expect that the task could be more stressful and demanding for custodial grandparents.

Transition to Custodial Grandparenting

The transition to custodial grandparenting is often a sudden and unexpected one. Family crisis, such as divorce, substance abuse, teen pregnancy, and child abuse and neglect, often leads to grandparents accepting the parenting role for their grandchildren. In 1991, it was estimated that 3.2 million (5%) children in the United States resided with grandparents or other relatives (Minkler, Roe, & Price, 1992). Research has indicated that resumption of the parenting role for grandparents is often experienced as a stressful and negatively evaluated event. It has been noted that grandmothers who care for a grandchild for extended periods of time report more ambivalence, dissatisfaction, and lowered morale (Johnson, 1988; Robertson,

1977). Resentment toward the parents of the grandchild, legal and financial concerns, and overburden due to multiple caregiving roles can all negatively affect the experience of the custodial grandparent and lead to a state of increased social isolation that furthers the cycle of stress (Shore & Hayslip, 1994).

Custodial grandparenting of normal children can be stressful due to a host of factors unrelated to the characteristics of the child, but this stress becomes all the greater when the child has behavioral problems (Hayslip et al., 1998). The is especially likely to be true of children with ADHD. A number of findings from research on custodial grandparenting have direct relevance to issues of the custodial grandparenting of children with ADHD.

Intergenerational Transmission

As ADHD has a strong familial component, it is likely that in many families there is a transmission of the disorder across generations. It may be that the grandparents, parents, and grandchildren have all struggled with the symptoms of the disorder either directly or in interaction with an affected family member. Similarly, the attributions and understandings of the disorder may change with each generation. Our understanding of the disorder and the ability to identify it have greatly improved over the past 20 years, and it is not at all unlikely that grandparents of today will have had little experience with current diagnostic and treatment procedures. Such grandparents may find themselves raising a child with ADHD who shares many of the behavioral problems that have existed in family members for generations and may attribute them to factors based on their understanding of the symptoms from the past. Thus, the problem behavior may be attributed to a family "trait" of laziness, wildness, stubbornness, and the likes. This intergenerational transmission of ADHD may in part explain the finding that troublesome parent-grandparent relationships have a negative impact on grandchild-grandparent relationships (Whitbeck, Hoyt, & Huck, 1993). It is also interesting to note that most children in custodial grandparenting arrangements are male (Shore & Hayslip, 1994). In addition, custodial grandparents reporting on raising problem grandchildren have been found to be twice as likely to report on male grandchildren

(Emick & Hayslip, 1999). Given that ADHD has a strong familial component and is found much more often in boys, it is likely that many of the behavioral problems that custodial grandparents are dealing with are related to manifestations of ADHD.

Social Support

Raising a child with ADHD can be an isolating experience. The characteristics of children with ADHD discussed earlier often create conflicts in educational, recreational, and social settings. Over time, repeated instances of conflicts in these settings can lead caregivers to withdraw from such contacts, thus reinforcing greater social isolation. Caregivers are in the uncomfortable position of not wanting their child to make a scene in public, and at the same time others are likely to reject the child and not want the child to participate in age-appropriate activities such as birthday parties and team sports. The net effect is that the caregiver and child are often isolated from others, a situation that can escalate conflicts between caregiver and child. These are salient issues for custodial grandparents of children with ADHD. Research has shown that custodial grandparents in general report more constraints on their social roles, as well as isolation from their friends, due to the resumption of parenting obligations (Shore & Hayslip, 1994). The problem is even greater for grandparents raising grandchildren with problem behaviors, who report even less available social support than traditional grandparents or custodial grandparents of children without problems (Emick & Hayslip, 1999). The importance of social support in aiding adjustment is widely recognized, and research has demonstrated the beneficial effects of social support for a variety of life stresses (Argyle, 1991; Cutrona, 1990).

Service Delivery

Getting custodial grandparents the services they need to help their grandchildren and themselves would appear to be a priority. Research on help-seeking behaviors of custodial grandparents is both hopeful and cautionary. Shore and Hayslip (1994) and Emick and

Hayslip (in press) found that traditional and custodial grandparents of grandchildren without problems were more likely to seek help for their own personal problems than were custodial grandparents of children with problems who were more likely to seek help for their grandchildren.

In the case of custodial grandparents raising grandchildren with ADHD, it is clear that service systems be available that meet the unique needs of this population. As Pinson-Millburn et al. (Pinson-Millburn, Fabian, Schlossberg, & Pyle, 1996) have suggested, mental health services for custodial grandparents should be flexible and intervene at the level of the grandchild, grandparent, and school through both direct and indirect means. One type of program that would be applicable would be in the form of grandparent training.

PARENT TRAINING FOR ADHD

From the information reviewed in this chapter we do know that custodial grandparents of children with problem behaviors experience more distress, social isolation, and overall burden than do traditional or custodial grandparents of normal children. Although further research is needed to better clarify the diagnostic status of problem grandchildren, there is sufficient reason to believe that many such children would meet the diagnostic criteria for ADHD and that they and their custodial grandparents could benefit from parent training for ADHD.

Parent training for ADHD represents a broad range of practice aimed at ameliorating the negative effects of ADHD on children and their families. Although there is a broad range of programs available (see Pelham et al., 1998), one type of program that can be easily adapted for use with custodial grandparents of children with ADHD will be presented. The program was developed by the author and is based on a review of the literature on treatment interventions for ADHD and a survey on parent needs in dealing with ADHD (Kottman et al., 1995). The goals of the program are to provide information/education, behavior management strategies, and social support.

The program consists of six weekly group-training sessions and can be easily adapted for use with custodial grandparents. Given the fact that custodial grandparents of problem children can experience significant social isolation, the group setting can be an asset in providing much needed social support. Typically 8 to 10 families are included. This size is large enough to stimulate interaction between participants and small enough to permit individual time and attention. Because custodial grandparents of problem children may be reluctant to seek services for themselves, it is imperative that the formation of groups be well advertised and explained. In speaking with grandparents about the program it may be helpful to emphasize that the program works to help grandparents help their grandchildren by becoming more knowledgeable about ADHD and its treatment.

In forming groups some screening is done to ensure that ADHD is the primary issue and that the group setting is appropriate. For some families there are multiple issues and stresses that can be more appropriately served through a more individualized or specialized program. Presenters are generally advanced doctoral students in psychology who have been working with children with ADHD and their families for a number of years. In making modifications to meet the needs of custodial grandparents, meetings could be scheduled at local facilities (schools, churches, activity centers, etc.) that would minimize travel and transportation costs. The availability of free child care through the use of student volunteers has been successful and popular with participants.

Meeting Times

Meetings are scheduled one evening a week for 90 minutes. The first 45 minutes of each meeting is didactic in nature, with a presentation on a selected topic, and the remaining time is reserved for questions and discussion. This time is consistently rated by participants as the most valuable aspect of the program. As children with ADHD are often the brunt of negative feedback and criticism, so too are their caretakers. They are often blamed for the misbehavior of their children and subjected to the anger and frustration of those who find their children's behavior difficult to tolerate. In addition, they must endure the pain of seeing their child rejected by peers and adults in social and educational settings. The group provides a safe place to talk about these and other issues. This time could be most helpful to custodial grandparents because it would provide a rare opportunity to interact with their peers who are experiencing similar problems and because there are so few people who are familiar with their struggles.

Session Topics

Session 1. The first session is devoted to defining ADHD. In addition to defining DSM-IV criteria (American Psychiatric Association, 1994), manifestations of ADHD across the life span are discussed. Because participants have children of varying ages, it is helpful to present as complete a developmental picture as possible.

Session 2. The second session provides an overview of treatment modalities and research on their efficacy. The goal is to provide information and resources that can be used in making treatment decisions.

Sessions 3 and 4. These sessions devote considerable time to planning and enacting positive behavior change. It is important to provide actual tools for effecting positive change in families. In Session 3, parent-child interaction patterns are discussed. Noncompliance is often a major issue between caregiver and child, and an attempt is made to show how caregivers get into coercive power struggles with their children and how this can maintain and escalate noncompliant behavior. Awareness of interaction styles is encouraged before moving on to Session 4, where learning theory and reinforcement principles are reviewed. The main goal is to convey that behavior can be directed and maintained through reinforcement.

An emphasis in this program is that *positives work better than negatives.* If punishment were an effective treatment for ADHD, that would certainly be known by now. Praise and attention can never be given enough. Children with ADHD need tremendous amounts of feedback; they do many things right during a day, and that can be recognized. Caregivers are asked to identify three target behaviors that they are the most concerned and/or frustrated about. They are then helped to develop a simple point system based on daily and weekly rewards.

The most common problem parents choose to work on with their children are getting ready in the morning and doing homework. Often these issues have become the frontlines in ongoing battles that make all concerned angry, frustrated, and upset. While it is easy to identify behaviors that are of concern, it is much more difficult to define them operationally. For example, to say, "What I would really like is for him to get ready by himself in the morning" leaves room for a lot of interpretation. Requests must be concrete, direct, and clear. So getting ready in the morning, might be phrased as "get out of bed when the alarm goes off, go directly to the bathroom, brush your teeth, and wash your hands and face." It may be that a child can do two of these steps with success, in which case that is the starting point and a place to build from.

Related to this is helping caregivers clarify what is realistic to expect. It is not uncommon for a caregiver to expect that a child should perform according to his or her chronological age. This is usually in the form of "At 10 years old they should be able to complete 30 minutes of homework on their own." Children are different, and the benchmark for any expectation should be based on what the individual child has shown the capacity to do, not what others their age do. Thinking in terms of a line between *can't* and *won't* can be helpful. On one side are those things that the child cannot yet do (remember and follow a four-step command), and on the other are those things that their child can do but chooses not to (follow a two-step command). It is often subtle, but when caregivers begin to think in these terms, it provides a baseline against which expectations can be determined.

To complete the point system, the use of rewards is discussed. Essentially, each day children are awarded 1 point (can be a check mark, token, etc.) for successful completion of each of the three target behaviors. A small reward is given for completion of two of the three target behaviors and a bonus for completion of all three target behaviors. The bonus can be made more exciting by having small wrapped presents to choose from or using a grab bag. As a rule of thumb, the rewards should cost no more than 25 cents (e.g., trading cards, action figures, stickers) or take more than 10 minutes (read a story, computer time, snack, etc.). At the end of the week the points are totaled and can be used toward major rewards. For example 100% of points achieved could earn a pizza party or a friend over for the night. No weekly rewards are given for any amount under 70%. Caregivers are asked to sit with their child and explain the point system and engage the child's cooperation in devising the list of rewards.

Such a system emphases the positive. It gives children a chance to be successful in a structured, consistent way that focuses on accomplishments. The time spent using the system should generally be positive, upbeat, and enjoyable. Second, it helps provide motivation where there is typically very little. Children with ADHD will do almost anything to avoid a task they perceive as aversive. This system acknowledges this and provides motivation that can increase task achievement and decrease task aversion and avoidance. Finally, it provides a tool that can empower caregivers to help their children and foster hope that problems that seem impossible can be dealt with.

Session 5. This session focuses on general house rules and the use of punishment. Two rules are suggested: (a) respond to first requests, and (b) play cooperatively with others. These rules are in effect both in and outside the home and can cover many of the issues that are likely to arise at home and in public places. Transitions are often difficult for children with ADHD, and it is recommended that the house rules be reviewed when entering a new situation. In terms of punishment, there is discussion of the use of time-out and logical consequences. Again, the provision of plenty of praise and feedback about appropriate behavior should help reduce the need for punishment.

Session 6. In the last session the focus is on communicating with schools and establishing methods for the completion of homework. Schools can vary considerably in their understanding of and ability to deliver services to children with ADHD. Meeting with school personnel before problems develop and providing them with information about ADHD and its manifestations in the school setting can reduce misunderstandings and conflicts. A home note system, which provides a daily communication between home and school, is recommended. Every attempt is made to make the home note system an aid rather than a punishment.

Homework can be a real flashpoint of conflict, and we encourage making homework a routine. To aid in the establishment of study as a habit it is necessary for the child to (a) have a set time to study each day (the amount of time is determined by the amount of work, the child's ability to focus attention, etc.), (b) study in the same place each day (preferably a desk with adequate lighting), and (c) have minimal distractions (e.g., no radio or TV). This final presentation generates considerable discussion of the success and failure that parents have experienced in dealing with the educational system. As this is the last session, time is given to bring closure to the program, and a follow-up session in 4 to 6 weeks is scheduled.

SUMMARY

Understanding and responding to the needs of custodial grandparents of children with ADHD is a topic worthy of greater attention both in research and in clinical practice. Custodial grandparents who struggle with these issues by themselves often experience a diminished quality of life, and their grandchildren suffer as well. Education and information about ADHD, guidance in managing problem behavior, and social support are but a few of the means of responding to these needs. The provision of such services through parent training for ADHD can be administered in a flexible and low-cost manner. National support groups such as Children and Adults with Attention Deficit Disorders (ChADD) and the Attention Deficit Disorder Association (ADDA) do an outstanding job responding to the needs of families struggling with ADHD and are accessible through Web pages and related links.

For many families, living with ADHD can at times be overwhelming. We recognize that there is much we can do to lessen that burden. Better understanding of the unique issues and challenges that confront custodial grandparents of grandchildren with ADHD can be instrumental in identifying, providing, and evaluating services that both custodial grandparents and grandchildren who struggle with ADHD need and deserve.

REFERENCES

Abidin, R. R. (1995). *Parenting Stress Index* (3rd ed.). Charlottesville, VA: Pediatric Psychology Press.

American Psychiatric Association. (1994). *Diagnostic and statistical manual of mental disorders* (4th ed., rev.). Washington, DC: Author.

Argyle, M. (1991). *Cooperation: The basis for sociability.* London: Routledge.

Baker, D. B. (1994). Parenting stress and ADHD: A comparison of mothers and fathers. *Journal of Emotional and Behavioral Disorders, 2,* 46–50.

Baker, D. B., & McCal, K. (1995). Parenting stress in parents of children with attention-deficit hyperactivity disorder and parents of children with learning disabilities. *Journal of Child and Family Studies, 4,* 57–68.

Baker, D. B., Knight, K., & Simpson, D. D. (1995). Identifying probationers with ADHD-related behaviors in a drug abuse treatment setting. *Journal of Criminal Justice and Behavior, 1,* 33–43.

Baker, D. B., & Pisecco, S. (1998). Building a parent support program and learning network. *Reaching Today's Youth: The Community of Circle of Caring Journal, 2,* 48–51.

Barkley, R. A. (1997). *ADHD and the nature of self control.* New York: Guilford Press.

Cunningham, C. E., & Sigel, L. S. (1987). Peer interactions of normal and attention deficit disordered boys during free play, cooperative task, and simulated classroom situations. *Journal of Abnormal Child Psychology, 15,* 247–268.

Cutrona, C. (1990). Stress and social support-in search of optimal matching. *Journal of Social and Clinical Psychology, 9,* 3–14.

Emick, M., & Hayslip, B. (1996). Custodial grandparenting: New roles for middle aged and older adults. *International Journal of Aging and Human Development, 43,* 135–154.

Emick, M. A., & Hayslip, B. (1999). Custodial grandparenting: Stresses, coping skills, and relationships with grandchildren. *International Journal of Aging and Human Development, 1,* 35–61.

Fischer, M., Barkley, R. A., Fletcher, K. E., & Smallish, L. (1993). The stability of dimensions of behavior in ADHD and normal children over an 8-year follow-up. *Journal of Abnormal Child Psychology, 21,* 315–337.

Hayslip, B., Shore, R. J., Henderson, C., & Lambert, P. (1998). Custodial grandparenting and grandchildren with problems: Impact on role satisfaction and role meaning. *Journal of Gerontology: Social Sciences, 3,* 1–10.

Hechtman, L. (1991). Resilience and vulnerability in long term outcome of attention deficit hyperactivity disorder. *Canadian Journal of Psychiatry, 36,* 415–421.

Johnson, C. L. (1988). Active and latent functions of grandparenting during the divorce process. *Gerontologist, 28,* 185–191.

Johnston, C., Pelham, W. E., & Murphy, H. A. (1985). Peer relationships in ADDH and normal children: A developmental analysis of peer and teacher ratings. *Journal of Abnormal Child Psychology, 13,* 89–100.

Kottman, T., Baker, D. B., & Roberts, R. S. (1995). Parental perspectives on ADHD: How school counselors can help. *School Counselor, 43,* 142–150.

Margalit, M. (1989). Academic competence and social adjustment of boys with learning disabilities and boys with behavior disorders. *Journal of Learning Disabilities, 22,* 41–45.

Minkler, M., Roe, K. M., & Price, M. (1992). The physical and emotional health of grandmothers raising grandchildren in the crack cocaine epidemic. *Gerontologist, 32,* 752–761.

Pelham, W. E., Wheeler, T., & Chronis, A. (1998). Empirically supported treatments for attention deficit hyperactivity disorder. *Journal of Clinical Child Psychology, 2,* 190–205.

Pinson-Millburn, M., Fabian, E., Schlossberg, N., & Pyle, M. (1996). Grandparents raising grandchildren. *Journal of Counseling and Development, 74,* 548–554.

Pisecco, S., Baker, D. B., Silva, P. A., & Brooke, M. (1996). Behavioral distinctions between children identified with reading disabilities and/or ADHD. *Journal of the American Academy of Child and Adolescent Psychiatry, 11,* 1477–1484.

Robertson, J. F. (1977). Grandmotherhood: A study of role conceptions. *Journal of Marriage and the Family, 33,* 165–174.

Shekim, W. O., Asarnow, R. F., Hess, E., Zaucha, K., & Wheeler, N. (1990). A clinical and demographic profile of a sample of adults with attention deficit hyperactivity disorder, residual state. *Comprehensive Psychiatry, 31,* 416–426.

Shore, R. J., & Hayslip, B. (1994). Custodial grandparenting: Implications for children's development. In A. Gottfried & A. Gottfried (Eds.), *Redefining families: Implications for children's development* (pp. 171–218). New York: Plenum.

Ward, M. F., Wender, P. H., & Reimherr, F. W. (1993). The Wender Utah Rating Scale: An aid in the retrospective diagnosis of childhood attention deficit hyperactivity disorder. *American Journal of Psychiatry, 150,* 885–889.

Weiss, L. (1990). *Attention deficit disorder in adults.* Dallas, TX: Taylor.

Weiss, G., & Hechtman, L. T. (1993). *Hyperactive children grown up: Empirical findings and theoretical considerations* (2nd ed.). New York: Guilford.

Weiss, G., Hechtman, L., Milroy, T., & Perlman, T. (1985). Psychiatric status of hyperactives as adults: A controlled prospective 15-year follow-up of 63 hyperactive children. *Journal of the American Academy of Child Psychiatry, 24,* 211–220.

Whitbeck, L. B., Hoyt, D. R., & Huck, S. M. (1993). Family relationship history, contemporary parent-grandparent relationship quality, and the grandparent-grandchild relationship. *Journal of Marriage and the Family, 55,* 1025–1035.

CHAPTER 10

Primary and Secondary Caregiving Grandparents: How Different Are They?

Robin S. Goldberg-Glen and Roberta G. Sands

D espite the proliferation of research, policy development, and clinical accounts on "skipped generation" families in the 1990s (e.g., Burton, 1992; Chalfie, 1994; Fuller-Thomson, Minkler, & Driver, 1997; Jendrek, 1994; Minkler & Roe, 1993; Pinson-Millburn, Fabian, Scholossberg, & Pyle, 1996), interest in these families was limited to the primary caregiver, typically the grandmother (Minkler & Roe, 1993; Sands & Goldberg-Glen, 1998), and the grandchildren (Shore & Hayslip, 1994; Solomon & Marks, 1995), disregarding the secondary caregiver, usually a spouse or partner. Over 50% of skipped-generation families are composed of married couples (Casper & Bryson, 1998; Fuller-Thomson et al., 1997; Pruchno, 1999; Saluter, 1992), who raise the grandchildren together. This chapter breaks new ground in describing a group of secondary grandparents who are spouses and partners of the primary caregiving grandparent.

PREVIOUS RESEARCH

Secondary caregivers are family members and friends who provide support, care, and backup assistance when the primary caregiver is not available. Research on various types of family systems has found that secondary caregivers provide supplementary care to recipients and replace primary caregivers when they are no longer able to offer assistance (Brody, 1985; Hooyman & Kiyak, 1999; Scanlon, 1988; Tennstedt, McKinlay, & Sullivan, 1989). Secondary caregivers of older adults—generally males—typically provide care with instrumental activities of daily living (e.g., finances, shopping, household work, financial management, etc.), whereas primary caregivers—generally wives, daughters, and daughters-in-law—provide direct, personal care (e.g., bathing, dressing, feeding, hygiene, etc.) (Cantor, 1991, 1994; National Alliance for Caregiving and AARP, 1997; Tennstedt et al., 1989). Gerontological research that makes gender rather than primary/secondary distinctions has found that males become involved with direct care when a female caregiver is unavailable to provide assistance to their relative (Finley, 1989; Foster & Brizius, 1993; Kaye & Applegate, 1990; Tennstedt et al., 1989) or when husbands are able to provide care for their chronically ill wives (Bengston, Rosenthal, & Burton, 1995). Men who have become primary caregivers of older adults have been characterized as "unsung or unrecognized heroes" (Brody, 1985; Kaye & Applegate, 1990; Scharlach & Kaye, 1997; Thompson, 1994).

Regardless of their gender, secondary caregivers have been given scant attention in the caregiving literature. Sometimes they are included in research as components of the primary caregiver's support system (Greenberg, Seltzer, & Greenley, 1993). As Bengston, Rosenthal, and Burton (1995) point out, "methodological individualism" produces studies that ignore secondary caregivers and attend to women caregivers and/or their care recipients (Fuller-Thomson et al., 1997). Given that over half of caregiving grandparents are married (Casper & Bryson, 1998; Fuller-Thomson et al., 1997; Pruchno, 1999; Saluter, 1992), there is a need to learn more about spouses who are secondary caregivers.

Like the previous studies on caregiving of other populations, research on grandparents who care for their grandchildren has provided limited coverage of caregivers other than the primary one. The four studies that will be described next make reference to secondary caregivers (Casper & Bryson, 1998; Fuller-Thomson et al., 1997; Goldberg-Glen, Sands, Cole, & Cristofalo, 1998; and Jendrek, 1993, 1994) but do not focus on this subgroup of surrogate parents in particular.

In an analysis of national census data from March 1997, Casper and Bryson (1998) show that the marital status of the grandparent affects the family's economic well-being. Grandchildren who live in households headed by grandmothers only (with the parents absent) are the most likely to receive public assistance and to be poor, whereas those who live with two grandparents are most likely to be uninsured, confirming their hypothesis that the larger the number of caregivers in the household, the more likely grandchildren were to be uninsured. Given this difference, children living in grandparent-headed households with secondary caregivers may have different needs and necessitate distinctive service interventions and policy decisions. This study of census data did not contain comparative information on the primary and secondary grandparents' perceptions of their situation.

Using the National Survey of Families and Households (NSFH) of Adult Americans, Fuller-Thomson, Minkler, and Driver (1997) make fleeting reference to the fact that of the of 173 primary caregiving grandparents who had cared for a grandchild for at least 6 months during the 1990s, 54% were married and 23% were grandfathers. This suggests that there are male and female secondary caregivers, but because the analysis was of primary caregivers only, nothing else was said about the secondary caregivers.

Goldberg-Glen et al.(1998) examine multigenerational patterns and internal structures in families in which grandparents raise grandchildren. This qualitative study utilizes genograms and the case study method, with three examples to illustrate variations in family structure and the interactional processes of these families. Although this article provides useful diagrams depicting detailed information on family patterns, including the presence of secondary caregivers, the generalizability of the findings is limited, given the method.

Jendrek (1993, 1994) studied the impact of surrogate caregiving on the lives of 114 predominantly White female grandparents who were either custodial, living with the grandchildren, or providing day care for them. Seventy-four percent of the 36 custodial grandparents were married when they began caring for their grandchildren. As a result of caring for the grandchildren for whom they had custody, 59% reported having less time for their spouse, 50% said they give less attention to their spouse, and 86% reported an increased need to change their routines and plans (Jendrek, 1993). Although this study focused on the primary caregiver, the findings suggest that the secondary caregiving grandparents/spouses are affected by the addition of grandchildren to their families.

This chapter is a beginning attempt to explore some of the differences between primary and secondary caregiving grandparents and to make suggestions for future research. The study described here extends the analysis of grandparent caregivers to include spouses and partners whom the primary informants identified as secondary caregivers. This exploratory study addresses the following questions:

- Who are the secondary grandparent caregivers?
- What are the primary grandparent caregivers' perceptions of the secondary caregiver?
- How do secondary caregivers compare to primary caregivers in their perceptions of family resources, including financial stability, external resources, family cohesion, and emotional control?
- How do secondary caregivers compare to primary caregivers on perceived stress?
- How do secondary caregivers compare to primary caregivers on psychological anxiety?
- How do secondary caregivers compare to primary caregivers on life satisfaction and well-being?

METHODS

This chapter is based on a larger study of stress, well-being, and life satisfaction among 129 grand- or great-grandparents who identified themselves as the primary caregivers of their biological or adoptive grandchildren (Sands & Goldberg-Glen, 1996).

Sample

The primary caregivers were recruited from schools, social service agencies, religious institutions, hospitals, and grandparent support groups in Philadelphia and surrounding counties. This sample was stratified by race and age, yielding approximately 51% who were African American; 49% who were Caucasian; 50% who were middle-aged (ages 50 through 59); and 50% who were older (60 and older). Among the 129 primary caregivers, only 6 were men.

Primary caregivers participated in one-time, face-to-face interviews that took about 1.5 hours. On these occasions, spouses or companions who were available in the house were asked to complete a pen-and-pencil questionnaire that included some of the same instruments used with the primary participants. Questionnaires with stamped return mailing envelopes were left behind for those secondary caregiving spouse/companions who were not at home. Among the 49 coupled grandparents, 33 secondary caregivers completed the form, yielding a response rate of 67%. The study described here focuses on the 33 secondary caregivers and their respective spouses/companions.

Table 10.1 describes the sample of 66 primary and secondary grandparent caregivers ($N = 33 \times 2$) who lived in the same household. The majority of primary caregivers were female ($n = 28$, 85%), whereas most of the secondary caregivers were male ($n = 28$, 85%). These findings are consistent with studies on caregiving that indicate that primary caregivers tend to be female (Brody, 1985; Older Women's League, 1989; Stone, Cafferata, & Sangl, 1987). There was a range of educational levels among both the primary and secondary caregivers. Seventy-six percent ($n = 25$) of the primary and 79% ($n = 26$) of the secondary caregivers had a high school degree or additional education. Approximately 97% ($n = 32$) of the sample were married, and 3% ($n = 1$) was widowed and was cohabitating. Eighty-five percent of the primary caregivers were White. With respect to religion, 61% ($n = 20$) were Catholic, 21% ($n = 7$) were Protestant, 12% ($n = 4$) were Jewish, 3% ($n = 1$) were Quaker, and 3% ($n = 1$) reported no religion.

Measures

Six standardized instruments were used to assess stress, life satisfaction, well-being, and resources. They are as follows.

TABLE 10.1 Comparison of Primary and Secondary Grandparent Caregivers

Primary			Secondary		
Characteristic	*N*	%	Characteristic	*N*	%
Gender			Gender		
Female	28	84.8%	Female	5	15.2%
Male	5	15.2%	Male	28	84.8%
Age			Age		
Range	50–73		Range	48–77	
Mean	60.12		Mean	62.15	
Median	61		Median	63	
SD	6.07		*SD*	8.16	
Education			Education		
< H.S.	(8)	24.2%	< H.S.	(7)	21.2%
H.S.	(16)	48.5%	H.S.	(17)	51.5%
Tech. school	(1)	37.0%	Tech. school	(0)	0%
Some college	(5)	15.2%	Some college	(4)	12.1%
College grad	(2)	6.1%	College grad	(4)	12.1%
Some grad	(1)	3.0%	Some grad	(0)	0%
Grad degree	(0)	0%	Grad degree	(1)	3.0%
How has physical health changed since caring for grandchild(ren)?					
Worse	(4)	12.1%	Worse	(13)	39.4%
Somewhat worse	(26)	78.8%	Somewhat worse	(0)	0%
Stayed the same	(3)	9.1%	Stayed the same	(20)	60.6%
Rating of physical health					
Excellent	(7)	21.2%	Excellent	(8)	24.2%
Good	(15)	45.4%	Good	(10)	30.1%
Fair	(10)	30.3%	Fair	(11)	33.3%
Poor	(1)	3.0%	Poor	(4)	12.1%
Relationship to grandchild					
Biological	(28)	84.8%	Biological	(23)	69.7%
Adoptive	(3)	9.1%	Adoptive	(3)	9.1%
Combination	(1)	3.0%	Combination	(1)	9.1%
Unrelated	(0)	0%	Unrelated	(5)	15.2%
Other	(1)	3.0%	Other	(1)	3.0%
Marital status					
Married	32	97%			
Widowed/ common law	1	3%			

TABLE 10.1   *(continued)*

Primary			Secondary		
Characteristic	*N*	*%*	Characteristic	*N*	*%*
Religion					
Catholic	(20)	60.6%			
Baptist	(2)	6.1%			
Episcopalian	(2)	6.1%			
Pentecostal/Holiness	(1)	3.0%			
Lutheran	(1)	3.0%			
Presbyterian	(1)	3.0%			
Quaker	(1)	3.0%			
Jewish	(1)	3.0%			
Other	(0)	0%			
None	(1)	3.0%			
Race					
White	(28)	84.8%			
Black	(5)	15.2%			

The FILE (Family Inventory of Life Events and Changes) was developed by McCubbin, Patterson, and Wilson (1983) to assess the pile-up of life events or stressors experienced by a family. The FILE is a 71-item self-report instrument that was designed to record a family's experience of normative and nonnormative life events and changes within the past year. Participants are asked whether a family life change, such as "increased strain of family money for food, clothing, energy, home care," occurred in the past year. McCubbin, Patterson, and Wilson (1983) assume that families typically deal with several stressors at any one time; therefore, the FILE serves as an index of the family unit's vulnerability as a result of stress pile-up.

McCubbin and Thompson (1987) found good overall scale reliability (Cronbach alpha = .81), construct validity, and test-retest reliability for the FILE. For the grandparent study, the wording of this scale was changed so that "grandmother" and "grandfather" replaced "mother" and "father." In addition, based on a pretest, each item was converted into a question, some items were modified for clarity, and small changes were made in the sequencing. For this analysis, the items were added to constitute a scale of pile-up of stressful life events.

The FIRM (Family Inventory of Resources for Management) was designed by McCubbin, Comeau, and Harkins (1981) to describe resources that predict how families adapt to stressful events. The FIRM assumes that families with a larger number of resources will "better" adapt to stressful events and manage stressful situations more effectively than those families with fewer resources. The FIRM inventory consists of 69 self-report items rated by the respondent, on a 0–3 scale, as to how well these items describe the respondent's family. It includes statements like "Family members understand each other completely." The FIRM has good internal reliability and correlates highly with the Moos Family Environment Scale.

Pretesting of the FIRM found that some of the questions were not sufficiently culturally sensitive or clear, and the questionnaire was too long. Accordingly, a number of questions (most of which were on scales that were not of theoretical interest or were peripheral to the purpose of the FIRM) were eliminated. The resulting instrument consisted of 37 questions. The Cronbach alpha on the total scale was .87.

Because the FIRM appeared to represent many dimensions, a principal components analysis with a Varimax rotation was conducted. Following a scree test, a 4-factor model was chosen, and items with loadings of .40 and above (or if more than one factor qualified, the factor with the highest loading for that item) were used to create subscales. The reliability coefficients for the subscales were as follows: .87 for Factor 1, Financial Stability; .81 for Factor 2, Family Cohesion; .66 for Factor 3, Open Communication; and .72 for Factor 4, Emotional Control. (See Sands & Goldberg-Glen, 2000, for a further discussion of these constructs.)

The Grandparental Perception of Stress Scale was adapted from Pearlin and Schooler's (1978) self-report questionnaire, which measures emotions associated with the perception of parental stress. The instrument consists of seven items that are measured along a 4-point Likert-type scale (Pearlin & Schooler, 1978). Pearlin and Schooler asked participants to rate their perceived emotions in response to the following question asked seven times with a different adjective inserted: "When you think of your experiences as a parent, how (worried) do you feel?" In this study, "grandparent who is raising your grandchild(ren)" was substituted for "parent." The Parental Stress Scale was created from a factor analysis that identified the presence of a single factor with loadings of from .69 to .84 (Pearlin & Schooler, 1978). The Cronbach reliability quotient for the scale that was used in the grandparent study was .84.

In this study, "distress" or "stress" was operationalized by using the Mental Health Symptoms Questionnaire (Veroff, Douvan, & Kulka, 1981). Questions comprising two factors developed by Veroff, Douvan, and Kulka in their comparative analysis of two national studies of mental health in a normal population were used here. Six items (e.g., shortness of breath, heart beats hard) comprised the factor Ill Health; five (e.g., trouble sleeping, nervousness), the factor Psychological Anxiety. The internal consistency reliability estimate on Ill Health, using Cronbach's coefficient alpha, ranged from .76 to .77; on Psychological Anxiety from .68 to .69 (Veroff, Douvan, & Kulka, 1981). The reliability coefficient for Psychological Anxiety on the grandparents was .72; for Ill Health it was .63.

Positive feelings are equated with "well-being" and measured by a subscale of the Valuation of Life Questionnaire developed by Lawton (1994) at the Philadelphia Geriatric Center. The scale consists of seven items that had loadings of .73 and above from a positive goals factor. Each item was rated on a scale from 1 (strongly agree) to 5 (strongly disagree). The Cronbach alpha coefficient on this scale in the grandparent study was .79.

The Satisfaction with Life Scale was designed to assess subjective life satisfaction (Dienner, Emmons, Larsen, & Griffin, 1985). The scale consists of five items, each of which is rated on a scale from 1 (strongly disagree) to 7 (strongly agree). An example of one of these items is "In most ways my life is close to my ideal." The Satisfaction with Life Scale has good reliability and validity (Fischer & Corcoran, 1994). The researchers changed the range of this scale from 1 to 7 ("strongly disagree" to "strongly agree") to 1 to 5 and obtained a Cronbach alpha coefficient of .81.

DESCRIPTIVE FINDINGS

Health

Primary caregivers reported that their health had changed since caring for their grandchildren. Ninety-one percent ($n = 30$) reported their health as becoming worse or somewhat worse since caring for their grandchildren. Over 39% ($n = 13$) of these same caregivers perceived their significant other's health as worse since they became caregivers. A closer look at physical health revealed that, overall, 67% ($n = 22$) of the primaries reported that their own health was good to excellent and perceived that 54% ($n = 18$) of their partners had a similar health status. Thus, they see their own health as better than that of their spouses/companions.

Relationships

Most of primary 85% ($n = 28$) and secondary 70% ($n = 23$) caregivers report being biologically related to the grandchildren they are caring for. The remaining primary caregivers included 3 adoptive grandmothers, 1 combination (biologically related and unrelated grandchildren), and 1 "other," whereas the remaining secondary caregivers included 3 adoptive grandparents, 1 combination, 5 unrelated, and 1 "other."

Household Income

As Table 10.2 shows, most of the families were living above the poverty line for a family of four in 1996. Sources of income came from a variety of places, mostly from employment, Social Security, and retirement/pensions. None of these coupled grandparents were living in subsidized housing, and about 94% owned their own homes outright. The data indicate that these caregiving dyads were financially stable. A little over half reported that an adult child's housing problem contributed to their taking in their grandchildren.

Household Characteristics

The average number of people living in the household ranged from 3 to 10, with a mean of 4.3 people. For the most part, the grandparents were taking care of 1 or 2 grandchildren, but some were taking care of more. Seventy-three percent ($n = 24$) of the households had

TABLE 10.2   Income of Primary Caregiver

	N	%
Income		
$417–833	(2)	6.1%
$834–1248	(2)	6.1%
$1250–1666	(5)	15.2%
$1667–2083	(7)	21.2%
$2084 –2499	(5)	15.2%
$2500–2926	(2)	6.1%
$2927–3333	(1)	3.0%
$3334+	(7)	21.2%
Missing	(2)	6.1%
Source of income		
Employment	(20)	60.6%
Social Security	(33)	66.7%
SSI	(4)	12.1%
Retirement/pension	(17)	51.5%
Savings	(10)	30.3%
Military benefits	(2)	6.1%
Unemployment compensation	(1)	3.0%
Contribution from parent	(6)	18.2%
Help from other family members	(4)	12.1%
Public assistance	(13)	39.4%
Other SW programs (food stamps)	(1)	3.0%
Investments	(8)	24.2%
Other sources	(1)	3.0%

SSI, supplemental security income; SW, social work.

a combination of grandparents and grandchildren only living in the family home. Sixty-one percent ($n = 20$) had legal custody of their grandchildren. Remarkably, close to 70% of the primary caregiving grandparents reported having conflicts with the parent of the grand-children for whom they were caring (see Table 10.3).

Family Dynamics

Table 10.4 shows how the family dynamics were affected by the grandchildren. The primary caregivers' perceptions of the secondary caregivers revealed that at least a third of the significant others

TABLE 10.3   Housing Characteristics

	N	%
Living in subsidized housing?		
No	(33)	100%
Did a housing problem contribute to your taking in your grandchild(ren)?		
Yes	(17)	51.5%
No	(16)	48.5%
Total number of people in household		
3	13	39.4%
4	9	27.3%
5	4	12.1%
6	6	18.2%
10	1	3.0%
Range	3–10	
Mean	4.3	
Median	4.0	
Mode	3	
SD	1.53	
Mix of children in household		
Combination of grandparent's child(ren) and grandchildren	9	27.3%
Only grandchild(ren)	24	72.7%
Total number of grandchild(ren)		
1	(20)	60.6%
2	(7)	21.2%
3	(3)	9.1%
4	(2)	6.1%
5	(1)	3.1%
Have legal custody		
Yes	(20)	60.6%
No	(13)	39.4%
Does grandparent have living children?		
Yes	(32)	97.0%
No	(1)	3.0%
Does grandparent have conflict with grandchild(ren)'s parent?		
Yes	(23)	69.7%
No	(10)	30.3%

played an equal role in spending time with the grandchildren. Over 50% of the primaries ($n = 17$) believed they spent the most time, whereas only 12% ($n = 4$) believed the secondary spent the most time with the grandchildren. Sixty-four percent ($n = 21$) reported having less privacy, while about 36% ($n = 12$) reported no change.

Only 9% of the primary caregiving grandparents reported having more financial disagreements with their partners as a result of caring for the grandchildren; most related that there was no such change. However, relationships appear to be somewhat affected by this new responsibility. Most of the grandparents reported that they expected the caregiving to continue for several years or until the grandchildren grew up.

Comparisons Between Primary and Secondary Caregivers

Paired *t*-tests were used to compare primary and secondary caregivers on the standardized scales that we used. As Table 10.5 shows, the comparison scores for the FILE indicate that the secondary caregivers experience more stressors than the primary caregivers do ($p < .05$).

There were also significant differences on the FIRM and two of the four subscales created from factors of the FIRM (Table 10.5). Overall, comparison scores for the FIRM indicate that the primary caregivers have greater resources than the secondary caregivers have ($p < .05$). With respect to the subscales, primary caregivers had more open communication resources than the secondary group had and greater financial stability (marginally significant). There were no significant differences in family cohesion and emotional control. Nor were there differences between primary and secondary caregivers with respect to perceived stress, well-being, psychological anxiety, and life satisfaction.

DISCUSSION

This study was an initial attempt to provide some descriptive information about secondary grandparent caregivers and compare them to their primary counterparts. Despite reports that over 50% of grandparent caregivers are married (Casper & Bryson, 1998; Fuller-

TABLE 10.4   Family Dynamics of Grandparent Caregivers

From Perspective of Primary Caregiver ($n = 33$)

	N	%
Who spends most time with grandchild(ren)?		
Primary	(17)	51.5%
Secondary	(4)	12.1%
Equal	(12)	36.4%
Has taking in grandchild(ren) caused financial disagreements?		
More	(3)	9.1%
Fewer	(2)	6.1%
No change	(27)	81.8%
Has caring for grandchild(ren) affected relationship with spouse?		
Closer	(7)	21.2%
More conflict	(6)	18.2%
Less time together	(10)	30.3%
No change	(5)	15.2%
Other	(5)	15.2%
How has taking care of grandchild(ren) affected your privacy?		
Less privacy	(21)	63.6%
No change	(12)	36.4%
How has taking care of your grandchild(ren) affected your sexual activity?		
Decrease	(14)	42.4%
No change	(19)	57.6%
Ever have time without children/grandchild(ren)? (empty nest)		
Yes	(17)	51.5%
No	(16)	48.5%
How helpful is spouse/companion in caring for grandchild(ren)?		
Very helpful	(28)	84.8%
Somewhat helpful	(3)	9.1%
Little	(1)	3.0%
Not very helpful	(1)	3.0%
Length of time expected to care for grandchild(ren)?		
Few months	(1)	3.0%
A year or so	(1)	3.0%
Several years	(26)	78.8%
Until grandchild(ren) grows up	(1)	3.0%
Combination (different children)	(2)	6.1%
Don't know	(2)	6.1%

TABLE 10.5 Comparison Between Primary and Secondary Caregiving Grandparents

Scale	Mean (Primary)	Mean (Secondary)	*t*-Value	*p*
FILE (stressors)	10.36	13.27	−2.38	<.05
FIRM (resources)	**73.45**	**67.94**	**2.38**	**<.05**
Open Communication	17.27	15.15	3.33	<.01
Financial Stability	18.42	16.36	2.01	.05
Family Cohesion	20.63	19.39	1.52	N.S.
Emotional Control	11.85	11.79	.10	N.S.
Perceived Stress	14.30	14.85	−.59	N.S.
Psychological Anxiety	4.18	3.97	.27	N.S.
Life Satisfaction	16.06	14.27	1.73	N.S.
Well-being	11.52	12.82	−1.38	N.S.

N.S., nonsignificant.

Thomson et al., 1997; Pruchno, 1999; Saluter, 1992), no one else has closely examined this sector of grandparents.

The participants in this study were predominantly White married couples who owned their own homes and had moderate incomes. Most were caring for one or two grandchildren. The major finding of the comparative analysis was that, with a few exceptions, the perceptions of secondary grandparents about caregiving and other aspects of their lives were similar to those of primary caregivers.

As an exploratory effort, this study has come up with some intriguing findings that can be investigated more thoroughly in future studies. It was interesting to note, for example, that the primary caregivers' perception of their spouses' change in health after taking in the grandchild was that it had become worse. These findings, combined with the fact that secondary caregivers appeared to have fewer resources (FIRM) and scored higher on experiencing greater stressful life events, may indicate that this newly acquired role with its added responsibilities may be more difficult for the secondary care provider than for the primary. If this is true, secondary caregivers in grandparent-headed families may have health and service needs that deserve special attention.

Another surprising observation was that the primary caregivers (mostly female) reported having fewer stressors and more resources than did secondary caregivers (mostly male). This finding deviates from the gerontological literature, which indicates that female caregivers (usually primary caregivers) perceive themselves as having fewer resources than male caregivers have and are more likely to modify their work schedules and career goals and even give up their jobs (Ingersol-Dayton, Starrels, & Dowler, 1996; Kramer, 1997; Kramer & Kipnis, 1995; Pavlko & Artis, 1997; U.S. Bureau of the Census, 1996).

Given that the primary and secondary caregivers live in the same household, one would expect their perceptions and experiences—family stressors (FILE) and resources (FIRM)—to be the same. The findings of significant differences may be the result of individual differences in primary and secondary caregivers, who live part of their lives separately and thus have some differences in perceived stressors and resources. The primary caregivers may have more resources (particularly "open communication" with the immediate and extended family) accrued from their previous experiences as caregivers of their children. They already learned how to manage the family (financially and emotionally) and to obtain the supports they need. The secondary caregivers may be experiencing more stressors from work. They may feel more pressured to provide financially for the "modified family" they now have.

Another intriguing observation is the high level of conflict between the grandparents and the parents of the grandchildren; this is not uncommon among grandparent caregivers (Shore & Hayslip, 1994). Considering that 39% of the grandparents do not have legal custody, conflict may have to do with rights over the child. Judicial determinations made for custody, guardianship, and adoption necessitate extreme modifications in the legal relationships between the grandchild and his or her parents (Karp, 1996), a change that is bound to be painful for everyone involved. Sometimes grandchildren are removed from their parents' home by child protective service agencies and placed in kinship care homes provided by their grandparents. When this occurs, child welfare agencies may distance parents from the grandparents and children themselves and, in turn, create interfamilial tensions (Crumbley & Little, 1997; Solomon & Marx, 1995; Takas, 1992) that affect the whole nuclear and extended family system, including secondary caregivers. Crumbley and Little (1997) attribute this conflict to the grandparent caregivers' ambivalence regarding the new caregiving role once they recognize that they must change their lifestyle and allegiance to certain family members and deal with the loss of freedom, as well as psychological, physical, and financial hardships. Although policy has focused on the provision of concrete services, legislation is needed to provide funding for family therapy that can assist the surrogate caregivers and the middle generation in dealing with their family conflict.

Finally, data revealed that the housing needs of the biological parents was a factor in the placement of a large portion of the grandchildren with the home-owning grandparents. This suggests a need for a close investigation of the impact of inadequate or unavailable housing on the placement of grandchildren with their kin.

These initial findings on primary and secondary caregivers highlight the need to consider more than one family member in research on grandparent-headed families. To more fully assess the role of secondary caregivers, future research should be on a larger, more representative sample. Future studies might investigate the contributions of secondary caregivers to the well-being of the family household, the effect of the secondary caregiver's health problems on the primary caregiving grandparent and grandchild, and how grandchildren who are brought up in single-grandparent-headed households compare with those raised in homes with two caregivers. Another promising avenue of research is nonspousal secondary caregivers (e.g., aunts, uncles, older siblings). It is hoped that research on grandparent-headed families in the 21st century will address the contributions of these secondary caregivers and the consequences of caregiving for their grandchildren, their spouses or partners, and themselves.

ACKNOWLEDGMENTS

This chapter is based on a paper presented at the 51st Annual Scientific Meeting of The Gerontological Association of America, Philadelphia, PA, November 1998. Funding for this research was provided in part by the AARP Andrus Foundation.

REFERENCES

Bengston, V., Rosenthal, C., & Burton, L. (1995). Paradoxes of families and aging. In R. H. Binstock & L. K. George, *Handbook of aging and the social sciences* (4th ed., pp. 253–282). San Diego, CA: Academic Press.

Brody, E. (1985). Parent care as a normative family stress. *Gerontologist, 25,* 19–30.

Burton, L. M. (1992). Black grandparents rearing children of drug-addicted parents: Stressors, outcomes, and social service needs. *Gerontologist, 32,* 744–751.

Cantor, M. (1991). Family and community: Changing roles in an aging society. *Gerontologist, 31,* 337–340.

Cantor, M. (1994). Family caregiving: Social care. In M. Cantor (Ed.), *Family caregiving: Agenda for the future.* San Francisco: American Society on Aging.

Casper, L. M., & Bryson, K. R. (1998). Coresident grandparents and their grandchildren: Grandparent-maintained families (Population Division Working Paper, no. 26). Washington, DC: U.S. Bureau of the Census.

Chalfie, D. (1994). *Going it alone: A closer look at grandparents parenting grandchildren.* Washington, DC: American Association of Retired Persons.

Crumbley, J., & Little, R. (Eds.). (1997). *Relatives raising children: An overview of kinship care.* Washington, DC: Child Welfare League of America.

Dienner, E., Emmons, R. A., Larsen, R. J., & Griffin, S. (1985). The satisfaction with life scale. *Journal of Personality Assessment, 49,* 71–75.

Finley, N. J. (1989). Theories of family labor as applied to gender differences in caregiving for elderly parents. *Journal of Marriage and the Family, 51,* 79.

Fischer, J., & Corcoran, K. (1994). *Measures for clinical practice: A sourcebook: Vol. 2. Adults* (2nd ed.). New York: Free Press.

Foster, S. E., & Brizius, J. A. (1993). Caring too much: American women and the nation's caregiving crisis. In J. Allen & A. Pifer (Eds.), *Women on the front lines: Meeting the challenge of an aging America* (pp. 47–73). Washington, DC: Urban Institute Press.

Fuller-Thomson, E., Minkler, M., & Driver, D. (1997). A profile of grandparents raising grandchildren in the United States. *Gerontologist, 37,* 405–411.

Goldberg-Glen, R. S., Sands, R. G., Cole, R. D., & Cristofalo, C. (1998). Multigenerational patterns and internal structures in families in which grandparents raise grandchildren. *Families in Society, 79,* 477–489.

Greenberg, J. S., Seltzer, M. M., & Greenley, J. R. (1993). Aging parents of adults with disabilities: The gratifications and frustrations of later-life caregiving. *Gerontologist, 33,* 542–550.

Hooyman, N. R., & Kiyak, H. A. (1999). *Social gerontology: A multidisciplinary perspective* (5th ed.). Boston: Allyn and Bacon.

Ingersoll-Dayton, B., Starrels, M., & Dowler, D. (1996). Caregiving for parents and parents-in-law: Is gender important? *Gerontologist, 36,* 694–700.

Jendrek, M. P. (1993). Grandparents who parent their grandchildren: Effects on lifestyle. *Journal of Marriage and the Family, 45,* 609–621.

Jendrek, M. P. (1994). Grandparents who parent their grandchildren: Circumstances and decisions. *Gerontologist, 34,* 206–216.

Karp, N. (1996). Legal problems of grandparents and other kinship caregivers. *Generations, 20,* 57–60.

Kaye, L. W., & Applegate, J. S. (1990). *Men as caregivers to the elderly: Understanding and aiding unrecognized family support.* Lexington, MA: Lexington Books.

Kramer, B. J. (1997). Differential prediction of strain and gain among husbands caring for wives with dementia. *Gerontologist, 37,* 218–232.

Kramer, B. J., & Kipnis, S. (1995). Eldercare and work-role conflict: Toward an understanding of gender differences in caregiver burden. *Gerontologist, 35,* 340–347.

Lawton, P. (1994). [Valuation of life questionnaire]. Unpublished report on pilot data, Senior Center Indices, Philadelphia Geriatric Center.

McCubbin, H. I., Comeau, J. K., & Harkins, J. A. (1981). FIRM: Family Inventory of Resources for Management. In H. I. McCubbin & A. I. Thompson (Eds.), *Family assessment inventories for research and practice.* Madison: University of Wisconsin–Madison.

McCubbin, H. I., Patterson, J. M., & Wilson, L. R. (1987). FILE: Family Inventory of Life Events. In H. I. McCubbin & A. I. Thompson (Eds.), *Family assessment inventories for research and practice.* Madison: University of Wisconsin–Madison.

McCubbin, H. I., & Thompson, A. I. (Eds.). (1987). *Family assessment inventories for research and practice.* Madison: University of Wisconsin–Madison.

Minkler, M., & Roe, K. M. (1993). *Grandmothers as caregivers: Raising children of the crack cocaine epidemic.* Newbury Park, CA: Sage.

National Alliance for Caregiving & American Association for Retired Persons. (1997). *Family caregiving in the U.S.: Findings from a national survey.* Washington, DC: Author.

Older Women's League. (1989). *Failing America's caregivers; A status report on women who care.* Washington, DC: Author.

Pavlko, E. K., & Artis, J. E. (1997). Women's caregiving and paid work: Causal relationships in late midlife. *Journal of Gerontology, 52B,* S170–S179.

Pearlin, L. I., & Schooler, C. (1978). The structure of coping. *Journal of Health and Social Behavior, 19,* 2–21.

Pinson-Millburn, N. M., Fabian, E. S., Schlossberg, N. K., & Pyle, M. (1996). Grandparents raising grandchildren. *Journal of Counseling and Development, 74,* 548–554.

Pruchno, R. (1999). Raising grandchildren: The experiences of Black and White grandmothers. *Gerontologist, 39,* 209–221.

Saluter, A. F. (1992). Marital status and living arrangements: March 1991 (Report No. 461). In *Current Population Reports, Population Characteristics,* Series P-20. Washington, DC: U.S. Government Printing Office.

Sands, R. G., & Goldberg-Glen, R. S. (Co-principal investigators). (1996). *The impact of surrogate parenting on grandparents: Stress, well-being, and life satisfaction.* Final Report submitted to the AARP Andrus Foundation.

Sands, R. G., & Goldberg-Glen, R. S. (1998). The impact of employment and serious illness on grandmothers who are raising their grandchildren. *Journal of Women and Aging, 10,* 41–58.

Sands, R. G., & Goldberg-Glen, R. S. (In Press). Factors associated with stress among grandparents raising their grandchildren. *Family Relations.*

Scanlon, W. J. (1988). A perspective on long term care for the elderly. *Health Care Financing Review* (Annual suppl.), 7–15.

Scharlach, A., & Kaye, L. W. (1997). Is aging more problematic for women than men? In A. E. Scharlach & L. W. Kaye (Eds.), *Controversial issues in aging* (pp. 125–135). Boston: Allyn & Bacon.

Shore, R. J., & Hayslip, B., Jr. (1994). Custodial grandparenting: Implications for children's development. In A. E. Godfried & A. W. Godfried (Eds.), *Redefining families: Implications for children's development* (pp. 171–218). New York: Plenum Press.

Solomon, J. C., & Marx, J. (1995). "To grandmother's house we go": Health and school adjustments of children raised solely by grandparents. *Gerontologist, 35,* 386–394.

Stone, R., Cafferata, G., & Sangl, J. (1987). *Caregivers of the frail elderly: A national profile.* Washington, DC: U.S. Department of Health and Human Services.

Takas, M. (1992). *Kinship care: Developing a safe and effective framework for protective placement of children with relatives.* Washington, DC: American Bar Association Center on Children and the Law.

Tennstedt, S. L., McKinlay, J. B., & Sullivan, L. M. (1989). Informal care for frail elders: The role of secondary caregivers. *Gerontologist, 29,* 677–683.

Thompson, E. H. (1994). Older men as invisible men in contemporary society. In E. H. Thompson (Ed.), *Older men's lives* (pp. 1–21). Thousand Oaks, CA: Sage.

U.S. Bureau of the Census. (1996). *Statistical abstract of the United States* (116th ed.). Washington, DC: U.S. Government Printing Office.

Veroff, J., Douvan, E., & Kulka, R. A. (1981). *The inner American: A self-portrait from 1957 to 1976.* New York: Basic Books.

Clinical Perspectives on Grandparents Who Raise Their Grandchildren

CHAPTER 11

The Physical, Mental, and Social Health of Custodial Grandparents

Jennifer Crew Solomon and Jonathan Marx

Good health facilitates independent living, quality social interaction, and financial stability. Poor health is synonymous with dependence, social isolation, and financial strain or even poverty. In this chapter we focus on the physical, mental, and social health of custodial grandparents and the relationship between surrogate parenting and health status. To critically examine the health of custodial grandparents and propose programs or policies, we must first create a shared understanding of the term *health*. We also need to assess whether custodial grandparents are at particular risk of experiencing poor health compared to their age peers.

We begin the chapter by discussing the concept of health and identifying factors related to the health of people middle-aged and older. We then review the research findings on the health of custodial grandparents. Next we compare the physical, mental, and social health of custodial grandparents with that of noncustodial grandparents who provide minimal hours of care for grandchildren. Finally, we suggest directions for future research and discuss policies and programs to address the health needs of custodial grandparents.

HEALTH: THE CONCEPT AND ITS MEASUREMENT

The World Health Organization (1958) defines health as a state of complete physical, mental, and social well-being, not merely the absence of disease or injury. The general term *health* can thus be divided into more specific components: physical, mental, and social health (Whitelaw & Liang, 1991). Physical health includes diseases (chronic and acute), functional ability (e.g., ADLs), and self-ratings of health. Mental health takes into account depression, anxiety, psychological problems, and life satisfaction. Social health reflects the quality and quantity of interaction with other people, particularly family and friends.

Moreover, these three aspects of health influence each other. For example, social health or social support affects both physical and mental health. Uchino, Cacioppo, and Kiecolt-Glaser (1996) report that a network of friends and/or family members who are available to provide emotional or personal assistance or information has a positive impact on both mortality and morbidity. That is, people with good social health live longer and have better physical health. Similarly, physical and mental health affect a person's ability to interact socially with others. People who have functional limitations may not be able to participate socially, and people with severe depression generally do not feel like socializing. High levels of depression are associated with poorer physical health and increased mortality (Roberts & Vernon, 1983). Along with the reciprocal relationships between physical, mental, and social health, other factors are also associated with health status.

FACTORS RELATED TO HEALTH

To assess the health of custodial grandparents and determine if they are particularly at risk for health problems, we need to understand the various influences on health in general and on the health of middle-aged and older people in particular. Research suggests that age, sex, race, and social class, as measured by education and financial well-being, influence health.

Age

With regard to physical health, younger people, ages 45 to 64, have much lower rates of hypertension, diabetes, arthritis, and heart disease than do people 65 and older (Adams & Marano, 1995). Older people (55+) are more likely to report chronic medical conditions. Verbrugge, Lepkowski, and Imanaka (1989) found that 60% of those 55 and older reported more than one chronic condition. Functional ability also shows a decline with increasing age. Only 6.0% of the 55–64 age group have difficulty with basic life activities such as walking, bathing, or dressing; however, 11.8% of the 65–74 age group and 26.5% of the 75–84 age group report functional limitations in activities of daily living (ADLs) (U. S. Bureau of Census, 1994).

Mental and social health also varies by age. Depression is one of the most common disorders among older adults. Some researchers suggest that geriatric depression is reactive or situational (Koenig & Blazer, 1992; Staudinger, Marsiske, & Baltes, 1995). For example, bereavement related to the death of a friend or spouse may lead to depression. These types of losses are more common in later life. Depression is also associated with medical problems such as chronic physical pain (Parmalee, Katz, & Lawton, 1991) and is a side effect of some medications used to treat diseases common to older people (LaRue, Dessonville, & Jarvik, 1985).

Social health also changes over the life course with the loss of friends and family members to death, as well as restricted social interaction due to illness. Studies comparing the social networks of younger and older adults indicate that older adults report fewer important people in their networks than do younger adults (Morgan & Kunkel, 1998). The results of longitudinal studies suggest that as people get older their contacts with friends declines (Hatch & Bulcroft, 1992). However, Antonucci and Akiyama (1987) found that older adults generally have a higher concentration of very close intimates relative to others who are less close in their networks.

Sex

Women have a health advantage over men, as reflected in longevity. Women's life expectancy exceeds men's by approximately 6 years. Women, however, tend to suffer more frequent illnesses and disability but not those that are life-threatening. For example, women experience higher rates of hypertension and arthritis than men do, but men are more vulnerable to heart disease than are women (Adams & Marano, 1995). Men also have more injuries and higher rates of life-threatening chronic diseases, such as heart disease and emphysema, than do women (Verbrugge, 1984).

There are, however, only two consistent differences between men and women in clinically diagnosed cases of mental illness. Women have higher rates of depression and anxiety disorders, and men have more personality disorders (Cockerham, 1996; Kessler et al., 1994). Furthermore, depression and anxiety below the clinical level of diagnosis are more common among women than men (Mirowsky & Ross, 1989, 1995).

Social health (e.g., relationships with friends and family) is also related to gender. Women appear to have more friendships than do men (Wright, 1989), and older women are better able than older men to make and keep friends (Hatch & Bulcroft, 1992; Matt & Dean, 1993). Keith, Hill, Goudy, and Powers (1984) found that older men tend to rely on their spouses and consider them their only close friends. In contrast, older women have close friends other than their spouses.

Race

African Americans at all ages are more likely to rate their physical health as fair or poor than are European Americans (Cohen & Van Nostrand, 1995), and the life expectancy of Blacks is lower than that of Whites. Some health conditions, such as sickle cell anemia and hypertension, may have a genetic basis. Blacks are only 12% of the U.S. populations but have 28% of the diagnosed hypertension (Hildreth & Saunders, 1992). Hypertension is related to other health problems such as kidney failure, heart disease, and strokes. Blacks are much more likely to suffer a heart attack and die than are Whites

(Becker et al., 1993) and also more likely to have activity limitations including ADLs and instrumental ADLs (Cohen & Van Nostrand, 1995)

Information about the relationship between mental health status and race is distorted by the possible influence of cultural factors (Fillenbaum, Heyman, Williams, & Burchett, 1990; Ford, Haley, Thrower, West, & Harrell, 1996) and social class (Barker, 1992). The prevalence of mental illness and related disabilities is not significantly different for Blacks and Whites; however, adults in poverty are 2.5 times more likely to have serious mental illness (Barker, 1992), and Blacks are more likely than Whites to be poor.

Factors associated with social health also show variation by race. Older Blacks tend to rely on a more diverse network, including both kin and fictive kin, for support. Fictive kin are people who are not legally related to each other but consider each other family. Blacks also have close community ties, for example, as church members (Sussman, 1985). Furthermore, Black women are more likely than White women to live in multifamily or extended-family households. Thirty-three percent of Black women, compared to only 14% of White women, live with other relatives, most commonly with adult children (U.S. Bureau of Census, 1994). According to Gold (1989, 1990), sibling relationships in later life among both Blacks and Whites tend to be positive and include emotional closeness and affection. However, older Black men have emotional ties with their brothers more than older White men do and seldom have apathetic or hostile sibling relationships.

Social Class/Income/Education

Physical health differences between African Americans and European Americans are intertwined with social class differences, as measured by education and income. According to Cockerham (1998), education is the single best predictor of health status. For example, educated people are generally well informed about preventive care and medical treatment (Ross & Wu, 1995).

Poverty and living conditions associated with poverty, such as poor nutrition, limited access to health services, including prenatal care, are negatively associated with both physical and mental health status.

Furthermore, the effects of poverty are lifelong and cumulative. Thus, the poor health of many older Blacks traces its origins to poor maternal health and inadequate prenatal care. Furthermore, people living in or near poverty level develop poor health at younger ages than do people with higher incomes (Butler & Newacheck, 1981).

Income is closely associated with self-rated physical health. For example, 52% of people in families with incomes of $50,000 or more per year rated their health as excellent, and only 28% of people in families with incomes less that $14,000 rated their health as excellent (U.S. Department of Health and Human Services, 1991). The relationship between social class and mental health shows a similar pattern (Parrillo, Stimson, & Stimson, 1999). People in lower social classes have poorer mental health than those of higher social classes. They have higher rates of schizophrenia and depression and are more unhappy, worried, and anxious.

Social class also accounts for some of the social health differences between African and European Americans. Mitchell and Register (1984) separated out the effects of race and social class and concluded that both Blacks and Whites displayed high levels of interaction among family members; however, slightly more Blacks than Whites shared a residence with a child or grandchild. In addition, Lopata (1979) found that working-class spouses maintain more rigid gender roles than do middle-class couples, and marital relationships have less impact on well-being.

Health: A Summary

Understanding the ways in which age, sex, race, and social class are related to physical, mental, and social health in the general population of middle-aged and older adults provides a basis for making predictions about the health of custodial grandparents. Older grandparents should have more health problems than younger grandparents. Grandfathers and grandmothers will have different types of physical and mental health problems, as well as different social networks. Racial and social class factors are more difficult to separate clearly; however, Black grandparents will probably have poorer physical and mental health than do White grandparents. Grandparents with less income and education will suffer more health problems than do wealthier and more educated grandparents. Older grandparents, grandfathers, and poorer grandparents will have less positive social health.

HEALTH OF CUSTODIAL GRANDPARENTS: LITERATURE REVIEW

The results of a number of studies suggest that the health of many custodial grandparents is poor (Burton, 1992; Minkler & Roe, 1993; Minkler, Roe, & Price, 1992; Smith, 1994; Solomon & Marx, 1998). For example, research on African American grandmothers and great-grandmothers raising grandchildren as a result of parental drug addiction indicates that some grandmothers experience disability and increased illness (Burton, 1992; Minkler & Roe, 1993; Minkler et al., 1992; Smith, 1994). Moreover, clinicians have found both physical (e.g., hypertension, back and stomach problems) and mental problems (e.g., depression) among grandparent caregivers (Miller, 1991). Slightly over one third of African American grandmothers in the Minkler, Roe, and Price (1992) study ($N = 72$) indicated that their health had worsened since beginning caregiving. Many attributed the change to the demands of their caregiving responsibilities. The study also found that grandmothers may downplay their health problems to protect grandchildren or because of fear that the children might end up in foster care.

In contrast, nearly half the grandmothers reported no change in health status, and one fifth stated that their health had improved. Some attributed the improvement to lifestyle changes produced by taking on the care of their grandchildren. Similarly, a study by Giarrusso, Feng, Wang, and Silverstein (1996), using the USC Longitudinal Study of Generations to compare the self-rated physical well-being of coparenting grandparents (at least one of the child's parents present), parenting grandparents (no parent present), and a grandparent control group, found that caregiving negatively affected few grandparents. The coparenting group had the worst health. Health differences between the parenting and the other groups were not statistically significant. Moreover, a 3-year follow-up revealed no significant deterioration in physical well-being. It is important to note that most grandparents (72%) in this study had household incomes above the national median income and nearly all (90%) were above poverty.

Using a more representative sample, we found health status differences between custodial and noncustodial grandparents. Data from the Health and Retirement Study (HRS), Wave 1 (1995), were used to compare demographic and physical health characteristics of custodial ($N = 123$) and noncustodial grandparents ($N = 1152$). Forty-five percent of custodial grandparents reported fair to poor physical health compared to only 24.3% of noncustodial grandparents. A higher proportion of noncustodial (57.6%) than custodial grandparents (39%) were satisfied with their financial status. Once again the relationship between income and well-being is evident.

Other factors, such as household composition, marital status, and characteristics of the grandchild, may influence the health of custodial grandparents. Solomon and Marx (1999) compared the health status of women 40 years old and older living in four different types of households: (1) single custodial grandmothers, (2) married custodial grandmothers, (3) single women living alone, and (4) married women living with a spouse. Health status was measured using self-rated health, number of health conditions, activity limitations, and restricted activities. Women living with husbands only had the best health, followed by married custodial grandmothers. Single women raising grandchildren had the poorest health compared to the other women. More of them rated themselves as being in poor health and as restricted in their daily activities in the past 2 weeks. They were also more likely to have health conditions.

The fact that married custodial grandmothers had much better health than single custodial grandmother suggests that other factors besides caring for grandchildren affects their well-being. For example, single grandmothers were not only in poorer health, they were also more likely to have incomes below the poverty line. The connection between social health and physical health is also evident here. One spouse can provide social, emotional, and physical support for the other. Single custodial grandparents not only lack the social support of a spouse, they may be restricted in their ability to develop or maintain other relationships. For example, custodial grandparents reported being limited in their other social roles, including decreased contact with family and lowered marital quality, leading to divorce (Jendrek, 1996; Minkler, Roe, & Robertson-Beckley, 1994;

Shore & Hayslip, 1994). "Sometimes a grandmother will leave a marriage to be able to take in and protect a small grandchild. Sometimes a grandfather will leave when the children arrive" (de Toledo & Brown, 1995, p. 38). Moreover, custodial grandparents stated that they had less time to get things done, less time with their spouses, less contact with friends, less privacy, and increased worrying and physical tiredness (Jendrek, 1996).

Factors related to the grandchildren, such as the number of grandchildren being cared for, their ages, and their behavior in school, may affect custodial grandparents' health. For example, taking on responsibility for two or more children is likely to mean more financial strain, more emotional stress, and more time in child care activities. Older children, especially teenagers, are often difficult and harder to please than younger children are (Cherlin & Furstenburg, 1986). In contrast, caring for children who are well behaved in school is associated with positive health outcomes for grandparents (Solomon & Marx, 1999). Good behavior in school may be an indication of good behavior in general and thus less stress for grandparents.

Related to social health, Shore and Hayslip (1994) suggest another source of stress and negative health consequences. Grandparents without legal guardianship experience uncertainty about whether the child's parents may return and remove the child from their care. The grandparents' concern is clearly justified when the parent has a drug or mental problem that would endanger the grandchild's well-being and safety.

Research has identified racial differences in health status. Several studies described the poor health status of African American custodial grandmothers (Minkler et al., 1992; Smith, 1994). Most single custodial grandmothers with poor health in the Solomon and Marx studies were Black. Although married custodial grandmothers' health was generally better than that of single custodial grandmothers, married custodial Black grandmothers had poorer health than their White counterparts. According to Mutchler and Burr (1991), stress associated with racism and discrimination may affect health status among Blacks.

It is clear from this literature review that the health of custodial grandparents is generally poor and that custodial grandparents have worse health than do noncustodial grandparents. This leads to the question of whether health vulnerability is partly a function of the number of hours spent caring for grandchildren. Solomon and Marx (1999) used the Health and Retirement Survey (HRS), Wave 1 (1995), to compare the health of coresiding and non-coresiding grandparents ($N = 1165$). Five categories, representing a grandparent-grandchild caregiving gradient (GGCG), were created by dividing the number of hours of care provided by non-coresiding grandparents over those provided by the custodial grandparents into quartiles. The CCGC was constructed by using non-coresiding grandparents who provided from 0 to over 5,000 hours of grandchild care in the past year. On the basis of previous research indicating differences between Blacks and Whites in the amount of time spent providing care for grandchildren, separate gradients were created for Blacks and Whites. The quartile categories for Blacks were as follows: 0–300 hours, 301–600 hours, 601–1,825 hours, and 1,826–5,824 hours. The quartile breaks for Whites indicate, as expected, much lower levels of hours caring: 0–150 hours, 151–392 hours, 393–995 hours, and 996–5,824 hours.

The results support racial differences in health outcomes. At every gradient level, including custodial, a larger proportion of White grandparents than of Black grandparents reported good health. For example, 70% of White custodial grandparents reported good health, but only 49% of African American grandparents did so. The impact of hours of caring also revealed notable racial differences. For Black grandparents, as the number of hours caring increased, the proportion reporting good health also increased until the fourth gradient level. At the fourth gradient the proportion reporting good health decreased and then decreased again for the category of custodial grandparents. In comparison, White grandparents' health declined as the number of hours caring increased. However, both Black and White grandparents' health showed negative associations with hours of care only at the highest levels of contact.

The number of hours of care does have an impact on well-being but also raises questions for further research. Notice that the upper quartiles for Whites (996–5,824) and Blacks (1,826–5,824) reflect very different levels of caring. Not only hours of providing care but also cultural differences concerning how much care is too much may influence the perception of stress and its consequences. Moreover, different hours of caregiving represent different types of care, such as baby-sitting for specific events, regular day care, and in the upper gradient (12–16 hours per day), possible coparenting situations. Clearly, the responsibilities and stresses differ by level of care. As Jendrek (1996) points out, day-care grandparents plan their days around caring for grandchildren. In contrast, occasional baby-sitting entails only specific disruptions to grandparents' normal schedules.

CUSTODIAL AND LOW-HOURS GRANDPARENTS

From previous research, we have some information on the well-being of custodial grandparents as indicated by physical health, mental health, and social health. In this section we systematically examine all three at the same time by comparing the physical, mental, and social health of custodial grandparents with that of noncustodial grandparents who provide minimal hours of care for grandchildren. We used grandparents providing 0–150 hours of care as a control group. This amount of care is intended to reflect the amount usually associated with being a grandparent and probably indicates occasional baby-sitting.

Physical Health

Physical health was measured by using three indices. The first index was created by using the respondents' reports of the ease with which he or she could do the following: run or jog a mile, climb several flights of stairs, or lift and carry 10 pounds. The second measure of physical health consisted of the number of reported ADLs requiring assistance: (1) bathing/showering, (2) eating, (3) dressing, and (4) getting in and out of bed. The third measure of physical well-being represents the number of reported chronic conditions: hypertension, heart problems, arthritis, or rheumatism.

Mental Health

Two indices were created to measure mental health. The first consisted of the following ratings: (1) emotional health, (2) psychological problems, (3) depression, (4) happiness, (5) enjoyment of life,

(6) sadness, (7) getting going, and (8) poor appetite. The second mental health measure addressed satisfaction with a number of aspects of the respondents' lives: house/apartment, neighborhood, health/physical condition, financial situation, friendships, marriage, job, family life, and life as a whole.

Social Health

The index for social health measured various dimensions of social support. Respondents' perceptions of social support was represented by their evaluations of loneliness as well as perceptions that people were unfriendly or didn't like the respondent. The availability of social support was indicated by whether they had relatives or good friends in the neighborhood, the number of neighbors known, and frequency of visits with neighbors. Finally, the quality of their relationships was addressed through questions evaluating their satisfaction with friendships, marriage, and family life.

Results

All items for the indices were coded so that higher numbers represented more positive outcomes. For ease of interpretation, each index was then dichotomized as good health or bad health and some or none, depending on the question. Demographics for the study can be found in Table 11.1. Nearly all respondents were female except in the Black low-hours category, which contained approximately 12% of the grandfathers. Marital status varied by race—most Whites were married and most Blacks were not. For both races, larger proportions of low-hours noncustodial grandparents than of custodial grandparents were married. Average age and education level differed only slightly among groups. Finally, fewer custodial grandparents (both Blacks and Whites) than low-hours grandparents were satisfied with their financial situation.

In Table 11.2, which illustrates the comparisons of the four categories of grandparents on physical, mental, and social health, the most obvious conclusion is that on every health measure but one a smaller proportion of Blacks than of Whites reported good health. The

TABLE 11.1   Demographics of Grandparents by Race and Caregiving

Race	Gender % Female	Marital % Married	Age (in years)	Education (in years)	Financial % Satisfied
	Background Factors				
White					
Custodial ($N = 43$)	97.7	60.5	55.1	11.5	39.5
Low hours ($N = 202$) (0–150 hr)	96.5	66.3	55.0	12.4	65.8
Black					
Custodial ($N = 58$)	98.3	20.7	55.8	11.0	37.9
Low hours ($N = 42$) (0–150 hr)	88.1	35.7	55.4	11.3	38.1

only exception is that Black grandparents in the low-hours-of-caring category were more likely than grandparents in the other three categories to report good physical health as measured by the ease of strenuous activity.

Focusing just on Whites, custodial grandparents were found to be less healthy on every index of physical, mental, and social health, compared to low-hours grandparents. A smaller proportion found it easy to run or jog a mile, climb several flights of stairs, and lift and carry 10 pounds. Only 25.6% percent reported no problems with chronic conditions such as hypertension, heart disease, or arthritis/ rheumatism. Nevertheless, most (60.5%) rated their physical health as good to excellent, and most (93%) reported no problems with basic activities of living (ADLs).

On measures of mental and social health, the custodial White grandparents also did less well than low-hours White grandparents. A smaller percentage (53.5% vs. 64.4%) indicated good emotional health on measures of self-rated emotional health; lack of psychological problems, including depression and depressive symptomatology such as sadness; inability to get going; and poor appetite and also expressed happiness and enjoyment of life. Fewer custodials (55.8%) than low-hours grandparents (79.7%) scored high on life satisfaction. Although most (65.1%) White custodial grandparents had good social health as indicated, by ties to other people as well as satisfaction

TABLE 11.2 Physical, Mental, and Social Health Status of Grandparents by Caregiving and Race

	Health Measures						
	Physical				Mental		Social
Race	% Good Activity Level	% No ADLs	% No Chronic Condition	% Good Current Health	% Good Emotional Health	% High Life Satisfaction	% Good Social Health
White							
Custodial (N = 43)	41.9	93.0	25.6	60.5	53.5	55.8	65.1
Low hours (N = 202) (0–150 hr)	64.9	98.0	43.6	87.1	64.4	79.7	79.2
Black							
Custodial (N = 58)	39.7	84.5	15.5	50.0	46.6	44.8	62.7
Low hours (N = 42) (0–150 hr)	66.7	90.5	16.7	57.1	52.4	71.4	54.8

with relationships, it was a smaller proportion (79.2%) than in the low-hours group.

The poorer health of custodial White grandparents was evident from the small percentage that found it easy to engage in strenuous activity and the large percentage (75%) that had at least one chronic condition. The most common chronic condition was arthritis/rheumatism (51.2%). Forty-six percent had had hypertension, and 33% currently had problems with high blood pressure. Nearly a quarter (23.3%) had had heart problems. Most, however, did not have any problems with ADLs, and more than half (60.5%) rated their current health status as good to excellent.

Positive mental and social health was relatively prevalent among White custodial grandparents. More than half of White custodial grandparents had good emotional health and life satisfaction. However, larger proportions of custodial than of low-hours White grandparents were depressed, unhappy, and sad. Custodial grandparents also enjoyed life less, had poor appetites, and were less satisfied with their houses, neighborhoods, physical health, jobs, and life as a whole. Although most (65.1%) custodial White grandparents scored high on positive social relationships, 44% of custodials were sometimes lonely, compared to 30% of low-hours grandparents. Fewer custodials reported good friends and family in the neighborhood. Moreover, they were less satisfied with their friendships.

Comparing categories of Black grandparents, custodial Black grandparents were less healthy than low-hours Black grandparents on all measures of physical health and also on mental health (i.e., emotional health, life satisfaction). The specific ADLs that gave custodial grandparents problems were getting dressed and getting in and out of bed. Interesting, though not surprising, low-hours Black grandparents were similar to Black custodial grandparents in chronic conditions. Only a minority in both groups reported no chronic conditions—16.7% and 15.5%, respectively. Over 60% of both low-hours and custodial Black grandparents had had hypertension, and half in both categories currently suffered from high blood pressure. Fifteen percent of low-hours and 27.6% of custodials had had heart problems. Finally, 43.4% and 55.2% of low-hours and custodial grandparents, respectively, suffered from arthritis or rheumatism.

The mental health of Black custodial grandparents also showed deficits, compared to low-hours grandparents. A larger percentage of Black custodial grandparents than of low-hours grandparents reported depression, unhappiness, and sadness (mental health). Fewer expressed satisfaction with various aspects of their lives (e.g., house/ apartment, neighborhood, job) and life as a whole. In addition, more were lonely even though they had friends and family in the neighborhood.

Other interracial comparisons also are interesting. For example, White custodial grandparents were similar to Black custodials on ease of physical exertion and social support but better in terms of ADLs, chronic conditions, current health status, emotional health, and life satisfaction. In contrast to the overall poorer mental health of custodial grandparents compared to low-hours grandparents, a larger proportion of both Black (81% vs. 64.3%) and White (62.8% vs. 51.5%) custodial grandparents rated their emotional health as good to excellent. Notice that Black custodial grandparents who, based on most health measures, could be viewed as the least healthy, nevertheless evaluated themselves as doing well emotionally.

Discussion

We can now interpret these findings, taking into account the factors discussed earlier as being associated with physical, mental, and social health—age, sex, marital status, social class (i.e., education and financial well-being). First, this sample is primarily age- and sex-homogeneous. The mean age for all categories was 55 years, and most grandparents were actually grandmothers. In spite of the relatively young age of the custodial grandparents, many had health problems. The aging process will probably only exacerbate these conditions.

Social class as measured by the average level of education also appeared to be similar across grandparent categories, with a high of 12.4 years of education (low-hours White grandparents) and a low of 11.0 years (Black custodial grandparents). However, an examination of the percentage that graduated from high school revealed that the best-educated grandparents were also the healthiest. Most (82.5%) White low-hours grandparents had at least a high school degree, and 67.4% of White custodial grandparents had at least a high school degree. Another, perhaps more revealing way to look at the influence of education on health is to report the proportion that did not finish high school. Among Blacks, 42.9% of low-hours grandparents and 46.6% of custodial grandparents did not graduate from high school. Nearly a third (32.6%) of White custodial grandparents also did not graduate. These percentages are in stark contrast to the low-hours White grandparents. Only 17.3% low-hours White grandparents did not finish high school.

Social class, as measured by financial well-being, reflected the now familiar pattern. The generally healthy low-hours White grandparents were more likely to be satisfied (65.8%) with their financial situation. Other categories of grandparents had similar proportions reporting financial well-being: 39.5% of White custodial, 37.9% of Black custodial, and 38.1% of Black low-hours grandparents.

The physical, mental, and social health of custodial grandparents is clearly poorer than that of their age peers. They have more chronic conditions and lower self-rated physical health, and they find strenuous activity more difficult. Although similar proportions of Black low-hours and custodial grandparents experienced chronic health problems, the implications of these conditions are quite different. Custodial grandparents suffering from hypertension, heart problems, and arthritis are responsible on a daily basis for grandchild care. Low-hours grandparents only infrequently assume such responsibility. By most measures, the emotional health and life satisfaction of custodial grandparents is lower than that of low-hours grandparents. They are more depressed and sad. They are unhappy with their living conditions, job, and life in general. Finally, the social health of custodials, as measured by both quantity and quality of relationships, is also worse than that of grandparents who do not have full-time responsibility for grandchild care. This means they have fewer people to rely on for assistance with child care, fewer people to turn to in emergencies, fewer people to confide in, and fewer sources of other types of social support.

LIMITATIONS OF THE RESEARCH

Before suggesting policies and services to help improve the health of custodial grandparents, we need to acknowledge the limitations of current research. The following questions highlight issues of specific concern: How adequate are the measures (e.g., health status, stress)? How do we determine the causes of health problems and separate out various influences? Are the samples appropriate for the questions?

How adequate are the measures of health and health-related factors? A number of studies have identified possible racial biases in measures of self-reported health (Anderson, Mullner, & Cornelius, 1987; Gibson, 1991). Some studies report that self-ratings of health overestimate poor health among Blacks (Ferraro, 1987; Maddox, 1962) and others find that it underestimates poor health (Cockerham, Sharp, & Wilcox, 1983; Linn, Hunter, & Linn, 1980). Researchers must therefore be sensitive to cultural differences.

How do we determine the causes of poor health and separate out various influences? Longitudinal research is necessary to address the issue of causation. For example, Minkler, Roe, and Price (1992) suggest that health status may be a criterion for choosing to become a surrogate parent or being chosen to care for grandchildren. Unfortunately, longitudinal research is costly in both time and money. In addition, certain stresses leading to poor health may begin long before grandparents assume total care of grandchildren, especially children of drug-addicted parents or children from abusive homes.

Moreover, separating out the effects of education, financial well-being, and race are difficult. Level of education influences financial well-being, and financial well-being has an impact on education from one generation to another. Race, racism, and discrimination are still currently intertwined with educational and financial opportunities. Moreover, poor health limits educational attainment and financial well-being. What is the direction of causation? A related issue is the grandparents' health history. Is the current poor health a recent event in an otherwise healthy life, or does it represent the continuation of lifelong struggles with disease and disability?

Finally, are the samples appropriate? Although we used the word *grandparents* in this chapter, it would have been more appropriate to use *grandmothers*. We know very little about custodial grandfathers. Real life is seldom as simple as scientific research pictures it. Who helps grandmothers? Do grandfathers help, or do they also require assistance from grandmothers? How helpful are other family members? These are all issues for future research to address.

PROGRAM AND POLICY IMPLICATIONS

Separating health status into physical, mental, and social health and recognizing their interrelationships helps us better understand what programs and services are needed to support and promote good health for custodial grandparents. The physical health of custodial grandparents could be improved by multilevel, community-wide programs that provide health services such as immunizations against influenza and pneumonia and regular checkups for both grandparents and grandchildren. Educational programs could encourage self-care for grandparents with chronic illnesses (Joslin & Brouard, 1995). Respite and child day-care services could serve a number of health-enhancing functions. Readily available child care would facilitate more opportunities for grandparents to meet their own health care needs.

In terms of mental health, educational programs should teach strategies for handling stress (Joslin & Brouard, 1995) and present ways of understanding the "emotional roller coaster" (de Toledo & Brown, 1995) and coping with emotions such as anger, guilt, fear, and doubt. Social health would be fostered in support groups that create a "safe second family" (de Toledo & Brown, 1995) where custodial grandparents can discuss their feelings with people who have had similar experiences and emotions. Marriage and family counseling services also would enhance social health.

Finally, the development of programs and services for custodial grandparents must take into account the fact that, for many of these grandparents, becoming surrogate parents to their grandchildren is just one more physical, mental, and social challenge. Their problems are not related only to raising their grandchildren. Low educational attainment, poor financial well-being, and for many, the effects of racism and discrimination from the past restrict their ability to meet this latest challenge successfully. In other words, the problems are long-term and broad; the solutions must likewise be long-term and broad.

REFERENCES

Adams, P. F., & Marano, M. A. (1995). *Vital health statistics* (vol. 10, pp. 83–84). Washington, DC: National Center for Health Statistics.

Anderson, R. M., Mullner, R. M., & Cornelius, L. J. (1987). Black-White differences in health status: Methods or substance? *Milbank Quarterly, 65,* 72–99.

Antonucci, T. C., & Akiyama, H. (1987). Social networks in adult life and a preliminary examination of the convoy model. *Journals of Gerontology, 42,* 519–527.

Barker, P. R. (1992). Serious mental illness and disability in the adult household population: United States, 1989. *Advance data,* no. 218. Washington, DC: Centers for Disease Control.

Becker, L. B., Han, B. H., Meyer, P. M., Wright, F. A., Rhodes, K. V., Smth, D. W., Barrett, J., & the Chicago Project. (1993). Racial differences in the incidence of cardiac arrest and subsequent survival. *New England Journal of Medicine, 329,* 600–606.

Burton, L. M. (1992). Black grandparents rearing grandchildren of drug-addicted parents: Stressors, outcomes, and social service needs. *Gerontologist, 32,* 744–751.

Butler, L. H., & Newacheck, P. W. (1981). Health and social factors relevant to long-term care policy. In J. Meltzer, F. Farrow, & H. Richman (Eds.), *Policy Options in Long-term Care* (pp. 38–76). Chicago: University of Chicago Press.

Cherlin, A. J., & Furstenberg, F. F. (1986). *The New American Grandparent.* New York: Basic Books.

Cockerham, W. C. (1996). *Sociology of mental disorder* (4th ed.). Englewood Cliffs, NJ: Prentice-Hall.

Cockerham, W. C. (1998). *Medical sociology* (7th ed.). Englewood Cliffs, NJ: Prentice-Hall.

Cockerham, W. C., Sharp, K., & Wilcox, J. A. (1983). Aging and perceived health status. *Journal of Gerontology, 38,* 349–355.

Cohen, R. A., & Van Nostrand, J. F. (1995). Trends in the health of older Americans: United States, 1994. In *Vital health statistics.* Washington, DC: National Center for Health Statistics.

De Toledo, S., & Brown, D. E. (1995). *Grandparents as parents: A survival guide for raising a second family.* New York: Guilford Press.

Ferraro, K. F. (1987). Double jeopardy to health for Black older adults? *Journal of Gerontology, 42,* 528–533.

Fillenbaum, G., Heyman, A., Wiliams, K., & Burchett, B. (1990). Sensitivity and specificity of standardized screens of cognitive impairment and dementia among elderly Black and White community residents. *Journal of Clinical Epidemiology, 43,* 651–660.

Ford, G. R., Haley, W. E., Thrower, S. L., West, C. A., & Harrell, L. E. (1996). Utility of Mini-Mental State Exam scores in predicting functional impairment among White and African American dementia patients. *Journal of Gerontology: Medical Sciences, 51A,* M185–M188.

Giarrusso, R., Feng, D., Wang, Q., & Silverstein, M. (1996). Parenting and co-parenting of grandchildren: Effect on grandparents' well-being and family solidarity. *International Journal of Sociology and Social Policy, 16*(12), 124–156.

Gibson, R. C. (1991). Race and the self-reported health of elderly persons. *Journal of Gerontology, 46*(5), S235–242.

Gold, D. T. (1989). Sibling relationships in old age: A typology. *International Journal of Aging and Human Development, 28,* 37–54.

Gold, D. T. (1990). Late-life sibling relationships: Does race affect typological distribution? *Gerontologist, 30*(6), 741–748.

Hatch, L. R., & Bulcroft, K. (1992). Contact with friends in later life: Disentangling the effects of gender and marital status. *Journal of Marriage and the Family, 54,* 222–232.

Hildreth, C. J., & Saunders, E. (1992). Heart disease, stroke, and hypertension in Blacks. In R. Braithwaite & S. Taylor (Eds.), *Health issues in the Black community* (pp. 90–105). San Francisco: Jossey-Bass.

Jendrek, M. P. (1996). Grandparents who parent their grandchildren: Effects on lifestyle. In J. Quadagno & D. Street (Eds.), *Aging for the twenty-first century: Readings in social gerontology* (pp. 286–305). New York: St. Martin's Press.

Joslin, D., & Brouard, A. (1995). The prevalence of grandmothers as primary caregivers in a poor pediatric population. *Journal of Community Health, 20*(5), 383–402.

Keith, P. M., Hill, K., Goudy, W. J., & Powers, E. A. (1984). Confidants and well-being: A note on male friendship in old age. *Gerontologist, 24,* 318–320.

Kessler, R. C., McGonagle, K. A., Zhao, S., Nelson, C. B., Hughes, M., Eshleman, S., Wittchen, H., & Kendler, K. S. (1994). Lifetime and 12-month prevalence of DSM-III-R psychiatric disorders in the United States. *Archives of General Psychiatry, 51,* 8–19.

Koenig, H. G., & Blazer, D. G. (1992). Mood disorders and suicide. In J. E. Birren, R. B. Sloane, & G. D. Cohen (Eds.), *Handbook of mental health and aging* (2nd ed., pp. 379–407). San Diego, CA: Academic Press.

LaRue, A., Dessonville, D., & Jarvik, L. (1985). Aging and mental disorders. In J. E. Birren & K. W. Schaie (Eds.), *Handbook of the psychology of aging* (2nd ed., pp. 664–702). New York: Van Nostrand Reinhold.

Lopata, H. Z. (1979). *Women and widows: Support systems.* New York: Elsevier.

Linn, M. W., Hunter, K. I., & Linn, B. S. (1980). Self assessed health, impairment and disability in Anglo, Black, and Cuban elderly. *Medical Care, 43,* 282–288.

Maddox, G. L. (1962). Some correlates of differences in self-assessment of health status among the elderly. *Journal of Gerontology, 17,* 180–185.

Matt, G. E., & Dean, A. (1993). Social support from friends and psychological distress among elderly persons: Moderator effects of age. *Journal of Health and Social Behavior, 34,* 187–200.

Miller, D. (1991, November). *The "Grandparents Who Care" support project of San Francisco.* Paper presented at the annual meeting of Gerontological Society of America, San Francisco.

Minkler, M., & Roe, K. M. (1993). *Grandmothers as caregivers: Raising children of the crack cocaine epidemic.* Newberry Park, CA: Sage Publications.

Minkler, M., Roe, K. M., & Price, M. (1992). The physical and emotional health of grandmothers raising grandchildren in the crack cocaine epidemic. *Gerontologist, 32,* 752–761.

Minkler, M., Roe, K. M., & Roberton-Beckley, R. (1994). Raising grandchildren from crack-cocaine households: Effects on family and friendship ties of African-American women. *American Journal of Orthopsychiatry, 64,* 20–29.

Mirowsky, J., & Ross, C. E. (1989). *Social causes of psychological distress.* New York: Aldine de Gruyter.

Mirowsky, J., & Ross, C. E. (1995). Sex differences in distress: Real of artifact? *American Sociological Review, 60,* 449–468.

Mitchell, J., & Register, J. C. (1984). An exploration of family interaction with the elderly by race, socioeconomic status, and residence. *Gerontologist, 24,* 48–54.

Morgan, L., & Kunkel, S. (1998). *Aging: The social context.* Thousand Oaks, CA: Pine Forge Press.

Mutchler, J. E., & Burr, J. A. (1991). Racial differences in health and health care service utilization in later life: The effect of socioeconomic status. *Journal of Health and Social Behavior, 32,* 342–356.

Parmalee, P. A., Katz, I. R., & Lawton, M. P. (1991). The relation of pain to depression among institutionalized aged. *Journal of Gerontology, 46,* P15–P21.

Parrillo, V. N., Stimson, J., & Stimson, A. (1999). *Contemporary social problems* (4th ed.). Boston: Allyn and Bacon.

Roberts, R. E., & Vernon, S. W. (1983). The Center for Epidemiological Studies Depression Scale: Its use in a community sample. *American Journal of Psychiatry, 140,* 41–46.

Ross, C. E., & Wu, C. (1995). The links between education and health. *American Sociological Review, 60,* 719–745.

Shore, J. R., & Hayslip, B. Jr. (1994). Custodial grandparenting: Implications for children's development. In A. E. Gottfried & A. W. Gottfried (Eds.),

Redefining families: Implications for children's development. New York: Plenum Press.

Smith, A. (1994). African-American grandmothers' war against the crack cocaine epidemic. *Arete, 19*(1), 22–36.

Solomon, J. C., & Marx, J. (1998). The grandparent grandchild caregiving gradient: Hours of caring for grandchildren and its relationship to grandparent health. *Southwest Journal of Aging, 14*(2), 31–39.

Solomon, J. C., & Marx, J. (1999). Who cares?: Grandparent/grandchild households. *Journal of Women and Aging, 11*(1), 3–25.

Staudinger, U. M, Marsiske, M., & Baltes, P. B. (1995). Resilience and reserve capacity in later adulthood: Potentials and limits of development across the life span. In D. Cicchetti & D. J. Cohen (Eds.), *Development psychopathology* (vol. 2, pp. 801–847). New York: Wiley.

Sussman, M. B. (1985). The family life of old people. In R. H. Binstock & E. Shanas (Eds.), *Handbook of aging and the social sciences* (2nd ed., pp. 415–449). New York: Van Nostrand Reinhold.

Uchino, B. N., Cacioppo, J. T., & Kiecolt-Glaser, J. K. (1996). The relationship between social support and physiological processes: A review with emphasis on underlying mechanisms and implications for health. *Psychological Bulletin, 119*, 488–531.

U.S. Bureau of Census. (1990). The need for personal assistance with everyday activities: Recipients and caregivers. *Current population reports,* Series P-70, no. 19. Washington, DC: U.S. Government Printing Office.

U.S. Bureau of Census. (1994). Marital status and living arrangements: March, 1993. *Current population reports.* Series P20-478. Washington, DC: U.S. Government Printing Office.

U.S. Department of Health and Human Services. (1991). *Current estimates from the National Health Interview Survey, 1990.* Washington, DC: U.S. Government Printing Office.

Verbrugge, L. M. (1984). Longer life but worsening health? Trends in health and mortality of middle-aged and older persons. *Milbank Memorial Fund Quarterly, 62*, 475–519.

Vergrugge, L. M., Lepkowski, J. M., & Imanaka, Y. (1989). Comorbidity and its impact on disability. *Milbank Quarterly, 67*, 450–484.

Whitelaw, N. A., & Liang, J. (1991). The structure of the OARS physical health measures. *Medical Care, 29*, 332–347.

World Health Organization. (1958). *The first ten years of the World Health Organization.* Geneva: Author.

Wright, P. (1989). Gender differences in adults' same- and cross-gender friendships. In R. S. Adams & R. Blieszner (Eds.), *Older adult friendship* (pp. 197–221). Newbury Park, CA: Sage.

CHAPTER 12

Grandparent Caregiving and Depression

Meredith Minkler, Esme Fuller-Thomson, Doriane Miller, and Diane Driver

Although grandparent caregiving is a widespread and growing phenomenon, there was, until recently, no nationally representative study examining the potential link between such caregiving and depression. Several cross-sectional studies based on small nonrepresentative samples (Burton, 1992; Jendrek, 1993; Minkler & Roe, 1993; Roe, Minkler, Thompson, & Saunders, 1996; Shore & Hayslip, 1994), as well as recent research utilizing the longitudinal Alameda County Study (Strawbridge, Wallhagen, Shema, & Kaplan, 1997), have suggested the possibility of elevated rates of depression and/or increased risk for depressive symptomatology among grandparents raising grandchildren. Although these reports give cause for concern, national data are needed that can shed further light on the mental health of grandparents fulfilling this role. The study described in this chapter was designed to meet this need by examining depression and grandparent caregiving, using a longitudinal, large national data set, the National Survey of Families and Households (NSFH).

SAMPLE AND METHODS FOR THE STUDY

The NSFH was conducted by the Center for Demography and Ecology at the University of Wisconsin–Madison. Of the 13,008 respondents originally interviewed during the first wave of data collection in 1987 and 1988, 10,008 respondents (77%) were reinterviewed during 1992, 1993, and 1994. (For a more detailed summary of study design and questions, see Sweet, Bumpass, & Call, 1988. For more detail on the methodology and results of the analyses discussed here, see Minkler, Fuller-Thomson, Miller, & Driver, 1997).

Of the more than 10,000 respondents in the original survey, during the second wave of data collection, 3,477 reported having one or more grandchildren. The primary focus of our analysis was on those grandparents who began or ended caregiving in the 1990s ($n = 144$) and the smaller group of those who had begun caregiving for their grandchildren within the past 5 years ($n = 79$). Grandparent caregiving status was defined by those who responded affirmatively to the question "For various reasons, grandparents sometimes take on the primary responsibility for raising a grandchild. Have you ever had the primary responsibility for any of your grandchildren for six months or more?" Grandparents who began caregiving during the past 5 years were defined as those who responded yes to the above question and who began caregiving after they were interviewed in the first wave of NSFH data collection.

Depression was measured by means of a modified 12-item version of the Center for Epidemiological Studies Depression Scale (CES-D). The CES-D is a widely utilized, easily administered self-report measure of current depressive symptomatology developed for use in large-scale community-based studies such as this one (Devins & Orme, 1985; Radloff, 1977). The traditional cut-point suggesting clinically relevant levels of depressive symptomatology in the full CES-D is a score of 16 or higher. Although the 12-item CES-D used in this study has a much smaller range than the full 20-item CES-D, we conservatively chose to retain the same cut-point of 16 to minimize the possibility of including false positives in our depression category.

ELEVATED RISK OF DEPRESSION IN GRANDPARENT CAREGIVERS

Bivariate chi-square analysis comparing recent grandparent caregivers with noncaregivers revealed that those who provide primary care for a grandchild are almost twice as likely to present levels of depressive symptomatology above the cut-point (25.1% vs. 14.5%, $p <$ .01). This finding is consistent with reports by clinicians (Davis, 1993; Miller, 1991; Raskin, 1990) and with findings of the Alameda County Study (Strawbridge et al., 1997) and of earlier, small nonrandom studies (Burton, 1992; Jendrek, 1993; Minkler & Roe, 1993; Roe et al., 1996; Shore & Hayslip, 1994), suggesting that elevated rates of depression may well exist among grandparent caregivers.

Although our cross-sectional data indicated that caregiving grandparents were more susceptible to depressive symptomatology, it was impossible, without a multivariate analysis, to determine whether this relationship was primarily due to caregiving status or to other differences between the two groups. For example, our research revealed that caregiving grandparents were more likely than noncaregivers to be female and to be younger ($p < .001$) than other grandparents and to have had higher rates of baseline (precaregiving) depression ($p < .05$). Each of these factors is associated with depression in previous studies of large community samples (George, 1995; Mirowsky & Ross, 1989). Of particular concern for our study was the finding by Strawbridge and his colleagues (1997) that individuals who raised their grandchildren had a difficult life course predating the onset of providing care for their grandchild. Because this factor, rather than the undertaking of caregiving responsibilities per se, may explain discrepancies in depression scores, it was important in the present study to conduct a multiple regression analysis of depression, using the modified CES-D score as the outcome variable.

In the multivariate analysis, the originally observed relationship held: Caregivers scored, on average, 2 points higher on the CES-D than did noncaregivers even when precaregiving depression and demographic characteristics were controlled. This finding is important in suggesting that grandparent caregiving itself is directly associated with higher levels of depression. It further supports earlier indications from small-scale qualitative and quantitative studies (Burton, 1992; Jendrek, 1993; Minkler & Roe, 1993; Roe et al., 1996; Shore & Hayslip, 1994; Strawbridge et al., 1997) and physician reports (Miller, 1991; Raskin, 1990) that grandparent caregiving may be an important contributor to depression and/or increased depressive symptomatology in midlife and older grandparents fulfilling this role.

As expected, we also found in the multivariate analysis that baseline levels of depressive symptomatology from the first wave of data collection were significantly associated with higher CES-D scores during the second wave ($p < .001$), as was being female ($p < .001$). Higher family income, older age, being married, and being in good or excellent health were significantly associated with lower levels of depression ($p < .01$). Contrary to expectation, however, neither high school completion nor our social support measure (socializing weekly with friends) was associated with depressive symptoms.

REASONS FOR THE ELEVATED DEPRESSION RATES: INSIGHTS AND UNANSWERED QUESTIONS

The finding of significantly elevated depression levels among grandparent caregivers in our study is interesting to consider within the broader context of research on the etiology of depression. Although numerous studies have confirmed the importance of recent severe events for most episodes of clinical depression in both patient and community populations, such events in and of themselves appear only rarely to trigger depressive episodes. (Brown, 1996; Brown & Harris, 1978; Brown, Harris, & Hepworth, 1995). The role of psychosocial factors suggesting vulnerability (e.g., low self-esteem, social isolation, and lack of sense of control) thus also must be taken into account. Finally, as noted below, the conceptual rating system of Brown et al. (1995), characterizing severe events in part in terms of the experience of humiliation and entrapment, together with measures of loss or danger and with the concept of "atypical events," may be particularly useful in the study of grandparent caregivers.

Although the NSFH data set did not enable an examination of the possible reasons for the elevated risk of depression among grandparent caregivers, earlier research (Burton, 1992; Jendrek, 1993; Minkler & Roe, 1993; Shore & Hayslip, 1994) has suggested that profound sadness over the circumstances surrounding the onset of care (e.g., an adult child's incarceration or incapacitation due to drug addiction or AIDS) may be more important than the caregiving itself as a contributor to the depression experienced. Such circumstances may indeed result in humiliation for parents, who may feel that they are perceived as having "failed" at child rearing and who also may feel considerable shame over the situation of their offspring (Minkler & Roe, 1993; Shore & Hayslip, 1994). Qualitative studies further have suggested that perceptions of entrapment may be common among grandparent caregivers, who describe their own lives as having been "stolen" from them as they embark on new and typically unwanted roles as "second time around parents" (Burton, 1992; Jendrek, 1993; Minkler & Roe, 1993). Finally, and especially among the youngest and oldest grandparents and those whose own child (the grandchild's parent) has died, perceptions of the assumption of caregiving as an atypical event and one that represents a "time-disordered role" (Selzer, 1976) in the life cycle may further increase the likelihood of depressive symptomatology (Burton, 1992; Burton & Bengtson, 1985; Jendrek, 1993; Minkler & Roe, 1993).

Hayslip and his colleagues (Hayslip, Shore, Henderson, & Lambert, 1998) have underlined the difficulties many children have in adjusting to the "often tragic circumstances under which custodial grandparenting comes about." In their study, grandparents raising grandchildren with physical, emotional or behavioral problems had higher levels of personal distress than their peers raising grandchildren without significant problems. Increased social isolation, the loss of a job or of economic security as a result of caregiving, the loss of a 'real' grandparental role as one becomes instead a surrogate parent, and the stresses associated with caring for children with special needs, infants, preschoolers and teens also have been observed among such caregivers and may be contributors to depression (Burton, 1992; Jendrek, 1994; Roe et al., 1996; Shore & Hayslip, 1994). As Brown and colleagues' (1995) schema suggests, combinations of such feelings and meanings attached to the new and generally "atypical" role of grandparent caregiver may increase the likelihood of depressive episodes.

SPECIAL VULNERABILITY FACTORS FOR DEPRESSION

Although we were able to demonstrate a higher risk for depression among grandparent caregivers, it is important from a clinical standpoint to identify characteristics of those caregivers most at risk. The final analysis we conducted (see Table 12.1) explored which factors among caregivers were associated with depression. For this analysis, we included only those grandparents who reported having begun or ended caregiving for a grandchild during the 1990s ($n = 144$). These included the 79 respondents who began caregiving during the preceding 5 years (used in the previous analysis) and an additional 65 respondents who began providing care 5 or more years earlier.

The multiple regression analysis indicated that those in good or excellent health reported significantly fewer depressive symptoms ($p < .001$). Those caregivers who had started caring for a grandchild relatively recently, as measured by the approximately 5 years since the first wave of data collection, scored significantly higher on the CES-D ($p < .05$). Two statistical trends ($p < .10$) were visible: age was negatively associated with depressive symptomatology, and women were more likely to have higher scores on the CES-D. Several factors that we had anticipated would be related to depression were not found to be so in this analysis. These nonsignificant variables included the following: being married, socializing at least weekly, being a high school graduate, having had a child die since the first wave of data collection, and having coresident children.

The finding of lower depression levels among grandparent caregivers with better self-reported health status is in keeping with numerous studies suggesting a strong link between depressive symptomatology and poorer self-assessed and objective health measures (Beckman & Leber, 1995; George, 1995; Kaplan, Roberts, Camacho, & Coyne, 1987). Similarly, the observed statistical trend of higher depression levels among female caregivers provides further support to the large body of evidence showing higher rates of depressive symptomatology among women than men (Beckman & Leber, 1995; George, 1995; Kaplan et al., 1987; Keith, 1993). The trend indicating lower depression levels among older grandparent caregivers is consistent with the fact that younger adults are more likely than their older counterparts to meet the criteria for a diagnosis of depressive disorder (Beckman & Leber, 1995; George, 1995). Further, a greater tendency

TABLE 12.1 Multivariate Analysis of Factors Predictive of Depressive Symptomatology (CES-D) Among Caregiving Grandparents of the 1990s ($n = 144$)

Variable	Unstandardized Regression Coefficients (b)	Standardized Regression Coefficients (Beta)	Statistical Significance of Hotelling's T
Assumption of caregiving	3.09	0.166	.047
Grandparents who started caregiving during the past 5 years (1)			
Grandparents who started caregiving 5 or more years ago (0)			
Race	−2.31	−0.108	.187
Black (1)			
Other (0)			
Age (in years)	−0.15	−0.18	.056
Education	−2.13	−0.11	.168
High school graduate (1)			
Less than high school completion (0)			
Marital status	−2.47	−.13	.140
Married (1)			
Widowed, divorced, separated, never married (0)			
Health status	−7.05	−.364	.000
Good to excellent health (1)			
Very poor to fair health (0)			
Gender	3.26	0.15	.062
Female (1)			
Male (0)			
Social integration	−1.27	−.06	.410
Socialize at least weekly (52 times/yr. or more) (1)			
Socialize less than weekly (0)			
Coresident dependent children	−0.39	−.02	.858
Respondent's children under the age of 19 still in home (1)			
No coresident offspring (0)			
Parental bereavement	1.11	.031	.680
Child died in previous 5 years ($n = 1$)			
No child died in previous 5 years ($n = 0$)			
Constant	23.53		.0001

Adjusted $R^2 = .259$
$F(10, 133) = 5.99$ ($p < .001$)

toward conflicting role demands and role strain may be experienced among younger grandmothers, many of whom are still working and/or have minor children still at home (Minkler & Roe, 1993).

The finding of significantly more depressive symptomatology among grandparents who had assumed primary caregiver responsibility during the past 5 years supports our hypothesis that the mental health consequences of this role may be more pronounced during the early stages of caregiving. Several factors support this interpretation, key among them the recency of the stressful circumstance (e.g., death, incarceration, or drug addition of offspring), which typically resulted in the grandparent's stepping in to raise his or her grandchildren.

Earlier qualitative research among grandparent caregivers has suggested a coming to terms over time with the situation of the adult child and with one's role as caregiver, with consequent improvements in self-assessed mental health (Minkler & Roe, 1993; Shore & Hayslip, 1994). Further, because grandparents often assume care when a child is very young (Chalfie, 1994; Fuller-Thomson, Minkler, & Driver, 1997; Joslin & Brouard, 1995; Minkler & Roe, 1993), it may be that the burden of care provision becomes somewhat easier as the child ages. This hypothesis is supported by recent research on the transition to parenthood in the traditional nuclear family. Cowan and her colleagues (Cowan, Cowan, Heming, & Miller, 1991) found that adaptation to the demands of a new baby can, even in the best of circumstances, cause difficulties in the realms of parenting stress, marital distress, role dissatisfaction and subsequent depression. Some of the new grandparent caregivers in our study may well have been experiencing similar difficulties in adjusting to the heavy physical and emotional demands of the infants and young children in their care.

NEEDS FOR FURTHER RESEARCH

The findings of our study suggest the need for much further research into the mental health of grandparent caregivers, with special attention to the factors that may increase their vulnerability to depression. More research is needed, for example, to test the above-mentioned hypothesis of a coming to terms with the grandparent caregiving role over time and to look in more detail at changes over time in depressive symptomatology and other mental health status indicators among grandparents who are primary caregivers. Attention also should be directed to teasing apart grief and depression; the former tends to be more episodic and less severe in its consequences. Research is needed, as well, on the special strains that may be associated with raising older grandchildren, particularly teenagers. Finally, further research is needed that more adequately assesses the role of marital status and living arrangements in relation to the mental health of grandparents who have assumed the role of surrogate parents.

IMPLICATIONS FOR CLINICIANS AND OTHER SERVICE PROVIDERS

Although much room exists for further investigation, the results of this initial study have important implications for clinicians and social service providers. First, the fact that undertaking care of a grandchild is associated with a significant increase in levels of depression suggests the need for exploring changing familial roles. Grandparents who suffer depression and other conditions related to their caregiving responsibilities may indeed be "hidden patients" in need of special attention (Joslin & Harrison, 1998; Minkler & Roe, 1993). Because depression among family caregivers has been shown to compromise immune functioning (Kiecolt-Glaser, Dura, Speicher, Trask, & Glaser, 1991; Schulz, Vistainer, & Williamson, 1990) and to manifest in insomnia and other complaints that in turn may interfere with caregiving (Biegel, Sales, & Schulz, 1991; Kiecolt-Glaser et al., 1991; Schulz et al., 1990), regimens for treating depressive symptomatology in grandparent caregivers should be introduced. Where possible, these regimens should include referral to grandparent caregiver support groups, respite programs, and other community-based services that have burgeoned over the past few years.

Particularly for new caregivers, who are at higher risk for depression, these programs and services may provide important sources of social support. As Burnette's (1998) recent pre- and posttest evaluation of a school-based grandparent caregiver group has demonstrated, moreover, that participants in such groups may experience significant improvement in depression scores. Burnette's study suggests cautious optimism in the potential of such groups for helping to improve the mental health of at-risk grandparent caregivers.

The need for psychological counseling in many grandparents who are raising their grandchildren also has been suggested (Burnette, 1998; Minkler & Roe, 1993; Shore & Hayslip, 1994). As Shore and Hayslip (1994) have pointed out, however, even grandparents who readily seek counseling and other mental health services for the grandchildren in their care have extremely low rates of such help seeking where their own mental health is concerned. Health and social service providers can play an important role in helping such caregivers address barriers (e.g., fear of stigma, lack of knowledge about how to access services, and financial costs) that have been shown to work against the seeking of needed mental health treatment in this population.

The continuing epidemics of drugs, AIDS, violence, teenage pregnancy, and high youth unemployment and divorce rates indicate that the phenomenon of grandparent caregiving is not likely to diminish in the near future (Burnette, 1997; Minkler, 1999). Continued awareness by service providers of the prevalence of grandparent caregiving and its potential negative mental health consequences should improve the identification of grandparent caregivers at risk and the provision of relevant health and social services to these grandparents, including, importantly, mental health services.

ACKNOWLEDGMENTS

The authors gratefully acknowledge the support of the Commonwealth Fund, a New York City–based national foundation that undertakes independent research on health and social issues. This chapter is based on an article by Meredith Minkler, Esme Fuller-Thomson, Doriane Miller, Diane Driver entitled "Depression in Grandparents Raising Grandchildren: Results of a National Longitudinal Study." The article appeared in the *Archives of Family Medicine, 6:* 445–452, 1997, and is abridged and updated here with the permission of the American Medical Association.

REFERENCES

Beckman, E., & Leber, W. (1995). *Handbook of depression* (2nd ed.). New York: Guilford Press.

Biegel, D., Sales, E., & Schulz, R. (1991). *Family caregiving and chronic illness.* Newbury Park, CA: Sage Publications.

Brown, G. W. (1996). Onset and course of depressive disorders: Summary of a research programme. In C. Mundt, M. J. Goldstein, K. Halweg, & P. Fielder (Eds.), *Interpersonal factors in the origin and course of affective disorders.* London: Gaskill. Academic Series.

Brown, G. W., & Harris, T. O. (1978). *Social origins of depression: A study of psychiatric disorder in women.* London: Tavistock Publications; New York: Free Press.

Brown, G. W., Harris, T. O., & Hepworth, C. (1995). Loss, humiliation and entrapment among women developing depression: A patient and non-patient comparison. *Psychological Medicine, 25,* 7–21.

Burnette, D. (1997). Grandparents raising grandchildren in the inner city. *Families in Society: The Journal of Contemporary Human Services, 78,* 489–499.

Burnette, D. (1998). Grandparents rearing grandchildren: A school-based small group intervention. *Research on Social Work Practice, 8,* 1–27.

Burton, L. (1992). Black grandmothers rearing children of drug-addicted parents: Stressors, outcomes and social service needs. *Gerontologist, 32,* 744–751.

Burton, L., & Bengtson, V. L. (1985). Black grandmothers: Issues of timing and continuity or roles. In V. L. Bengtson & J. F. Robertson (Eds.), *Grandparenthood* (pp. 61–77). Beverly Hills, CA: Sage Publications.

Chalfie, D. (1994). Going it alone: A closer look at grandparents parenting grandchildren. Washington, DC: American Association of Retired Persons.

Cowan, C. P., Cowan, A. P., Heming, G., & Miller, N. B. (1991). Becoming a family: Marriage, parenting and child development. In P. A. Cowan & E. M. Hetherington (Eds.), *Family transitions: Advances in family research* (vol. 2, pp. 79–109). Hillsdale, NJ: Lawrence Erlbaum.

Devins, G. M., & Orme, C. M. (1985). *Center for Epidemiological Studies Depression Scale: Test critiques* (vol. 2). Kansas City, MO: Westport Publishers.

Fuller-Thomson, E., Minkler, M., & Driver, D. (1997). A profile of grandparents raising grandchildren in the United States. *Gerontologist, 37,* 406–411.

George, L. (1995). Social factors and illness. In R. H. Binstock & L. K. George (Eds.), *Handbook of aging and the social sciences* (4th ed., pp. 229–252). New York: Academic Press.

Hayslip, B., Jr., Shore, R. J., Henderson, C. E., & Lambert, P. (1998). Custodial grandparenting and the impact of grandchildren with problems on role satisfaction and role meaning. *Journals of Gerontology, 53B,* S164–S173.

Jendrek, M. P. (1993). Grandparents who parent their grandchildren: Circumstances and decisions. *Gerontologist, 34,* 206–216.

Joslin, D., & Brouard, A. (1995). The prevalence of grandmothers as primary caregivers in a poor pediatric population. *Journal of Community Health, 5,* 383–401.

Joslin, D., & Harrison, R. (1998). The "hidden patient": Older relatives raising children orphaned by AIDS. *Journal of the American Women's Medical Association, 5,* 65–71, 76.

Kaplan, G. A., Roberts, R. E., Camacho, T. C., & Coyne, J. C. (1987). Psychosocial predictors of depression: Prospective evidence from the Human Population Laboratory studies. *American Journal of Epidemiology, 125,* 206–220.

Keith, V. M. (1993). Gender, financial strain and psychological distress among older adults. *Research on Aging, 15,* 123–147.

Kiecolt-Glaser, J. K., Dura, J. R., Speicher, C. E., Trask, J., & Glaser, R. (1991). Spousal caregivers of dementia victims: Longitudinal changes in immunity and health. *Psychosomatic Medicine, 53,* 345–362.

Miller, D. (1991, November). *The "Grandparents Who Care" support project of San Francisco.* Paper presented at the annual meeting of the Gerontological Society of America, San Francisco.

Minkler, M., Fuller-Thomson, E., Miller, D., & Driver, D. (1997). Depression in grandparents raising grandchildren: Results of a national longitudinal study. *Archives of Family Medicine, 6,* 445–452.

Minkler, M., & Roe, M. (1993). *Grandmothers as caregivers: Raising children of the crack cocaine epidemic.* Newbury Park, CA: Sage.

Minkler, M. (1999). Intergenerational households headed by grandparents: Contexts, realities, and implications for policy. *Journal of Aging Studies, 13,* 199–218.

Mirowsky, J., & Ross, C. E. (1989). *Social causes of psychological distress.* New York: Aldine de Gruyter.

Radloff, L. S. (1977). The CES-D scale: Self-report depression scale for research in the general population. *Applied Psychological Measurement, 1*(3), 385–401.

Raskin, V. D. (1990). Postpartum depression in a caretaking grandmother: Case report. *Jefferson Journal of Psychiatry, 8,* 18–21.

Roe, K. M., Minkler, M., Thompson, G., & Saunders, F. F. (1996). Health of grandmothers raising children of the crack cocaine epidemic. *Medical Care, 34,* 744–751.

Schulz, R., Vistainer, P., & Williamson, G. M. (1990). Psychiatric and physical morbidity effects of caregiving. *Journal of Gerontology, 45,* 181–191.

Selzer, M. (1976). Suggestions for the examination of time-disordered relationships. In J. F. Gubrium (Ed.), *Time, roles and self in old age* (pp. 111–125). New York: Human Sciences Press.

Shore, R. J., & Hayslip, B. (1994). Custodial grandparenting: Implications for children's development. In A. Godfried & A. Godfried (Eds.), *Redefining families: Implications for children's development.* New York: Plenum.

Strawbridge, W. J., Wallhagen, M. I., Shema, S. J., & Kaplan, G. A. (1997). New burdens or more of the same? Comparing grandparent, spouse, and adult child caregivers. *Gerontologist, 37*(4), 505–510.

Sweet, J., Bumpass, L., & Call, V. (1988). *The design and content of the National Survey of Families and Households* (NSFH working paper no. 1). Madison: University of Wisconsin, Center for Demography and Ecology.

CHAPTER 13

School-based Interventions for Children in Kinship Care

Anita Rogers and Nancy Henkin

Schools are an untapped and natural resource for dealing with the needs of children being raised in kinship care. However, most schools are unprepared to deal with the needs of this alternative family constellation and have not been proactive in identi-fying and/or responding to the special needs of this population. School administrators, teachers, and counselors often do not know how to interact with the caregivers and may lack sensitivity to these children and their new families. Strategies must be developed to meet the educational, psychological, and emotional needs of these children and their kinship families.

SCHOOL RISK FACTORS FOR CHILDREN IN KINSHIP CARE

Children being raised in kinship care, particularly those who are low-income, face a variety of issues that affect their ability to function at school and at home. Children who lack healthy relationships with their primary caregiver may demonstrate delays in areas critical for school success, such as social and emotional skills, self-esteem, language, and cognitive functioning (Bowlby, 1988). Studies by Craig (1992), Putnam (1993), and Terr (1991) suggest that children who have experienced abuse or violence may demonstrate significantly lower developmental levels, dysfunctional learning processes, inappropriate socialization skills, and an inability to focus on specific tasks. Behaviors such as hyperarousal, hypervigilance, and impulsivity are also common among these students (van der Kolk, 1987).

Children in kinship care often experience feelings of loss, anger, and rejection, making it difficult for them to form trusting relationships with their caregivers, teachers and peers (Kennedy & Keeney, 1988). They may experience "split loyalties" among the kinship caregiver, the parent, siblings, and professionals and feel they have to choose between loved ones (Crumbley & Little, 1997; Solomon & Marx, 1995). Embarrassment is another emotion felt by this population, particularly when their caregiver is significantly different in age or ability from other parents and cannot participate in some parent-child activities. Confusion regarding roles of parents and caregivers and fears about the mortality of their caregivers are additional issues confronting the children (Crumbley & Little, 1997). The children also are sometimes the objects of ridicule by their friends, particularly if the absentee parent still resides in the neighborhood and engages in antisocial behaviors. Their tendency to "defend" their parent often results in fights with their peers.

Some qualitative studies have suggested that children being raised by grandparents also have significant health-related problems. These include high rates of asthma and other respiratory problems, weaker immune systems, poor eating habits, inadequate sleep, physical disabilities, and attention deficit disorders (Dowdell, 1995). These findings may partly account for the high rate of school absenteeism among children in kinship care.

The problems that children in kinship care face are intimately intertwined with the issues facing their caregivers. Research (Burton, 1992; Minkler, Roe, & Price, 1992) suggests that grandparents are beset with a myriad of problems related to the care of their grandchildren, particularly those of drug-addicted parents. An exploratory study by Goldberg-Glen (1992) found that older adults who had become primary caregivers for children felt frustrated, overwhelmed, and anxious. Often grandparents are particularly frustrated because they are unable to help their grandchildren with homework. This may be because of their lack of familiarity with current subject matter or their own limited literacy skills. Attendance at school conferences and activities is often minimal, due to feelings of embarrassment and intimidation as well as a reluctance to share private information with school district personnel. Some of the kin providers also cite the lack of available time, patience, and energy as deterrents in helping their children succeed academically.

"GRANDMA'S KIDS": A MODEL SCHOOL-BASED PROGRAM

Program Overview

In 1995, Temple University's Center for Intergenerational Learning in Philadelphia received a federal grant from the Center for Substance Abuse Prevention to implement a drug abuse prevention program for children in kinship care. The program, "Grandma's Kids," has the following major objectives: (1) increase in student's academic performance, attachment to school, knowledge of harmful effects of ATOD (alcohol, tobacco, and other drugs) use, and problem-solving skills; (2) decrease in the negative behaviors and mental health problems of participating students; (3) increase in the social support networks, parenting skills, and access to community resources of caregivers; (4) increase in the frequency of positive contact between caregivers and school personnel; and (5) increase in the capacity of schools to meet the special needs of the target population.

Target Population

The "Grandma's Kids" program targeted children, older relative caregivers, and school personnel in three elementary schools each school year. The schools are located in low-income areas and serve predominantly African Americans.

Student Population

The children, whose primary custodial caregiver was usually a grand-parent, were selected from third and fourth grades and ranged in age from 8 to 11 years old. Many of the children have been drug-exposed (exposed to drugs in utero, affected by their birth parents' drug use, or drug users themselves). The project served approximately 60 youth per year, 20 per school. Roughly an equal number of males and females participated. Poor grades, uneven attendance, tardiness, and behavior problems have marked the children's school experiences. Their erratic school performance may be attributed to the children's movement from one relative to the next in order to avoid foster care placement or a return to substance-abusing parents.

According to counselors at the participating schools, the children who participated in "Grandma's Kids" had a great deal of anger, which was reflected in their relationships with school staff and peers. They were prone to fighting and tended to be disrespectful to adults. Many had unresolved issues of loss and grief; several in the program were struggling with the death of a parent or sibling. School staff described some children as "flat," having lost their "spark for life." Others were characterized as overemotional, crying endlessly or showing fear of an impending crisis. Counselors also reported that these children tended to be more defensive and insecure than other students were. A surprising number required intensive mental health intervention and were referred for psychological assessment.

Caregiver Population

Caregivers in "Grandma's Kids" were predominantly female, African American, and over 50 years of age. They each cared for an average of three children, ranging in age from newborn to 12 years. These children were usually from multiple birth parents. Most caregivers in the program had had responsibility for their children for at least 2 years and doubted seriously if the birth parent would assume full custody again. Many caregivers had poor literacy skills and were not active in their grandchildren's schools. They also showed high levels of stress, as reflected by their scores on the project-administered Parenting Stress Index (PSI). Of the caregivers tested in the first program year, 58.3% scored above the 90th percentile for total parenting stress. These scores are considered to be clinically significant. Older caregivers were found to have a significantly lower level of stress than younger ones, perhaps because younger caregivers are still working and may have more trouble assuming this new role than the older ones do. The caregivers in the program attributed their elevated stress levels to assumed parental responsibilities, financial difficulties, and lack of family and organizational resources.

Because of limited funds, many of the caregivers did not seek sufficient medical care for themselves. Several of the caregivers appeared to have alcohol abuse problems. It was a challenge for program staff to help caregivers face their own substance abuse issues without scaring them away from the program. The intergenerational cycle of substance abuse was apparent and generally not acknowledged by the kinship caregivers.

Primary Program Components

The "Grandma's Kids" program had three major components: (1) student support, (2) caregiver support, and (3) school support.

Student Support

Before- or after-school programs for children provide a valuable resource to caregivers (Turner, 1995). Besides providing a needed respite for the caregiver, often these programs offer breakfast and snacks, a welcome benefit, particularly to low-income families. "Grandma's Kids" offered a 4-day-per-week after-school program that addressed the psychosocial and academic needs of the children. It consisted of the following activities: (1) life skills/drug education, (2) academic tutoring, and (3) group counseling. In addition, a 2-week summer camp provided recreation, cultural activities, and intergenerational community service.

Life Skills/Drug Education. The promotion of social competence has been identified as a promising prevention approach (Caplan et al., 1992). This involves teaching personal and social skills as well as age-appropriate information and creating environmental supports to help students apply these skills to real-life situations. The after-school sessions used the "Second Step" curriculum, which focused on empathy training, impulse control, and anger management. The curriculum is designed to reduce impulsive and aggressive behavior in children ages 9 to 12 and to increase their level of social competence. The curriculum includes 46 lessons that are highly interactive, including photo stories, posters, role plays, audiovisual aids, and homework assignments. To increase the lesson's cultural content, school coordinators used props and scheduled trips and activities that were reflective of the children's environment. Hands-on, high-interest, interactive strategies were used, such as arts and crafts, storytelling, mask making, and theater arts. Sessions also dealt with peer and family pressures and decision-making skills. The smooth delivery of the lessons was often interrupted by the behavioral problems of the children.

Academic Tutoring. Academic support is clearly linked to improved school achievement. Solomon and Marx (1995) found that children raised in grandparent-grandchild households did not perform academically as well as those children in traditional two-family households but about the same as in one-parent households. Aquilino (1996) found that children raised by grandparents had a greater likelihood of not completing high school than those raised in traditional or one-parent families. Hawkins et al. (1992) identified school failure in the fourth, fifth, and sixth grades as a major risk factor for later substance abuse. Tutoring was provided daily to help students in "Grandma's Kids" complete their schoolwork and develop study skills. Each child's academic work was individualized and based on the child's educational needs as identified by his or her teacher. High school and college students were recruited from area schools to serve as the tutors and to assist with behavioral management. The tutorial assistance provided to children was cited by caregivers as one of the program's primary benefits to them and their children.

Group Counseling. Recent research (Kelly, 1993; Poe, 1992) suggests that counseling and other mental health services are needed to help children deal with their feelings of abandonment, anger, and confusion. Group counseling, in particular, can reduce the isolation children feel and reinforce the message that they are not alone. Once a week certified therapists conducted a 1 1/2-hour counseling session at each school. Sessions were designed to help children expand their repertoire of positive conflict resolution skills, build their self-esteem, learn peer resistance skills, develop a future orientation, improve their daily coping skills, adjust to their alternative family environment, and reinforce the topics discussed in the life skills curriculum. Therapists also focused on issues that seem to be of immediate concern or need to children, such as personal hygiene and sexuality.

Each session had the following format: (1) check-in time for students to identify any pressing concerns, (2) warm-up activity, (3) main exercise connected to life skills curriculum, and (4) closing or wrap-up activities. To accommodate the short attention span of many of the children, the main activities were divided into segments of no more than 10 minutes each. Therapists focused on experiential exercises rather than long group discussions. Movement activities gave children a legitimate outlet to move around and expel energy. Each child also developed his or her own "Grandma's Kid Book" that chronicled personal thoughts, concerns, and issues.

Therapists maintained group process notes to chronicle topics discussed and the individualized issues and needs of children. They noted that children in "Grandma's Kids" seemed overwhelmed by their circumstances, saddened by their lack of control to change their environment, ready for violence at any time, and in need of constant attention, even if it is negative. Therapists suspected that most of the children were suffering from mild to severe posttraumatic stress syndrome as a result of their indirect and direct exposure to violence in their family and neighborhoods as well as to physical and sexual abuse. The children's discussions of violence were graphic and matter-of-fact. Violence had become an acceptable, though frightening, part of their daily lives. The group counseling sessions served as a vehicle for assessing children's coping skills and determining if additional mental health services were needed. Program staff reported that the sessions helped children bond better with each other and subsequently with their grandparents. The sessions also allowed children to begin to deal more openly with their problems and face the fact that their parents may not return to care for them.

Summer Program. The 2-week, all-day summer program provided a needed respite for the caregivers and reinforced the skills children gained throughout the school year. Because caregivers often have other options available to them in the summer months, the total number of children involved was lower. Therefore, the program was offered in one location for all three participating schools. In addition to continuing the life skills curriculum and group counseling, the summer program provided cultural and recreational activities and opportunities for community service. For youth that have low self-esteem and have had little success in traditional learning environments, community service activities seemed to enhance their investment in school and the community. Children in the summer program visited area nursing homes and senior centers, where they participated in arts and crafts, spelling bees, and discussions with residents/members. Children were sensitized to the needs of the elders and the setting before they began their visits. Such sensitivity gave children a greater understanding of the issues facing their own grandparents.

Caregiver Support

Social ties and support have been shown to protect people from pathological states during a crisis and help maintain their self-esteem and life satisfaction (Cobb, 1976; Cohen & Syme, 1985; Pilisuk, 1982). Caregivers who perceive themselves as having few supports are especially vulnerable to emotional strain and other stresses related to the consequences of caregiving (George & Gwyther, 1986). When family and friends cannot provide the needed support to a new caregiver, it is extremely important to provide such a network (Burton, 1992; Minkler & Roe, 1993). Caregivers need opportunities for networking and problem solving in conjunction with information on resources and effective parenting strategies (Burton, 1992; Goldberg-Glen, 1992; Minkler & Roe, 1993). The primary interventions for caregivers in "Grandma's Kids" included (1) resource and referral assistance and (2) caregiver workshops and special events.

Resource and Referrals. At the beginning of each project year, a caregiver intake interview was conducted by the kinship coordinator to assess caregiver and child. These interviews were conducted in a variety of ways to accommodate caregivers: on site at schools, in the homes, and by telephone. As an intermediary between the caregivers and other agencies, the coordinator facilitated referrals for individual and family counseling, physical examinations, mental health assessments and hospitalizations, housing, and legal custody. Project staff had a hands-on approach to problem solving that resulted in a positive reputation among caregivers and school personnel. Caregivers inquired about managed care, access to benefits under welfare (TANF), the Electronic Benefit Transfer, where to find information for children with mental health disorders, how to seek help without terminating the parent's rights, employment and educational opportunities, housing options, and substance abuse concerns.

If a social worker or case manager is from another agency assigned to the kinship care family, he or she can work with school personnel to help the caregiver address the special educational needs of the child in care (Crumbley & Little, 1997). This may include arranging for school transportation, early intervention services and other educational supports, and obtaining information on a child's past educational history. In many instances the caregivers will have to be educated about how different types of learning disabilities manifest themselves. The professional worker can also assess the caregiver's educational level to determine if she or he needs assistance in school-related tasks.

Workshops and Special Events. Older caregivers in "Grandma's Kids" cited a sense of isolation and a lack of information about how to make the school, legal, and health care systems work in the best interest of their grandchildren and themselves. Although traditional support group structures were tried at the beginning of the project, attendance at the school-based neighborhood sessions was low. This was true whether the sessions were held bimonthly or monthly. When asked why they did not attend, caregivers cited the following reasons: (1) they feared punitive action when inquiring about child welfare sources regarding children in their care; (2) they wanted specific information relative to their issues, not generic discussions; and (3) they needed to develop trust with the staff before they would commit to attending and discussing their issues. Ultimately, what brought out the caregivers was the promise of entertainment, a meal, and/or gifts. Consequently, most activities integrated parent education and resource information into a social event. These events were usually held just for caregivers, providing them with much needed respite and an opportunity to socialize.

Successful activities included a luncheon jazz program with donated door prizes (e.g., television, video recorder, haircuts, toilet-
ries), a gospel brunch at a local restaurant, and a "Shop til' You Drop"
giveaway of clothing, toys, and equipment. When grandparents had
to bring their child(ren) to one of the events, baby-sitting was provided. There were some specific workshops that focused on the
following topics: disciplining children, split loyalties, housing resources, financial support, and stress management. Participation was
fairly high in these workshops because caregivers received varied
bonus points that resulted in a gift certificate to the local supermarket
at the end of the workshop series.

School Support

As research has indicated, there is clearly a need to enhance the
ability of school personnel to work with older caregivers and children
who have been drug-exposed (Goldberg-Glen, 1992; Pitman, 1990).
How a teacher organizes tasks for kinship children can be a major
determinant of children's school success or failure. Although children in kinship care may not be in a special education class, some
of the strategies employed in such classes are helpful. Research
(Delapena, 1991) suggests that these children need organized classrooms and routines that minimize disturbances, foster consistent
responses from school staff, support orderly transitions within and
between classrooms, and offer support to children who are stressed
by the demands of different environments. This is often difficult
when a teacher has a class of 35 children, many of whom have other
problems. Teaching appropriate coping strategies, helping students
understand that their actions will have an affect on others, and
showing children how to communicate their needs and feelings are
all tasks that will benefit the entire classroom.

Principals of the selected site schools identified the following areas
for staff training: exploring problems faced by older caregivers and
the children they are raising, understanding how family dynamics can
affect school achievement, and developing strategies for reaching out
to older caregivers. In response, the program provided staff (1)
sensitivity workshops, (2) ongoing feedback to classroom teachers
about the issues facing their students in the program, and (3) invitations to program-sponsored family events.

Sensitivity Workshops. During each school year, the project offered two training workshops for teachers and other personnel to enhance their capacity to work more effectively with the children participating in the program. Three ingredients were necessary to attract and ensure teacher attendance at these sessions: (1) in-service hourly payment, (2) sessions held immediately after school closing, and (3) refreshments. Workshop sessions included videos on the dilemma of kinship caregivers and their children, presentations by the therapists on the issues facing the children, the provision of resource materials on kinship, and problem-solving discussions. In many instances, teachers were unaware of the many obstacles facing the children in the program. Their increased understanding of kinship care issues translated into their reported greater sensitivity to the needs of the children and their caregivers.

Feedback to Teachers. Ongoing communication between teachers and project staff was an essential ingredient of "Grandma's Kids." At the beginning of each project year, teachers were asked to complete an academic and behavioral assessment of each child participant. These assessments helped the after-school coordinators to design individualized tutorial sessions and to better handle behavioral problems. Additionally, teachers were asked to provide academic worksheets in the children's areas of needs. Regular contact between project staff and teachers ensured that appropriate support was provided. At the end of the project year, teachers assessed the children's progress relative to academic and behavior changes.

Invitations to Family Events. Rarely do school personnel have the opportunity to socialize with the caregivers in a nonthreatening environment. The project-sponsored luncheons and trips provided an opportunity for school personnel to talk casually with caregivers. Because most of the events were held during school time, the personnel in attendance at these events were usually the counselors and the school principals.

Staffing

The optimal staff for a program serving three schools includes a full-time project director, a part-time kinship coordinator, a part-time school coordinator and aide at each participating school, one stipended grandparent advocate at each school, part-time therapists, and tutorial volunteers. The project director provides oversight for administrative and program development activities. The kinship co-ordinator is the primary link to the caregivers and their needs. The school coordinators, with the assistance of aides, are responsible for implementing the life skill curriculum, communicating with teachers, and organizing tutorial services. The grandparent advocate calls caregivers on a regular basis to identify any immediate concerns, encourage caregivers to attend workshops and/or special events and help to coordinate school resources for caregivers. The therapists are contractual and conduct the weekly group counseling sessions. The tutors from area colleges and high schools assist the children academically and provide needed behavioral management assistance.

Program Evaluation

The evaluation was designed and implemented by Temple University's Institute for Survey Research (ISR), an independent research center that has no direct ties to the Center for Intergenerational Learning. Both an outcome and a process evaluation of the "Grandma's Kids" program was conducted.

The *outcome* evaluation examined program effectiveness through measurements taken on children and caregivers. Each year, three Philadelphia schools were chosen as the "treatment" or experimental schools, and three others were chosen as the "comparison" schools, making this a quasi-experimental design. The following variables were assessed to determine the project's impact on children: (1) knowledge, attitudes, and behavior related to drugs; (2) academic grades; (3) behavior grades; (4) attendance; and (5) tardiness. The Parenting Stress Index (Abidin, 1983) was administered to caregivers at the beginning and end of each program year.

The *process* evaluation described the history and context of the project, documented the delivery of interventions, and examined barriers associated with implementation. Data were collected continuously throughout the project and reviewed by both program and evaluation staff. The after-school coordinators maintained a portfolio on each child, containing the following: (1) participation contract, signed by students and project staff; (2) individual record of attendance; (3) intake interview, including expectations and personal goals; (4) participation/interest inventory for Second Step curriculum (Beland, 1997); (5) counseling notes and records of referrals completed by the therapists; (6) sample collection of child's work/progress notes from individual tutors; and (7) personal reflections on program satisfaction from interviews.

For the caregivers, an intake interview was conducted by the kinship coordinator to assess needs and determine what referrals should be made. The number and type of referrals made and appointments kept was documented, as well as the individual's experience with the particular activity. This information was utilized to track use of existing services, coordinate referral mechanisms, and initiate increased support if necessary. Caregiver attendance at group activities also was recorded.

School staff's perception of project impact on students and the extent of their participation in training also was assessed and included (1) a questionnaire-interview administered quarterly on teacher's perception of each student's participation and behavior in class, (2) a questionnaire-interview administered quarterly to other school personnel regarding perception of student's behavior and functioning in school, (3) a quarterly assessment of the number and nature of interactions with older caregivers, and (4) interviews with school staff regarding expectations and satisfaction with training.

PROGRAM CONSIDERATIONS AND FINDINGS

Although the final evaluation of "Grandma's Kids" has not been completed, the following learnings may be helpful to others interested in developing programs for children in kinship care.

- *Turf issues.* When a school-based kinship program is being directed by an outside agency, often turf issues arise, particularly in relation to school counselors. Many school counselors have an enormous caseload and therefore tend to operate on an emergency rather than a prevention basis. Kinship care families need prevention to address ongoing problems as well as assistance with crisis situations. Sometimes an outside agency can expedite a referral relative to custody, mental health services, entitlement programs, and other social service resources. To minimize turf conflicts, the outside agency should include the school counselor in all decisions relative to the children and families they serve. *Project staff should provide regular updates to counselors regarding any educational, mental health, or social service needs that have been identified and addressed.*

- *Space.* Although classrooms are virtually empty after school, many teachers are reluctant to have people use and change their space. It is preferable for an after-school program to have its own space, where children can display their work on an ongoing basis rather than changing meeting places on a daily basis. It is also important to avoid competition with other after-school initiatives for space, especially if community residents operate those programs. *Working out space arrangements at the beginning of the program by meeting with school administration and community stakeholders is essential.*

- *Program scheduling.* Children in kinship care are often mobile, traveling back and forth to other relatives or their biological parents on weekends. Absenteeism is often high on Mondays because children may not have returned to their regular kinship environment. On Fridays, children may be getting ready to leave for the weekend. *After-school programs for these populations are best scheduled from Tuesday to Thursday.*

- *Trust relationships with families.* Like any other program, it takes time for families to develop trust in service providers. Kinship care families are particularly wary of persons prying into their lives for fear that the children may be taken away from them, that they may lose their entitlements, or that other family secrets may get unearthed. *Assurances of confidentiality must be repeated often, and program relationships must be sustained for at least 1 year for families to feel secure enough to share information with providers.*

- *Shared resources.* Kinship programs in schools should coordinate the resources within and outside the school environment. School and project personnel should identify for each other the full range of resources that are available to children and families. *Any resource list should be a compilation of coordinated services from all parties involved.*

- *Caregiver incentives.* Often low-income caregivers will not attend educational programs solely for the intrinsic value of these sessions. In many instances, low-income caregivers are more likely to participate in programs that offer them tangible resources (food, coupons, gifts, etc.). Although this caregiver attitude may seem offensive to some, the overall goal is to provide them with information that can improve the quality of life for children in their care. *Programs should include a line item in their budget for caregiver incentives.*
- *Cultural competence.* In "Grandma's Kids," cultural competence was fostered through the employment of an African American staff that was aware of the cultural nuances of the kinship care families. The following are strategies help ensure that services are culturally appropriate:

  - Regular telephone calls to kinship care providers in lieu of just sending written updates on their children foster trust and accommodates those providers who have literacy issues.
  - Planned social events draw on the cultural experiences of the caregivers (gospel brunch, jazz lunch) and the children ("rap" contests, African American arts).
  - Using stipended grandparent advocates from each of the targeted schools builds trust with caregivers.
  - Strength-based approaches that focus on the caregivers' and children's assets, not deficits, raise the self-esteem of both groups.

Much more still needs to be learned regarding successful interventions for children being raised in kinship care. "Grandma's Kids" has not only provided insight into many of the challenges faced by children, caregivers, and school personnel, it has also tried out a number of promising strategies for supporting this very special population. An 8-minute video about "Grandma's Kids" is currently available; a manual on kinship care for school personnel and a final evaluation report will be completed by fall 1999.

REFERENCES

Abidin, R. (1983). *Parenting Stress Index.* Charlottesville, VA: Pediatric Psychology Press.

American Association of Retired Persons (AARP). (1993). *Grandparents raising their grandchildren: What to consider and where to find help.* Washington, DC: Author.

Aquilino, W. (1996). The life course of children born to unmarried mothers: Childhood living arrangements and young adult outcomes. *Journal of Marriage and the Family, 58,* 293–310.

Barth, R. (1991). Educational implications of prenatally drug-exposed children. *Social Work in Education, 13,* 130–136.

Beland, K. (1997). *Second Step.* Seattle, WA: Committee for Children.

Benard, B. (1991). *Fostering resiliency in kids: Protective factors in the family, school, and community.* San Francisco: Far West Laboratory for Educational Research and Development.

Bowlby, J. (1988). *A secure base: Parent-child attachment and healthy human development.* New York: Basic Books.

Burton, L. (1992). Black grandmothers rearing children of drug-addicted parents: Stressors, outcomes and social service needs. *Gerontologists, 32,* 744–751.

Caplan, M., Weissberg, R. P., Grober, J. S., Sivo, P. J., Grady, K., & Jacoby, C. (1992). Social competence promotion with inner city and suburban young adolescents: Effects on social adjustment and alcohol use. *Journal of Consulting and Clinical Psychology, 60,* 56–63.

Cobb, S. (1976). Social support as a moderator of life stress. *Psychosomatic Medicine, 38,* 300–314.

Cohen, S., & Syme, S. L. (Eds.). (1985). *Social support and health.* San Diego, CA: Academic Press.

Craig, S. F. (1992). The educational needs of children living with violence. *Phi Delta Kappan, 74*(1), 67–71.

Crumbley, J., & Little, R. (Eds.). (1997). *Relatives raising children: An overview of kinship care.* Washington, DC: CWLA Press.

Delapena, I. (1991). *Strategies for teaching young children prenatally exposed to drugs.* Chicago: National Association for Perinatal, Addiction, Research and Education.

de Toledo, S., & Brown, D. E. (1995). *Grandparents as parents: A survival guide for raising a second family.* New York: Guilford Press.

Dowdell, E. B. (1995). Caregiver burden: Grandparents raising their high-risk children. *Journal of Psychosocial Nursing, 33,* 27–30.

George, L., & Gwyther, L. (1986). Caregiver wellbeing: A multi-dimensional examination of family caregivers of demented adults. *Gerontologists, 26,* 253–259.

Goldberg-Glen, R. (1992). [Grandparents as caregivers in contemporary American society]. Unpublished research data.

Hawkins, J., Catalano, R. F., & Miller, J. (1992). Risk and protective factors for alcohol and other drug problems in adolescence and early childhood: Implications for substance abuse prevention. *Psychological Bulletin, 12,* 64–105.

Kelley, S. J. (1993). Caregiver stress in grandparents raising grandchildren. *Journal of Nursing Scholarship, 25,* 331–337.

Kennedy, J., & Keeney, V. (1988). The extended family revisited: Grandparents rearing grandchildren. *Child Psychiatry and Human Development, 19,* 26–35.

Minkler, M., & Roe, K. (1993). *Grandmothers as caregivers: Raising children of the crack cocaine epidemic.* Newbury Park, CA: Sage.

Minkler, M., & Roe, K. (1996). Grandparents as surrogate parents. *Generations,* spring, 34–38.

Minkler, M., Roe, K., & Price, M. (1992). The physical and emotional health of grandmothers raising grandchildren in the crack cocaine epidemic. *Gerontologist, 32,* 752–761.

Minkler, M., Roe, K. M., & Robertson-Beckley, R. (1994). Raising grandchildren from crack cocaine households: Effects of family and friendship ties of African-American women. *American Orthopsychiatric Association, 64,* 21–29.

Murphy, J. P. (1984). Substance abuse and the family. *Journal for Specialists in Group Work, 9,* 106–112.

Pilisuk, M. (1982). Delivery of social support: The social inoculation. *American Journal of Orthopsychiatry, 52,* 20–31.

Poe, L. M. (1992). *Black grandparents as parents.* Berkeley, CA:

Putnam, F. W. (1993). Disassociative disorders in children: Behavioral profiles and problems. *Child Abuse and Neglect, 17,* 39–45.

Rothenberg, D. (1996). Grandparents as parents: A primer for schools. *ERIC Digest* (PS-96-8).

Saltzman, G., & Pakan, P. (1996). Feelings . . . in the grandparent raising grandchildren triad (or relationship). *Parenting Grandchildren: A Voice for Grandparents, 2*(1), 4–6.

Shore, R. J., & Hayslip, B. (1994). Custodial grandparenting: Implications for children's development. In A. Godfried & A. Godfried (Eds.), *Redefining families: Implications for children's development.* New York: Plenum.

Solomon, J. C., & Marx, J. (1995). To grandmother's house we go: Health and school adjustment of children raised solely by grandparents. *Gerontologists, 35,* 386–394.

Terr, L. C. (1991). Childhood traumas: An outline and overview. *American Journal of Psychiatry, 148,* 10–20.

Turner, L. (1995). Grandparent-caregivers: Why parenting is different the second time around. *Family Resource Coalition Report, 14*(1–2), 6–7.

Vander Kolk, C. J. (1987). Psychosocial interventions with visually impaired persons. In B. W. Heller, L. M. Flohr, et al. (Eds.), *Psychosocial Interventions with Sensorially Disabled Persons: Mind and Medicine* (pp. 33–52). Orlando, FL: Grune and Stratton.

Weissberg, R., & Caplan, M. (1990). *Social problem solving module.* Unpublished document.

Wells, K. C., & Forehand, R. (1985). Conduct and oppositional disorders. In P. Bornstein & A. Kazdin (Eds.), *Handbook of clinical behavior therapy with children* (pp. 218–265). Homewood, IL: Dorsey.

CHAPTER 14

Using a Microanalysis of a Videotaped Interview to Understand the Dynamics of a Grandparent-headed Household

Roberta G. Sands and Robin S. Goldberg-Glen

This chapter presents an analysis of an interaction between a caregiving grandmother and an interviewer in which the grandmother revealed a family secret. Family secrets—information about events and stories that are withheld from some family members and/or outsiders because it is perceived to be embarrassing, disgraceful, or damaging—are frequently observed by family therapists (e.g., Imber-Black, 1993, 1998). Events such as imprisonment, mental illness, alcoholism, and out-of-wedlock pregnancies are examples of the secrets that some families keep. Secrets such as these rarely emerge in research interviews, and methods to analyze data of this sort are few and far between. This chapter illustrates how microanalytic techniques can be used to examine closely how such sensitive information is disclosed in a research interview.

MICROANALYSIS

Microanalysis is the detailed examination of verbal and nonverbal behavior, usually using data from audiotapes or videotapes. It evolved from work begun in the 1950s in Palo Alto, California, where an interdisciplinary group of scholars associated with the Center for Advanced Study in the Behavioral Sciences developed *context analysis*, in which interactions recorded in film were viewed and analyzed (Kendon, 1990).

A book that was an outgrowth of one of the authors' association with the Palo Alto Group, *The First Five Minutes* (Pittenger, Hockett, & Danehy, 1960), is an early example of the microanalysis of a tape-recorded interview. This book contains an annotated transcription of every word and sound that was spoken during the first 5 minutes of an initial psychotherapy session. The transcription is complete with codes to denote prosody (the texture or quality of the voice) and phonemes (meaningful sound units). Labov and Fanshel (1977) moved this line of research further along by examining the verbal text and paralinguistic cues, expanding the implicit meaning of the text and deriving interaction rules.

Two other scholars associated with the Palo Alto Group, Birdwhistell and Scheflen, went on to develop the field of nonverbal communication (Kendon, 1990). Scheflen's (1973) analysis of psychotherapy sessions found that these therapeutic interactions had a consistent structure, with stages that could be identified by observing posture and the use of space. Similarly, Erickson and Shultz (1982) identified nonverbal indicators of changes in the structure of events in counseling interviews. Kendon (1990) has systematically studied changes in gaze direction, move coordination, and greetings.

Scholars of discourse, ethnography of communication, interactional sociolinguistics, and conversation analysis closely and systematically examine verbal and nonverbal language in use. Methods derived from these fields have been used to examine classroom interaction (Green & Wallat, 1981a), medical discourse (Mishler, 1984), and legal encounters (Fisher & Todd, 1986), as well as face-to-face interactions in other institutional and work settings (Boden & Zimmerman, 1991; Drew & Heritage, 1992) and psychotherapy (Ferrara, 1994; Ribeiro, 1994).

The authors of this chapter were influenced by Erickson's (1992) work on the ethnographic microanalysis of interpersonal interactions. Erickson uses ethnographic methods such as participant observation to gain knowledge of the range of events that occur in a particular setting, as well as which events are typical or expected and which are rare. The ethnographic component provides a context for a close examination of events that are of theoretical interest. Atypical events, for example, may be subject to a microanalysis to help understand why they are rare and what they mean. Viewing interactions as coordinated events, Erickson microanalyzes simultaneous verbal and nonverbal behavior of multiple participants over time. The authors also were influenced by Green and Wallat's (1981b) conceptualization of message units, chunks of texts that constitute semantic units. Like Green and Wallat they draw from Gumperz's (1982) description of "contextualization cues," such as pauses, variations in prosody, and other paralinguistic and nonverbal indicators that mark the beginning and endings of lines.

BACKGROUND AND METHODS

In 1995 the authors conducted a survey of 129 individual grandparents who were caring for their grandchildren. These primary caregiving grandparents were interviewed about their situations and how their responsibilities affect their mental health and well-being. The interview contained many standardized instruments that were subjected to a quantitative analysis. A year later a qualitative follow-up study of 20 grandparent-headed families was initiated. These interviews took place in the grandparents' homes, where they were simultaneously audiotaped and videotaped. Two master's-level social workers conducted the interviews. The interviewers were trained to ask questions that would help them construct *ecomaps* and *genograms*. Ecomaps are assessment tools used by social workers to obtain a picture of families' supports and stressors (Hartman & Laird, 1983). To create an ecomap, the interviewer asks informants to identify the social systems that are involved in their lives (e.g., schools, churches, extended family, and health care providers) and to describe the extent to which these systems are supportive and/or stress-generating. Genograms are drawings of the family tree, usually over at least three generations (McGoldrick, Gerson, & Schellenberger, 1999). They include generational lines, names, birth and death dates, the quality of the relationships, and descriptions such as alcoholic, heart condition, and so forth.

After the interviews were completed, the interviewers transcribed them, and the authors reviewed and indexed them topically. In addition, the authors asked the interviewers to describe their most significant interviews and why they were meaningful. The videotapes of the interviews identified as significant were viewed by the authors and interviewers several times and discussed thoroughly. One of these contained a segment in which the grandmother revealed a family secret. This was one of 2 among the 20 interviews in which a family secret was revealed. In the example presented here, the grandmother revealed that her estranged husband was the father of one of the grandchildren for whom she was caring.

After viewing the videotape (90 minutes) and reading the transcription of the entire interview several times, the authors divided the interview into the major sections described in Table 14.1. The times on this table were obtained from the videotape, which had the time imprinted on it. The 2-minute segment that was selected came toward the end of the interview, within the genogram interview.

Subsequently, the authors revised the initial transcription of the identified segment to include the details that came from multiple playing of an audiotape of the interview. Next they closely observed the selected segment, as well as sections that came before and after it, innumerable times and revised the message units (Green & Wallat, 1981b) initially discerned from the audiotape. During some viewings they attended to hand and arm movements; on other occasions, head movements and gaze. In the end they reconstructed the transcription to include verbal and nonverbal behaviors over time. The authors took separate notes on their observations and the times in which they occurred; where they disagreed, they rewatched these segments until they came to an agreement about what they saw and at what time. The total transcription, viewing, and discussion time was approximately 20 hours.

TABLE 14.1   **Structure of Videotaped Interview**

Minutes	Sequence of Events Within Interview
00:00–7:00	Introduction Review of changes in household since last interview Describe a typical day in your family
7:01–48:00	Ecomap interview (mapping of household's social systems) David Alvin Grandmother
48:01–1:09	Genogram interview (family tree) Grandmother's family of origin
(51:50–53:43)	**"Um were you married?"** (beginning of section that is microanalyzed) Grandmother's children and grandchildren
1:10–1:30	Wrap-up Family discussion about their relationships Grandmother's perspective on caregiving Ending

Ochs (1979) asserted that decisions about transcription are dictated by theory, although the theory is not always acknowledged. Many researchers, for example, foreground verbal behavior over nonverbal or include only the verbal. The authors included both verbal and nonverbal communication of the participants; but by placing the verbal communication to the left, they have highlighted the verbal. Placement of the nonverbal to the right helps the reader interpret the underlying meaning of what is expressed overtly. The authors also have foregrounded time—the 2 minutes, broken into units of seconds, in which an interaction selected from the C family took place.

THE C FAMILY

Monica C., a heavy-set, 57-year old, separated African American woman was caring for two grandsons, Alvin, 17, and David, 16, each by a different one of Mrs. C's daughters. Alvin had previously lived in foster homes, where, he said, he was abused. More recently, he dropped out of a Job Corps program in which he was enrolled. David, who is mentally challenged, was in school. Alvin, who was described as a loner, hinted that he smokes and drinks. Mrs. C. reported that she had high blood pressure, arthritis, and angina and drank from age 16 to 3 or 4 years ago, when she began to recover.

The ecomap interview imparted the following. The younger grandson spoke positively of school and sports. The older grandson found some support from religion and said that he enjoyed sports and listening to music. The grandmother received support from the health care system and religion (but not the church). She was estranged from most of her children but had friendly relations with neighbors and was in touch with friends from other neighborhoods by telephone.

The genogram interview revealed that Mrs. C's mother was an unmarried teenager when Monica was born. Monica was raised by an aunt until she was eight, when she returned to her mother. Monica married in 1956 and was separated 10 years later. She had eight children (two boys, six girls) of whom three died during childhood and a fourth died the previous year from HIV disease. Six of the children (including two who are deceased) had substance abuse problems.

The interviewer found the home disorganized. The grandchildren (especially Alvin) did not accept their grandmother's authority. David demanded more attention than she was willing to give. The grandmother openly complained about the grandchildren and declared that she would rather be in the work force than caring for her grandchildren.

DESCRIPTION OF THE INTERACTION

Table 14.2 presents the transcribed segment of the interview in which the grandmother reveals the family secret about David's father. It is recommended that readers review this table prior to reading the analytic description that follows. As noted earlier, the segment that was microanalyzed was part of the genogram interview, in which the interviewer elicited information needed to construct a family tree. It occurred almost an hour into the interview, when rapport had been established.

TABLE 14.2 Microanalysis of Interaction

Start Time	Sp	Verbal	Nonverbal
51:50	INT	Um were you married?	Interviewer (INT) faces grandmother (GM), but the video camera sees her from the back.
51:51	GM	OO:OH BOY hey was I ever.	GM's hands are on her lap and she is twiddling thumbs. When she speaks, she shakes head from side to side.
51:53	INT	Okay	
51:54		Tell me heh about that	
51:56	GM	Still is	GM's head is still.
51:57	INT	Okay you're still married?	
51:58	GM	Oh yeah.	GM turns head left toward interviewer, then turns head down.
51:59	INT	And your husband?	
52:01	GM	I don't know (1.4-second pause)	GM shakes head.
52:02		I don't know	GM looks ahead.
52:03		*where that bugger at*	GM turns head to the right (away from interviewer)
52:04	INT	What's his name?	
52:05	GM	Andrew.	GM slightly looks up at interviewer.
52:06	INT	Andrew	
52:07		and so he's living.	
52:08	GM	Mmm hmmm heh heh heh (laughing)	GM looks away from interviewer.
52:10	INT	Do ya know how old he is?	
52:11	GM	Oh boy	
52:12		Maybe HE's about 67.	GM smiles and looks toward interviewer.
52:15	INT	Okay.	
52:16		But you don't know where he is.	
52:17	GM	*Ah he's in North Philly*	GM shakes head and looks forward, making eye contact with interviewer.
52:19	INT	So ya don't have any contact?	

(continued)

TABLE 14.2   *(continued)*

Start Time	Sp	Verbal	Nonverbal
52:21	GM	Whenever I go try to see hi- *See how he is* *See how he's doing*	GM looks toward interviewer, then forward, then away from interviewer into space (dreamy).
52:29	INT	So sometimes you do see him.	
52:30	GM	U-huh.	GM looks at interviewer, nodding, still twiddling thumbs.
52:31	INT	What year were you married?	
52:33	GM	Uh (pause)	GM looks at interviewer, nodding.
52:35		'56	
52:37		February	GM looks straight ahead (not at interviewer).
52:39	INT	And so you're still married.	
52:41		You jus' separated?	
52:42	GM	U-huh.	GM looks at interviewer and nods.
52:44	INT	When did you separate?	GM stops twiddling her thumbs.
52:45	GM	Oh (.9-second pause) 30 (1.6-second pause)	GM turns head forward, staring into space.
52:47	GM	About 30 years	GM turns head toward interviewer.
52:50	INT	Thirty years ago?	
52:51	GM	Mmm hmm (pause)	Interviewer writes response.
52:58	INT	*Okay* (pause) So you s-try to see him but he—he's not someone you're real close to? Or are you would you say you're close with him?	
53:05	GM	When we meet it's it's all right (pause)	
53:09		There's—there's no um	GM throws popcorn into bowl.
53:11		thing (pause)	GM slides right hand across thigh, pinches towel, and raises right arm and hand straight onto couch.

TABLE 14.2   *(continued)*

Start Time	Sp	Verbal	Nonverbal
53:14	INT	No conflict.	
53:16	GM	Uh um (pause) that's his.	GM points to grandchild with left hand and returns left hand to arm of couch. (Grandchild is out of the visual range of the camcorder.)
53:19	INT	Hmm?	Interviewer looks in direction GM pointed.
53:20	GM	*That's his.*	Interviewer looks again.
53:21	INT	What was? (long pause)	
53:24	GM	Diablo.	GM nods head.
53:27	INT	OO:OH (long pause)	
53:33		*his his*	
53:35	GM	*offspring.*	
53:36	INT	Okay.	
53:37		That's Andrew's child?	
53:39	GM	Mmm hmm.	
53:40	INT	*Obviously these are not your children.*	
53:42	GM	Uh uh.	GM shakes head.
53:43	INT	Tell me about your children Who your children were You said you had . . .	
53:47	GS	I'll be back	Grandson tries to leave.

Transcription Key:

Sp, speaker; GM, grandmother; GS, grandson; INT, interviewer.

Italics indicate that the voice became softer.

Colon (:) within a word (OO:OH) is a stretched-out word.

Capitalized words and expressions denote emphasis.

Sounds such as "heh heh" and "mmm" were written out.

The division of lines within turns at speaking was determined by the presence of contextualization cues (Gumperz, 1982), such as pauses and the voice dropping.

Punctuation is used as it is used in written English, that is, . denotes a pause; ? indicates a raised voice; and . . . means there is an elision.

The transcription begins after a discussion about the grandmother's family of origin, and a new topic ("Were you married?") is introduced. When this question is asked, the grandmother responds with energy and sarcasm in her voice, hinting at an eventful marital history. The interviewer picks up and mimics some of the humor that was in the grandmother's statement and invites the grandmother to speak about her marriage. The grandmother does not, however, accept the invitation to talk further on this topic. She simply says, "Still is." But throughout this exchange the grandmother responds with her head, shaking it from side to side at 51:51, keeping it stationary at 51:56, and directing it toward the interviewer at 51:58. From her head shaking, it can be inferred that there was something unpleasant about the marriage, but it is unknown at this point what made it so.

The interviewer then inquires about Mrs. C's husband ("And your husband?"), but it is not clear what the interviewer wanted to know about him. It may be that the interviewer was confused about the status of the husband, as the grandmother said that they were married, and by this time in the interview it was obvious that her husband did not live with her. The grandmother next declares that she does not know where he is, but there appears to be a subtext underlying this text. Similar to what she did at 51:51, she shakes her head and moves it forward, suggesting that there was something not right about this man. She reinforces this idea when she refers to him as a "bugger" at 52:03.

At this point the interviewer seeks factual information about the grandmother's husband, beginning with his name. When the interviewer establishes that Andrew is living, the grandmother utters a sound (*mmmm*), laughs, and looks away from the interviewer, without explaining what makes this humorous. After the interviewer learns Andrew's age, she restates the grandmother's previous statement about not knowing where he lived. This time, however, Monica reveals that she *does* know where he lives. When the grandmother states his whereabouts, she again shakes her head and looks forward and then makes eye contact with the interviewer.

Apparently picking up on the grandmother's earlier statement, "I don't know. . . . I don't know . . . ," the interviewer phrases the next question negatively, "So ya don't have any contact?" Again, Monica indicates that what she said or implied earlier was not the case. She said that there is some contact at her initiative, but she says this looking into space and in a tone that sounded dreamy to the authors. As during 52:01–52:02, Monica repeats herself in lines 52:21–52:28. According to Tannen (1989), repetition is a rhetorical device that has a number of functions in conversations. A rhythmic pattern of repetition that becomes expanded, which occurred in these two examples, conveys the speaker's attitude, stimulates listener involvement, and establishes a theme (Tannen, 1989). Erickson (1984) notes that African Americans use a great deal of repetition in their speech.

Continuing along the same lines, the interviewer asks when the grandmother was married and establishes that she is still legally married but has been separated for 30 years. During this exchange, the grandmother looks at the interviewer and away, looking away when the grandmother appeared to be thinking about her response. When the interviewer probes about when the separation occurred, the grandmother gives brief verbal responses followed by long pauses (52:45–52:47 and 52:51–52:57).

At this point the interviewer appears to be confused, perhaps by these pregnant pauses. The interviewer reiterates that the grandmother is in contact with the man from whom she is separated but wonders whether they are emotionally close. The grandmother responds by saying that when they meet "it's all right," pauses, and restates this idea in different words. During this interaction, the grandmother changes the position of her right hand and arm in stages—first throwing popcorn into a bowl, then moving her hand across her thigh to a towel, where she seems to be wiping her hand, and then raises her arm and hand onto the top of the couch. After a long pause, the interviewer states, "No conflict."

Again the grandmother's overt statements belie her meaning. She points to her younger grandchild (David) and says after pausing, "That's his." At this climactic moment, the interviewer looks in the direction the grandmother was pointing but seems confused. When she asks, "Hmm?" the grandmother repeats her previous statement, but the interviewer still does not seem to understand what is being said. After the grandmother nods her head and uses an alternative name for the grandchild (Diablo), the interviewer finally realizes what the grandmother means. When the interviewer next says "his, his," the grandmother completes the sentence with "offspring." The

interviewer reiterates what she finally understands, that the grandmother's estranged husband (Andrew) is the grandchild's father,
from 53:36–53:37, which the grandmother confirms at 53:39, thus
ending this narrative.

The transcription includes a few lines past the resolution of the
above interaction (called coda) to show the interviewer's transi-
tioning to her next set of questions, which are about the grandmother's adult children. It also includes a statement by one of the
grandchildren that he was leaving, to show that the "family secret"
was disclosed in the presence of the grandchildren. After the grandchild's utterance, the grandmother raised her voice angrily and told
that grandchild that he could not leave.

DISCUSSION

This microanalysis of a segment of a transcript depicted the process
in which a grandmother who was raising two grandsons revealed
that one of the grandsons for whom she was caring was her stepchild
through her estranged husband, as well as her grandchild through
her daughter. This information did not surface in the initial interview
with this grandmother, even though questions were asked about the
composition of the household and how the members were related
to the grandmother. Clearly, Mrs. C. must have suffered great anguish when she realized, some time in the past, that her husband
had impregnated her daughter. To be raising the child of this liaison
would seem to compound pain from the past many times over. In
this case, the grandchild is "mentally challenged," probably mentally
retarded, a likely consequence of incest. It is no wonder that Mrs.
C. does not want to be in the caregiving role, particularly with
this child.

The discovery of this fact within this second interview raises questions about the completeness of other interviews in which questions
are not asked about every family relationship. In child welfare, for
example, where permanent placements with relatives like grandparents are actively sought, complicated relationships like those depicted in this microanalysis need to be identified. If children are
placed in homes where there are secrets from the past, old issues
can contaminate the present and adversely affect the caregiver and

child. Similarly, placement of an older adult with an adult child with whom there was a difficult relationship can fail. Clinicians should be sensitive to these possibilities and prevent their becoming reactivated.

The language that the grandmother used to depict the secret is in itself telling. When she said, "That's his," she was suggesting that David is a thing ("that") who belongs to her estranged husband, not to her. The words suggest a disowning and rejection of the child. The interviewer reacted to this strange use of language by asking the grandmother to restate and interpret what she meant. The interviewer's nonverbal response was literally a "double-take."

This interview highlights the need for sensitivity to nonverbal and verbal cues that suggest underlying issues on the part of the research interviewer and those who are analyzing interview data. The person who interviewed this family was a recent graduate of a master's-level social work program; her clinical experience was limited. A retrospective examination reveals that she attended well to the task of obtaining concrete information that would help her create a genogram but seemed to miss hints that there was a family secret. She did not appear to realize that the informant was dodging questions and sending mixed signals about what must have been a highly emotionally charged relationship. Instead, the interviewer sought answers that would help her define the relationship as close or conflictual so that she could draw either a straight (denoting a close) or crooked (denoting conflictual) line between the two individuals on the genogram. When the grandmother did provide "answers," the interviewer had a difficult time decoding the message. Finally, the grandmother explained her communication directly.

The examination of this interview underscores how difficult it is to anticipate and respond to the unexpected in research interviewing. Even qualitative interviewers are trained to follow research procedures in a systematic manner and to elicit answers. In the interview that was microanalyzed, the search for answers diverted the interviewer from the most compelling goal of research—discerning the underlying meaning.

This chapter has shown what can be learned by microanalyzing a brief, 2-minute segment of a longer interview. Like a microscope that magnifies the size of something small, microanalysis allows one to zoom in on the elements of a social interaction, determine its components, and determine what makes it works. Used to assess critical moments of interaction, it is a promising tool for the clinical gerontological researcher.

ACKNOWLEDGMENTS

Based on a paper presented at the 51st Annual Scientific Meeting of the Gerontological Society of America, Philadelphia, November 1998.

REFERENCES

Boden, D., & Zimmerman, D. H. (Eds.). (1991). *Talk and social structure: Studies in ethnomethodology and conversation analysis.* Cambridge: Polity Press.

Drew, P., & Heritage, J. (Eds.). (1992). *Talk at work: Interaction in institutional settings.* Cambridge: Cambridge University Press.

Erickson, F. (1984). Rhetoric, anecdote, and rhapsody: Coherence strategies in conversation among Black American adolescents. In D. Tannen (Ed.), *Coherence in spoken and written discourse* (pp. 81–154). Norwood, NJ: Ablex.

Erickson, F. (1992). Ethnographic microanalysis of interaction. In M. D. Le Compte, W. L. Millroy, & J. Preissle (Eds.), *The handbook of qualitative research in education* (pp. 201–225). San Diego, CA: Academic Press.

Erickson, F., & Shultz, J. (1982). *The counselor as gatekeeper: Social interaction in interviews.* New York: Academic Press.

Ferrara, K. W. (1994). *Therapeutic ways with words.* New York: Oxford University Press.

Fisher, S., & Todd, A. D. (Eds.). (1986). *Discourse and institutional authority: Medicine, education, and law.* Norwood, NJ: Ablex.

Green, J. L., & Wallat, C. (Eds.). (1981a). *Ethnography and language in educational settings.* Norwood, NJ: Ablex.

Green, J. L., & Wallat, C. (1981b). Mapping instructional conversations: A sociolinguistic ethnography. In J. L. Green & C. Wallat (Eds.), *Ethnography and language in educational settings* (pp. 161–205). Norwood, NJ: Ablex.

Gumperz, J. (1982). *Discourse strategies.* Cambridge: Cambridge University Press.

Hartman, A., & Laird, J. (1983). *Family-centered social work practice.* New York: Free Press.

Imber-Black, E. (Ed.). (1993). *Secrets in families and family therapy.* New York: W. W. Norton and Co.

Imber-Black, E. (1998). *The secret life of families: Truth-telling, privacy, and reconciliation in a tell-all society.* New York: Bantam Books.

Kendon, A. (1990). *Conducting interaction: Patterns of behavior in focused encounters.* Cambridge: Cambridge University Press.

Labov, W., & Fanshel, W. (1977). *Therapeutic discourse: Psychotherapy as conversation.* New York: Academic Press.

McGoldrick, M., Gerson, R., & Shellenberger, S. (1999). *Genograms: Assessment and intervention* (2nd ed.). New York: W. W. Norton.

Mishler, E. G. (1984). *The discourse of medicine: Dialectics of medical interviews.* Norwood, NJ: Ablex.

Ochs, E. (1979). Transcription as theory. In E. Ochs & B. B. Schieffelin (Eds.), *Developmental pragmatics* (pp. 43–72). New York: Academic Press.

Pittenger, R. E., Hockett, C. F., & Danehy, J. J. (1960). *The first five minutes.* Ithaca, NY: Paul Martineau.

Riviero, B. T. (1994). *Coherence in psychotic discourse.* New York: Oxford University Press.

Scheflen, A. E. (1973). *Communicational structure: Analysis of a psychotherapy transaction.* Bloomington: Indiana University Press.

Tannen, D. (1989). *Talking voices: Repetition, dialogue, and imagery in conversational discourse.* Cambridge: Cambridge University Press.

CHAPTER 15

Determinants of Custodial Grandparents' Perceptions of Problem Behavior in Their Grandchildren

Bert Hayslip Jr., Persephanie Silverthorn, R. Jerald Shore, and Craig E. Henderson

In the United States approximately 11% of grandparents have provided custodial care for their grandchildren at some point in time (Fuller-Thomson, Minkler, & Driver, 1997). Furthermore, over 2 million children are reared in three-generation households, often with the biological parent sporadically present, leaving the grandparent to provide primary custodial care (Woodworth, 1996). Such figures represent a 44% increase over those in 1980 (Flint & Perez-Porter, 1997).

Many of the children raised by grandparents exhibit behavioral and emotional problems, but it is unclear whether their difficulties result from disturbances in their families of origin, from their reaction to the transition from one caregiving arrangement to another, or from residing with grandparents. It also has been demonstrated that a history of troublesome parent-grandparent relationship seems to negatively affect the grandchild-grandparent connection (Whitbeck, Hoyt, & Huck, 1993). As integenerational relationships and caregiving are reciprocal (Parke, 1988), the actual return of the grandparent to the role of a full-time parent is likely to have an impact not only on the middle-aged or older person but also on the child for whom he or she is now responsible.

Given that grandchildren often faced adverse circumstances in their original homes, it is sometimes believed that such children, who present with a host of mental and behavioral problems (Schwartz, 1994), may require mental health intervention. However, little research exists as to the prevalence of mental health problems in grandchildren raised by custodial grandparents or on psychological treatments obtained for these children. In general, childhood disorders are classified into two major dimensions of behavior problems (Achenbach, 1995). The first dimension has been labeled *undercontrolled* or *externalizing* and includes various acting-out, disruptive, delinquent, hyperactive, and aggressive behaviors. The second broad dimension of childhood behavior problems has been labeled *overcontrolled* or *internalizing* and includes such behaviors as social withdrawal, anxiety, and depression (Achenbach, 1995). Given that externalizing problems tend to be much more disruptive to others, it is not surprising that these problems account for one third to one half of referrals to psychologists (Kazdin, Siegel, & Bass, 1990) and school mental health facilities (Atkins, McKay, Talbott, & Arvantis, 1996).

Behavioral problems in children are relatively common. In general, boys are more often diagnosed than girls, beginning in preschool and lasting throughout childhood (Costello et al., 1996; Costello, Farmer, Angold, Burns, & Erkanli, 1997), although this pattern shifts in adolescence to more equal rates of disorders between boys and girls or with girls showing higher rates of psychopathology (Simonoff et al., 1997; Verhulst, van der Ende, Ferdinand, & Kasius, 1997).

Although data from a large epidemiological sample indicate that children living with their custodial grandparents are at a greater risk of experiencing problems at school, compared to children residing with two biological parents, this does not appear to be due to living with a grandparent, as children living with one biological parent were more likely to experience school problems than children living with their grandparents (Solomon & Marx, 1995). No other study has explicitly investigated whether or not behavior and school problems are more prevalent in children living with custodial grandparents; thus, the prevalence in this population is unknown.

In addition, little is known about grandparents' perceptions of behavior problems in their grandchildren or in grandparents' willingness to obtain psychological services. The prevailing belief is that increasing numbers of grandparents are seeking psychological help for their grandchildren (e.g., Emick & Hayslip, 1996). Indeed, a community-recruited sample found that 40% of custodial grandparents had obtained therapeutic services for their grandchildren, with an additional 25% planning to seek mental health services in the immediate future (Shore & Hayslip, 1994). However, custodial grandparents may also minimize the need for intervention, hoping that the behavior problems will cease on their own (Emick & Hayslip, 1996).

Significantly, data show that grandparent-headed families are more likely to be African American, to be nonemployed, and to have fewer years of education compared to two-parent families and one-parent families (Solomon & Marx, 1995). In addition, both grandparent-headed households and single-parent households are more likely to live below the poverty line and have older children, compared to two-parent households (Solomon & Marx, 1995). Often, the consequences of these multiple stressors is a deterioration in the quality of life as well as the physical and mental health (Fuller-Thompson et al., 1997; Minkler, Roe, & Price, 1992; Shore & Hayslip, 1994) of the grandparents. Although some investigators have focused on the positive aspects of grandparenting (see Emick & Hayslip, 1996, for a review), the majority of the literature has focused on the stressors and negative consequences associated with custodial grandparenting.

As more research is devoted to the phenomenon of custodial grandparenting, more can be understood about the emotional and physical toll that grandparenting can take. However, several questions remain unanswered. First, few investigations have focused on the behavioral and emotional problems found in grandchildren living with custodial grandparents. Both Baker (chap. 9, this volume) and Silverthorn and Durrant (chap. 4, this volume) discuss the treatment of problem behaviors in grandchildren; and grandparenting self-help books (e.g., de Toledo & Brown, 1995; Takas, 1995) discuss what to do if grandchildren exhibit emotional or behavioral problems, but data are limited as to how many grandchildren are actually in need of such services. Although the perception is that more grandparents are seeking help for their grandchildren, this has not been empirically confirmed. A further problem in studying help-seeking and problematic grandchild behavior is a lack of precision; Solomon and Marx (1995) looked at broad categories, such as "obedient in school" and "behaved with teachers." A second and related unanswered question is whether behavior problems in grandchildren are related to grandparent sociodemographic factors, including physical health, social support, seeking services for the grandchild, and seeking services for themselves.

Research by Hayslip, Shore, Henderson, and Lambert (1998) and by Emick and Hayslip (1999) suggests that role meaning, role satisfaction, the quality of relationships with grandchildren, and coping skills are differentially affected by whether or not grandparents are raising their children. Importantly, grandparents raising problem grandchildren exhibiting a variety of behavioral, emotional or neurological problems were more negatively affected in the above ways than those raising grandchildren with few problems.

In this light, the purpose of the present study was to explore the determinants of custodial grandparents' perceptions of problems in their grandchildren, on the assumption that an understanding of such antecedents can better enable both researchers and service providers to identify more accurately both grandparents and grandchildren who are likely to have difficulties in their adjustment to a new family form, as well as to better enable such persons to design interventions that are either preventive or ameliorative in nature and that might help both generations.

SUBJECTS AND PROCEDURE

Participants in this study were drawn from 193 male and female grandparents solicited from the Dallas–Fort Worth area of Texas (see Hayslip et al., 1998). Those who parented their grandchildren were considered the custodial group ($n = 101$, M age = 54.6 years,

$SD = 8.2$). They were defined as those who had assumed physical and financial responsibility for a grandchild who was age 18 or younger and who lived in the grandparent's home. In no case, when queried, did respondents in the custodial grandparent group describe the extent of their caregiving responsibilities as "part-time" or "casual" in nature.

The custodial group of grandparents raising grandchildren who were in this study consisted of 21 males and 80 females. Eighty-three were Caucasian, 14 were African American, and 4 were Hispanic. Respondents ranged in age from 30 to 71 ($M = 54.82$, $SD = 7.87$). Self-rated health ranged from 1 (very poor) to 5 (very good) ($M = 3.72$, $SD = .95$). The age of the grandchild about whom the respondents completed the survey ranged from less than 1 year of age to 14 ($M = 7.20$, $SD = 2.34$). Sixty-nine of the grandchildren were male, and 32 were female. Eleven of the 101 grandparents in this group coresided with their adult children as well as the grandchild they were raising. They had been raising their children for an average of approximately 4.5 years ($M = 4.32$, $SD = 2.47$).

The circumstances under which grandparents assumed responsibility for their grandchildren included divorce; incarceration; mental, emotional, or physical impairment of the parent; death of the parent; child abuse; or parents' drug abuse. Divorce, child abuse, and parents' emotional disturbance and drug abuse were the most common.

A measure of social support from the adult child, other family, and friends was created by summing perceptions of the extent (1 = none, to 5 = a great deal) to which such persons provided 11 different types of assistance, resulting in a 33-item scale assessing the extent of such support from others (alpha = .82).

Motives for the grandparent's assuming the parental role were operationally defined in terms of Likert ratings for 8 items defined in terms of 3 subsets: (1) *self-oriented* (4 items): making up for past mistakes as a parent, wanting to demonstrate that one had learned how to parent over the years, wanting to show that one was a better parent than the adult, feeling obligated to take the child when no one else would; (2) *child-oriented* (2 items): wanting to keep the child in the family in lieu of foster care, wanting to nurture the relationship with the grandchild; and (3) *parent-oriented* (2 items): wanting to allow the parents to get back on their feet before they resumed parenting, wanting to get back at the parents for the pain they had inflicted.

Respondents also were asked about the nature of professional help they had sought to cope with difficulties associated with raising a grandchild (e.g., formal grandparent support groups, individual or family therapy).

Antecedent conditions that were seen by the grandparent as giving rise to the assumption of the grandchild's care were operationalized in terms of (1) parental impairment, in a physical, emotional, or intellectual sense; (2) incarceration of the parent; (3) parental divorce; (4) parental death; (5) abuse of the child (child neglect, sexual abuse, physical abuse); and (6) parental self-abuse via drugs or alcohol. For parental impairment (3 items), parental self-abuse (2 items), and child abuse (3 items), scores were created by adding the dichotomous ratings (applies/does not apply) together; for parental divorce, death, or incarceration, single dichotomous items defined each.

Of central concern to the present study were the grandparent's responses to questions regarding the extent to which their grandchildren manifested nine specific problem behaviors and one additional general category in which grandparents wrote in problems and behaviors not listed in the questionnaire. Respondents rated the problem behaviors (9 specific problems in addition to an "other" category) on a continuum of severity (1 = no problem, to 5 = severe problem) (see Hayslip et al., 1998).

RESULTS

Utilizing the Likert ratings (outlined above) of the severity/intensity of behavioral, emotional, and neurological problems as dependent variables, a series of stepwise regression analyses were carried out to explore the determinants of such ratings by custodial grandparents in this sample ($N = 101$). Independent variables were, in each case, the grandparent's level of education (in years), grandparent self-rated health, grandparent age, grandparent gender, perceived social support in carrying out parental responsibilities, whether the grandparent had sought help for himself or herself, whether the grandparent had sought help for the grandchild, antecedents giving rise to the assumption of parenting (see above), and motives for becoming a parent again (see above). For each perceived problem variable, the overall regression equation was statistically different from zero (minimum $F = 7.09$, $p < .01$), suggesting that the predictors as a set were, in each case, substantively related to grandparents' perceptions of problem behaviors in the grandchildren they were raising.

These analyses specifically suggested (see Table 15.1) that for alcohol problems and drug use, self-oriented reasons for becoming a custodial grandparent best predicted ($p < .05$) such difficulties, whereas having sought help for the grandchild and poorer grandparent health predicted ratings of oppositional behavior. Having sought help for the grandchild also best predicted the severity/intensity of hyperactivity, learning difficulties, and altercations with the law.

TABLE 15.1   Predictors of Problem Behaviors in Grandchildren ($N = 101$)

Dependent Variable	Predictor	Beta
Alcohol	Motives: self-improvement	.26**
Drugs	Motives: self-improvement	.26**
Oppositional behavior	Seek help—Gc	.49**
	GP health	−.20*
Mental retardation	Social support	.31**
Hyperactivity	Seek help—Gc	.53**
	Reasons: child abuse	.21*
	GP health	−.17*
Sexual identity	Reasons: jail	.42**
	Reasons: parent impairment	.24**
Learning difficulties	Seek help—Gc	.48**
	GP health	−.27**
	Motives: self-improvement	.31**
	Social support	.17*
	Reasons: Gc's parent	−.17*
Depression	GP gender	−.33**
	Reasons: parent abuse	.23*
GC-law	Seek help—Gc	.26**
Other	Seek help—GP	.33**
All behaviors	Seek help—Gc	.49**
	GP health	−.34**
	Motives: self-improvement	.25**

*$p < .05$.
**$p < .01$.

Poorer grandparent health was also related to hyperactivity and learning difficulties. Reasons giving rise to the assumption of the parental role (related to the inability of the parent to function for a variety of reasons) predicted difficulties in the grandchild's sexual identity and depression, and negative feelings regarding the grandchild's parent predicted learning difficulties. Only for hyperactivity did child abuse predict problem severity. Regarding grandparent demographic characteristics, male grandparents were less likely to perceive depression as a problem in their grandchildren than were females. For the overall index incorporating all problem behaviors (computed as a linear sum of each), having sought help for the grandchild, poorer grandparent health, and wanting to be a better parent predicted problem intensity.

In a smaller, independent sample of 51 custodial grandparents (12 males, 39 females; M age = 56.41) (see Emick & Hayslip, 1999), results (see Table 15.2) were somewhat similar to those reported above, especially regarding the overall index of problems; having sought help for the grandchild also best predicted ($p < .05$) problem

TABLE 15.2   Predictors of Problem Behaviors in Grandchildren ($N = 51$)

Dependent Variable	Predictor	Beta
Alcohol	Reasons: parental impairment	.32*
Drugs		
Oppositional behavior	Gc's parent	.40**
	Health	−.32*
Mental retardation		
Hyperactivity	Seek help—Gc	.52***
	GP age	−.33**
	Social support	−.26*
Sexual identity	Reasons: parental impairment	.47**
Learning difficulties	Motives: self-improvement	−.31*
Depression	Reasons: parental divorce	.49**
GC-law	Gc's parent	.31*
Other	Seek Help—Gc	.29*
All behaviors	Seek Help—Gc	.51**
	Reasons: parental divorce	.28*
	Motives: self-improvement	.25**

*$p < .05$.
**$p < .01$.

severity. This was also true for hyperactivity and the other miscellaneous problem category. Parental impairment best predicted problems with alcohol and sexual identity, and poorer grandparent health predicted oppositional behavior. However, in contrast to the above, positive feelings toward the grandchild's parent predicted problem severity for oppositional behavior and altercations with the law, and less social support was related to higher hyperactivity ratings. Additionally in this regard, wanting to improve as a parent negatively predicted the severity of learning difficulties. Interestingly, in this smaller sample, parental divorce was related to perceived severity of grandchild depression and greater overall problem severity. In this sample, younger grandparent age was related to greater perceived hyperactivity.

Given the salience of help seeking in the above regression analyses, we further explored its role in influencing perceptions of grandchild problems via treating—having sought help for either one's grandchild or oneself—in dichotomous terms, utilizing a one-way MANOVA. These analyses suggested that for the linear combination of problem behaviors, the effects of having sought help for a grandchild were substantial, multivariate $F(10, 91) = 8.82$, $p < .01$, as were the effects of having sought help for oneself, multivariate $F(10, 91) = 1.92$, $p < .05$. The effects of having sought help for the grandchild (favoring those who had done so) were strongest for oppositional behavior, hyperactivity, learning difficulties, depression, and altercations with the law.

For help seeking regarding the grandparent, such effects were most substantive for oppositional behavior, learning difficulties, and other miscellaneous problems, favoring those who had sought help. For the overall index of problem behaviors, the effects of help seeking for the grandchild, $F(1, 100) = 46.23$, $p < .01$, were substantial, favoring having done so ($M = 18.14$ vs. $M = 12.06$). This was also true for having sought help for oneself, $F(1, 100) = 7.79$ ($M = 16.17$ vs. $M = 13.29$).

When this MANOVA was replicated for the smaller sample of 51 custodial grandparents, the multivariate effect of help seeking for the grandchild was again a powerful one, $F(10, 41) = 6.43$, $p < .01$, with greater problem severity scores linked to having sought help for drug use, oppositional behavior, hyperactivity, learning difficulties, difficulties with the law, and other miscellaneous problems. For having sought help for oneself, such effects were considerably attenuated at the multivariate level ($p > .05$). For overall problem behaviors, severity ratings favored those who had sought help for the grandchild, $F(1, 50) = 17.29$ ($M = 17.30$ vs. $M = 11.71$), whereas such effects were weakened considerably regarding having sought help for oneself ($p < .07$), though they still favored those who had sought help.

DISCUSSION

These findings, utilizing both the larger ($N = 101$) and smaller ($N = 51$) samples, suggest that a variety of factors are associated with the rated severity and intensity of problem behaviors among grandchildren being raised by their grandparents. Perhaps most apparent is the relationship between having sought help for the grandchild and the greater perceived severity of difficulties whose manifestations are externalized (e.g., learning difficulties, hyperactivity, and oppositional behavior). This was also the case when an overall index of problems was created, wherein having sought help for the grandchild was related to greater overall problem severity in both samples. This may reflect the extent to which such behavior problems actively interfere with the grandchild's relationships with either peers or teachers or with the grandparent himself or herself. Thus, such problems are more likely to warrant a decision to seek professional help for the grandchild to the extent that such behavior brings the child into conflict with others at school or in the community at large, interferes with school performance, or makes more difficult the task of raising the grandchild.

Significantly, greater perceived severity of such behaviors, as well as overall problem severity, is associated with poorer grandparent health, substantiating the negative impact on grandparents of having to deal with such grandchildren, a finding that has been observed by Burton (1992), Minkler, Roe, and Price (1992), Emick and Hayslip (1999), and Hayslip et al. (1998) in both African American and Caucasian samples of custodial grandparents.

In contrast, having sought help for oneself was less strongly related to perceptions of problem severity in the larger sample of custodial grandparents and unrelated to problem severity in the smaller sample. This not only likely exacerbates the personal impact on role satisfaction, relationship quality, and well-being of having to raise a grandchild with a variety of behavioral or emotional difficulties (see Emick & Hayslip, 1999), but it also intensifies the negative impact on one's health (see above).

That having sought help for the grandchild and not oneself predicted problem severity may also reflect the suitability of turning to others outside the family for help or the perceived availability of such help. In this respect, older persons are believed to be notoriously reluctant to seek help for themselves (see Knight, 1996). This may further isolate them from their age peers who are not raising their grandchildren (Shore & Hayslip, 1994). In addition, they may lack knowledge about appropriate sources of professional help regarding both the diagnosis and treatment of behavior disorders in their grandchildren, as well as being unskilled in behavior management techniques (see Emick & Hayslip, 1999).

At the same time, both a desire to be a better parent and feeling a personal obligation to raise the grandchild was related to greater drug/alcohol abuse problem severity and overall problem severity; this was more apparent in the large sample than in the small sample. In concert with the fact that the circumstances giving rise to custodial grandparenting also related to problem severity, one can easily understand why persons may feel that they have failed as parents yet are desirous of doing a better job with their grandchildren. Moreover, they may feel somewhat responsible for raising an adult child whose very behavior undermines the well-being of the grandchildren, leading to the adult child's being unable to parent adequately.

These data are, of course, limited in that they lacked independently gathered, confirmatory data speaking not only to the presence or absence of difficulties in the grandchildren but also to the severity of such difficulties if they existed at all. Moreover, sampling error, particularly with regard to the smaller sample, may explain the inconsistencies between studies regarding the predictors of problem severity, as well the direction of such relationships.

Despite the above limitations, these data clearly suggest that the determinants of grandparents' perceptions of problems in the grandchildren they are raising are best understood in the context of the availability of help for problems whose manifestations are in varying degrees externalized in nature, as well as the grandparent's views about the emotional, relationship, and health-related costs and benefits of custodial grandparenting. These data also clearly signal the necessity for greater efforts at educating grandparents about the mental health system so that both accurate and timely diagnosis and treatment of their grandchildren's difficulties can be realized. They also argue for research establishing the efficacy of therapeutic interventions that are aimed at either the grandparent or the grandchild. Last, they suggest that greater attention to the development and coordination of community-based services that provide grandparents with a respite from their parental roles (Burton, 1992; Grant, Gordon, & Cohen, 1997) so that they might lead more enriching lives is clearly warranted.

REFERENCES

Achenbach, T. M. (1995). Empirically based assessment and taxonomy: Applications to clinical research. *Psychological Assessment, 7,* 261–274.

Atkins, M. S., McKay, M. M., Talbott, E., & Arvantis, P. (1996). DSM-IV diagnosis of conduct disorder and oppositional defiant disorder: Implications and guidelines for school mental health teams. *School Psychology Review, 25,* 274–283.

Burton, L. M. (1992). Black grandparents rearing children of drug-addicted parents: Stressors, outcomes, and social service needs. *Gerontologist, 32,* 744–751.

Costello, E. J., Angold, A., Burns, B. J., Stangl, D. K., Tweed, D. L., Erkanli, A., & Worthman, C. M. (1996). The Great Smoky Mountains study of youth: Goals, design, methods, and the prevalence of DSM-III-R disorders. *Archives of General Psychiatry, 53,* 1129–1136.

Costello, E. J., Farmer, E. M., Angold, A., Burns, B. J., & Erkanli, A. (1997). Psychiatric disorders among American Indian and White youth in Appalachia: The Great Smoky Mountains study. *American Journal of Public Health, 87,* 827–832.

de Toledo, S., & Brown, D. E. (1995). *Grandparents are parents: A survival guide for raising a second family.* New York: Guilford.

Emick, M., & Hayslip, B. (1996). Custodial grandparenting: New roles for middle aged and older adults. *International Journal of Aging and Human Development, 43,* 135–154.

Emick, M., & Hayslip, B. (1999). Custodial grandparenting: Stresses, coping skills, and relationships with grandchildren. *International Journal of Aging and Human Development, 48,* 35–61.

Flint, M. M., & Perez-Porter, M. (1997). Grandparent caregivers: Legal and economic issues. *Journal of Gerontological Social Work, 28,* 63–76.

Fuller-Thompson, E., Minkler, M., & Driver, D. (1997). A profile of grandparents raising grandchildren in the United States. *Gerontological Society of America, 37,* 406–411.

Grant, R., Gordon, S. G., & Cohen, S. T. (1997). An innovative school-based intergenerational model to serve grandparent caregivers. *Journal of Gerontological Social Work, 28,* 47–61.

Hayslip, B., Shore, R. J., Henderson, C., & Lambert, P. (1998). Custodial grandparenting and the impact of grandchildren with problems on role meaning. *Journal of Gerontology: Social Sciences, 53B,* S164–S174.

Kazdin, A. E., Siegel, T. C., & Bass, D. (1990). Drawing on clinical practice to inform research on child and adolescent psychotherapy: Survey of practitioners. *Professional Psychology: Research and Practice, 2,* 1189–1198.

Knight, B. (1996). *Psychotherapy with older adults.* Thousand Oaks, CA: Sage.

Minkler, M., Roe, K. M., & Price, M. (1992). The physical and emotional health of grandmothers raising grandchildren in the crack cocaine epidemic. *Gerontologist, 32,* 752–761.

Parke, R. (1988). Families in lifespan perspective: A multilevel, developmental approach. In M. Hetherington, R. M. Lerner, & M. Perlmutter (Eds.), *Child development in the lifespan perspective* (pp. 49–68). Hillsdale, NJ: Erlbaum.

Schwartz, L. L. (1994). The challenge of raising one's nonbiological children. *American Journal of Family Therapy, 22,* 195–207.

Shore, R. J., & Hayslip, B. (1994). Custodial grandparenting: Implications for children's development. In A. Gottfried & A. Gottfried (Eds.), *Redefining families: Implications for children's development* (pp. 171–218). New York: Plenum.

Simonoff, E., Pickles, A., Meyer, J. M., Silberg, J. L., Maes, H. H., Loeber, R., Rutter, M., Hewitt, J. K., & Eaves, L. J. (1997). The Virginia twin study of adolescent behavioral development: Influences of age, sex, and impairment of rates of disorders. *Archives of General Psychiatry, 54,* 801–808.

Solomon, J. C., & Marx, J. (1995). "To grandmother's house we go": Health and school adjustment of children raised solely by grandparents. *Gerontologist, 35,* 386–394.

Takas, M. (1995). *Grandparents raising grandchildren: A guide to finding help and hope.* Crystal Lake, IL: Brookdale Foundation Group.

Verhulst, F. C., van der Ende, J., Ferdinand, R. F., & Kasius, M. C. (1997). The prevalence of DSM-III-R diagnoses in a national sample of Dutch adolescents. *Archives of General Psychiatry, 54,* 329–336.

Whitbeck, L. B., Hoyt, D. R., & Huck, S. M. (1993). Family relationship history, contemporary parent-grandparent relationship quality, and the grandparent-grandchild relationship. *Journal of Marriage and the Family*, *55*, 1025–1035.

Woodworth, R. S. (1996). You're not alone . . . you're one in a million. *Child Welfare*, *5*, 619–635.

CHAPTER 16

When Grandparents Raise Grandchildren Due to Substance Abuse: Responding to a Uniquely Destabilizing Factor

Barbara A. Hirshorn, Mary Jane Van Meter, and Diane R. Brown

In many cases grandparents or grandparent figures, some as young as their early 30s and as old as their late 80s, are raising grandchildren by themselves when the parents of the children are substance-abusing and either unable or unwilling to rear their offspring (e.g., Anglin, 1990; Burton, 1992; Minkler & Roe, 1993; Minkler, Roe, & Price, 1992). As with many parenting grandparents in the United States, they experience personal developmental issues related to life course change and identity as well as challenges regarding complex social networks and lack of formal support from the public and nonprofit sectors. However, for this population of grandparents, such issues often are intensified by additional stressors stemming from the behavior of the substance-abusing adult child whose offspring they are raising. Indeed, because of the adult child's behavior, they may be perpetually off-balance, prevented from acting in a planful, purposeful way and forced to react continually to situations beyond their own control.

These grandparent caregivers are the target population of an intervention, described in this chapter. The intervention was piloted for 2 years (mid-1995 to mid-1997) at three sites in the Detroit, Michigan, metropolitan area and for 1 year in Columbia, South Carolina, and is now being finalized for national dissemination.

This chapter explores (a) the theoretical underpinning of the project's intervention, (b) the project's design components, (c) the outcome of the intervention on participating grandparent and grandparent figures, and (d) the mechanics of implementing the intervention—issues related to "fit."

APPLYING A CONCEPTUAL FRAMEWORK IN AN INTERVENTION

Boundary Ambiguity

Minuchin (1974) argued that boundaries must be well defined to allow members to carry out their functions without interference. Uncertainty regarding boundaries in the family generally indicates a pattern of unclear and possibly ambiguous norms, roles, rules, and relationships (Boss, 1988; Boss & Greenburg, 1984). This uncertainty may reflect any or all of the following: the individual's lack of organizing skills, uncertainty regarding how to exert control, not knowing how to set rules and responsibilities for others, an inability to plan one's own present or future because of unexpected circumstances of unknown duration, or the loss of self as a result of role engulfment—as when a care provider gives up other important roles and loses social contacts because of the urgency and primacy of the care role (Skaff & Pearlin, 1992).

Generally, for the families in this intervention, boundary ambiguity existed in three areas:

1. *The psychological and/or physical presence of the adult child who parented the grandchildren.* The existence and degree of family members' boundary ambiguity is determined by the congruence between their perception of who is in and who is outside the family with the physical reality of who is in or out of that family system (McCubbin & Patterson, 1983). Boss (1988) points out that the issue of ambiguous family boundaries is most salient at times of transition or change, especially when an individual leaves the family. Equilibrium is then restored either physically—when that individual returns to resume a former position (e.g., a POW father) or when someone else replaces that individual (e.g., mother's remarriage brings a new father)—or perceptually, when family members reconcile themselves to the loss or vacated roles are reassigned to other members.

In contrast, in families in which grandparents are raising the children of substance-abusing adult offspring, hope may exist indefinitely that the adult child will overcome the addiction and resume the role of a functioning parent. Furthermore, the situation may include periods of either perceptual or physical presence. The adult child may continue an on-again/off-again physical presence by periodically appearing at the grandparent's home, particularly when funds are low. Psychologically, at these times the adult child may reengage emotional feelings of loyalty and love from both children and parent(s) despite an inability or unwillingness to assume any real commitment to them. In short, the child-rearing grandparent in this family is never certain when the adult child may reappear or how that individual will play upon the emotions of the young children or upset household rules and routines. Because there is neither a distinct presence nor absence, either physically or perceptually, of the drug-addicted middle generation, boundaries regarding family roles, norms, and the allocation of resources remain ambiguous for all in the household unit, including the grandchildren.

2. *The duration of the child-rearing role for the grandparent.* Although periods of boundary ambiguity are inevitable over the life course of most families, there is an expected duration and outcome to this ambiguity. Even when grandparents raise grandchildren because parents are looking for employment in another geographic area or

as a result of mental illness or death, they typically can assume the new parenting role with some degree of confidence as to its duration. In contrast, grandparents with drug-abusing adult children are often unsure when they can expect to reach closure on their child-raising responsibilities. Indeed, part of the ambiguity lies in *not knowing* whether or not the adult child will bear additional children for whom the grandparent may feel compelled to provide care at some undefined future point(s). This precludes any anticipation of how long the child-raising role will last.

An additional layer of ambiguity lies in *not knowing* if the substance-abusing adult child will come to terms with her or his addiction at some point and attain the level of stability that would allow her or him to assume parenting responsibilities again. For the grandparent, then, these contingent behaviors of the substance-abusing adult child preclude any anticipation of how long the child-raising role will last.

3. *The uncertain existence and level of formal or informal support.* These grandparents often are unsure that they can rely on either the formal health and social service sector or other family members or friends for varied forms of assistance. Many in preliminary focus groups described diminished contact with friends and relations who were wary of involvement in situations with nonrecovering addictive individuals and were even disparaging of the grandparents for assuming the roles and responsibilities that they had. Also reported were government bureaucracies often indifferent or even hostile to their efforts at seeking assistance. Thus, for many, the caretaking role is not only physically demanding and emotionally stressful but also socially isolating and financially depleting.

Self-Management

Rule setting as well as goal setting and goal accomplishment are necessary to reduce boundary ambiguity and are enhanced by organizational capabilities and intentional assertive behavior directed at promoting one's own welfare. Self-management is a process by which these grandparents can set the necessary household rules and goals for the family and self. An adaptation of the concepts of management and family management (Deacon & Firebaugh, 1981; Gross, Crandall, & Knoll, 1973), self-management is purposeful behavior employed in the development or use of resources (personal qualities and material) to achieve one's goals.

In this context, where "self" refers to the grandparent, these tasks must include organizing (preparing the self) as well as planning (rule and goal setting) and implementation. A second program goal, then, is to assist grandparents to achieve a new sense of self-management, both as full-time caretakers of young children and as architects of their own lives. In this way, they may develop a new perception of their responsibilities that may be less stressful.

A command of these processes is especially important in situations involving others who are substance-abusing and who may never alter their own behavior. Indeed, grandparents assuming responsibility for raising the offspring of substance-abusing adult children may find themselves in circumstances that deplete personal and material resources. Moreover, they are unlikely to have anticipated the extent and kinds of stresses these responsibilities would introduce into their own lives.

A practical, adaptive response, therefore, is for these individuals to learn self-management skills that enable them to assess and alter, if necessary, aspects of their own lives, thereby enhancing their own well-being and that of the young children they are raising. These aspects include: behavior toward the addicted adult child, the perspective these grandparents have of their roles and responsibilities within the extended network of family and friends, how they organize and use time and other resources, and their personal goals.

Self-management skills, by reducing boundary ambiguity and promoting the ability of grandparents to take charge of their own lives, can enhance the personal well-being of the grandparent directly, the interactions between the grandparent and the children she or he is raising, the atmosphere in the home environment, and interactions between the family unit and members of the outside world (extended family, friends, schools, social service providers, etc.). Indeed, the acquisition of these personal skills, by leading to greater clarity regarding family roles and resources and greater internal locus of control for the grandparent, can produce a greater feeling of security among the young children in the household.

Family and Neighborhood Systems

Systems theory served as the general theoretic framework for both the grandparent-headed household and the extended multigenerational family. First, the grandparent was viewed as the "entry point" to the interpersonal dynamics in a three- (or more) generation family system in which one individual, the substance-abuser in the middle generation, was having a very destabilizing impact on the larger multigenerational family unit. Thus, potentially, family members across more than one household unit may be affected and destabilized.

Additionally, key to the establishment and sustainability of the project was anchoring the family system in its respective environmental context—a specific neighborhood/community's geographic and social setting. This larger neighborhood system is the context in which the family carries out the majority of its daily social and resource exchange activities. Moreover, informal social networks, local community agencies, and church-based organizations are most likely to be in the immediate geographic environment. The intervention utilized these social units to (a) serve as a base from which to access other local units for participant recruitment (e.g., schools, local news media), (b) provide a mechanism for enhancing program institutionalization over the long run, and (c) provide "home grown" program advisors and "boosters" during the developmental stage (Hirshorn, Van Meter, & Sanders, 1997).

PROJECT DESIGN COMPONENTS

The 10-Week Core Learning Program

The program was designed to meet once weekly for 2 hours. Because the participants were adults and had varying educational backgrounds, sessions were interactive rather than didactic. Group leaders, or facilitators, who were either staff members or affiliates of the participating community-based organizations, posed questions, elicited experiential information from participants, and directed discussion by introducing new concepts and ideas. Throughout the 10-session program the emphasis was on developing problem-solving skills that can be generalized to applications in future situations. The curriculum focused on the following issues:

Family Roles: Exploring the roles of individual family members in the grandparent-headed household; the disparity between expected and existing behaviors of individual family members; and attendant feelings when those roles are unfulfilled.

Clarification of Boundary Ambiguity: Developing an understanding of boundaries related to family roles, rules, and norms and the steps necessary to assure that personal and familial boundaries are clear, particularly in applications supporting the healthy functioning of grandparent-headed households formed as a result of substance abuse.

Assertiveness—Self-Management: Developing the ability to set and maintain boundaries by using assertiveness skills in the context of a caring family while also meeting one's own needs and maintaining personal rights.

Positive Home Environment: Creating an understanding of the importance of a caring family environment and the ways to achieve it. Emphasis is placed on how praise, communication, and observation can reduce unacceptable behavior; identifying some of the behaviors of children who have been abused and/or neglected; dealing with anger; effective listening techniques, especially concerning children; and steps in problem solving.

Developing Support: Analyzing one's current social support network and the possible need for change, as well as finding new sources of support.

Setting Personal Goals: Encouraging participants to learn the steps of good decision making, as these apply to goal setting, and to recognize barriers to achievement and learn techniques for overcoming those barriers.

Expanding Personal Horizons: Developing problem-solving skills related to finding new opportunities for employment, retirement, education, self-enrichment, and learning how to access resources to further personal endeavors.

During the 2-year pilot phase, class size was limited to a maximum of 12 participants to permit optimal group interaction. However, most iterations of the intervention during the pilot phase contained between 7 and 10 participants. Free child care (either on-site or through a baby-sitter) and transportation to and from the intervention site were options for all participants. A "graduation luncheon" for those who had completed at least 8 of the 10 program sessions, celebrated the accomplishment with certificates of completion, symbolic gifts, such as mugs or T-shirts, and, in one instance, extensive media coverage.

During the first year of the pilot the intervention was offered in the Detroit, Michigan, metropolitan area in three ethnically distinct settings (Latino, African American, and Caucasian) to allow for cultural customization, if and when needed, and the sharing of confidences within cultural subgroups. During the second pilot year the intervention was offered in Detroit as well as in Columbia, South Carolina, in ethnically heterogeneous settings for reasons discussed presently.

Partnership with Community-based Organizations

For the project design phase, underpinning the choice of community-based organizational partners was the need to find appropriate venues to recruit grandparents of particular cultural backgrounds. Three community-based social service organizations in the Detroit area worked with the project during its first pilot year, each identifying program participants and a facilitator to implement the learning program intervention and designating staff members responsible for local recruitment through the organization's client base or outreach efforts. These organizations, although all community-based, had varied goals: the provision of community mental health services, church-based community development, and emergency services provision. During the second pilot year, in Detroit, two of these organizations continued to work with the project, and another was added.

In contrast, the Columbia, South Carolina, site, added during the second pilot year, was the county department of social services. Working through this site offered the singular opportunity of partnering with a complementary program that focused on substance-abusing women, 15 to 44 years old, with offspring typically living with grandparents or grandparent figures. Therefore, at this site all but one of the participants were recruited directly from relatives of this client base.

Advisory Board Input

At the onset of the first pilot year, getting the project on sound footing required forming and meeting with an advisory board composed of representatives of the three community-based sites, additional representatives from each specific culture (Latino, Caucasian, and African American), and project investigators. These meetings provided essential feedback validating the design of the learning program's basic curriculum, its pace and timing, issues to consider regarding its potential reception by individuals of different cultural backgrounds, the recruitment process, and the content of resources provided to participants (e.g., an annotated local directory of formal services).

Evaluation Procedure

The intent of the project's formative evaluation was to record and analyze the impact of various components of the project on the design and implementation of the learning program—the intervention. Formative evaluation tasks included collecting information from site-based staff regarding intervention implementation and from learning program facilitators regarding presentation and content; getting feedback from program participants regarding course organization, content, delivery, and so on; and getting input from advisory group members regarding learning program development (Herskovitz, 1996).

The purpose of the outcome evaluation was to document the extent to which participation in the learning experience provided grandparents with skills that reduce boundary ambiguity and promote self-management, thereby enhancing personal well-being.

The outcome evaluation design included a pre- and posttest collection of information that tested the following hypotheses:

1. *The learning program will improve grandparent self-management skills.* The analysis will ascertain significant differences on indicators of self-management skills at T1 (pretest) in comparison with T2 (posttest).

2. *The learning program will reduce boundary ambiguity among grandparents.* Scores on boundary ambiguity measures will also be compared at T1 and T2.

3. *The learning program will improve personal well-being among grandparents.* Measures of mental health will be examined to determine significant differences between T1 and T2.

This study could have been designed so that a control group of at-risk grandparents was administered both the pretest and posttest instruments. However, that structure also would have provided participating researchers with distinct ethical challenges given the known crisis-ridden lives these grandparents lead.

THE OUTCOME EVALUATION

The pretest instrument included measures in five major areas: (1) demography and household structure, including a household roster and family network for each child 18 years old or younger in the participant's household; (2) personal and family background; (3) mental and physical health, including the National Center for Health Statistics' 1992 checklist of physical conditions, Radloff's 1977 CES-D mental health scale, and measures of the physical health and disabilities of resident offspring of the substance-abusing adult child; (4) boundary ambiguity measured by an adaptation of a scale developed by Boss, Greenberg, and Pearce-McCall (1990); and (5) self-management skills, measured by a newly developed scale.

Forty-five of the 50 participants over the 2-year period were female. Participants were normally distributed between 30 and 60 years of age, although 23 (46%) were in their 40s. Half (25) were self-identified as African American, 30% (15) as Caucasian, 7 (14%) as Hispanic; and two others as American Indian. Forty-two percent had completed high school; equal proportions had either less than a high school education (28%) or more than a high school education (30%). Nearly one-half (23 participants) were currently married.

The pretest instrument was reviewed by the advisory board and piloted with grandparents from each target ethnic group who would *not* be participants in the learning program. The instrument was then administered to program participants by central project staff during an approximately 1-month period prior to the onset of the 10-week program implementation. Project staff scheduled individual appointments for pretest administration at the community-based site at a time convenient to the grandparent and provided transportation and day care if necessary.

Following the 10th and last session of the learning program, central project staff reinterviewed participants by telephone, asking a subset of the questions in the pretest. (These interviews were always conducted prior to the focus group assessment of the curriculum, as indicated above in the formative evaluation.) The posttest instrument measured change in (1) household composition and parenting circumstances, (2) current mental and physical health, (3) boundary ambiguity, and (4) self-management skills.

RESULTS

The primary outcome of 2 years of piloting the intervention was evidence of the success of the learning program curriculum as a mechanism for assisting this particular population of grandparents, those with substance-abusing adult children, in managing their lives. Data analyses indicate that the intervention was successful. (See Tables 16.1–16.3.)

For measures of boundary ambiguity, self-management skills, and mental health, mean scores were computed at the two points in time (T1 within 1 month of the first session of the intervention and T2 within 2 weeks of the last session) to assess program impact. Table 16.1 presents the means differences in three scaled measures of participant well-being (boundary ambiguity, self-management skills, and mental health as measured by the CES-D) for Year 1 participants. Table 16.2 presents the same information for Year 2 participants; Table 16.3, for both pilot years' participants combined.

The following hypotheses were tested:

TABLE 16.1   Project Year 1 Mean Differences in Participant Measures of Well-Being from Pretest (Time 1) to Posttest (Time 2) ($n = 22$)

| Variable | Pretest | | Posttest | | | | | |
	M	*SD*	*M*	*SD*	*t*	*p* Value	r_{12}	*p* Value
BA[a]	50.90	9.76	43.64	7.58	−3.62	<.01	.46	<.05
SM[b]	46.34	6.44	48.24	6.50	1.27	n.s.	.41	<.1
CES-D[c]	17.48	11.69	13.27	12.96	1.94	<.1	.66	<.05

[a]BA, boundary ambiguity. Responses are within the range 1 to 5 for a total possible score of 85 for 17 items. Higher scores indicate greater BA.
[b]SM, self-management. Responses are within the range 1 to 4 for a possible total of 64 for 16 items. Higher scores indicate a better sense of SM.
[c]CES-D is a measure of stress experienced during the previous week. Responses are within the range 0 to 3 for a possible total of 60 for 20 items. Higher scores indicate more stress.

TABLE 16.2   Project Year 2 Mean Differences in Participant Measures of Well-Being from Pretest (Time 1) to Posttest (Time 2)

| Variable | Pretest | | Posttest | | | | | |
	M	*SD*	*M*	*SD*	*t*	*p* Value	r_{12}	*p* Value
BA[a] ($n = 26$)	47.95	6.72	45.12	6.99	1.91	<.1	.39	<.05
SM[b] ($n = 25$)	46.59	8.56	48.84	8.02	2.11	<.05	.80	<.01
CES-D[c] ($n = 26$)	21.91	8.84	20.23	7.18	1.16	n.s.	.59	<.01

[a,b,c]See footnotes for Table 16.1

TABLE 16.3   Project Years 1 and 2 Combined Mean Differences in Participant Measures of Well-Being from Pretest (Time 1) to Posttest (Time 2)

| Variable | Pretest | | Posttest | | | | | |
	M	*SD*	*M*	*SD*	*t*	*p* Value	r_{12}	*p* Value
BA[a] ($n = 48$)	51.87	9.28	48.55	8.08	2.53	<.05	.47	<.01
SM[b] ($n = 47$)	46.42	7.25	48.11	6.93	1.87	<.1	.62	<.01
CES-D[c] ($n = 48$)	19.88	10.37	17.04	10.71	2.24	<.05	.66	<.01

[a,b,c]See footnotes for Table 16.1

1. *The learning program will improve grandparent self-management skills.* This was true for the Year 2 grandparents as a group ($p < .05$). For the combined Year 1 and Year 2 group of participants, self-management skills improved but at a lower level of statistical significance, ($p < .10$), due to two Year 1 outlier individuals whose personal lives became markedly worse during the time of the intervention.
2. *The learning program will reduce boundary ambiguity among grandparents.* For Year 1 participants as a group this was true ($p < .1$). It was true, as well, for Year 2 grandparents as a group but statistically significant at only the $p < .10$ level. However, the impact was greater for the combined group of Year 1 and Year 2 participants ($p < .05$).
3. *The learning program will improve personal well being among grandparents.* For Year 1 participants as a group this was true for emotional well-being ($p < .10$). There was no statistically significant change in emotional health for the Year 2 participants alone, but for the combined group of Year 1 and Year 2 participants a positive impact was statistically significant ($p < .05$).

An indirect measure of impact on participants was the information gained from focus groups held by an independent evaluator, with each group of participants following the 10-week learning program implementation. Although these were exploratory and actually implemented as part of the formative evaluation, results were extremely consistent. To a 5-point scaled question rating the program "overall," in which 1 was "poor" and 5 was "excellent," response was unanimous: "excellent" across ethnicity, site, geographic locale, and gender. Exemplary comments included: "good to find others in the same situation," generated "bonding," generated "sharing," "reinforces our own values" (Herskovitz, 1996).

Results indicated that personal empowerment was enhanced by an understanding of the concepts of individual and familial boundaries and the application of these concepts to one's own family context. Participants also learned to use effective listening skills and to implement assertive behavior to diffuse anger and aggressiveness among family members in situations that might otherwise escalate into more serious conflict. Moreover, they learned how to make purposeful decisions regarding self and the family unit; to solve complex problems related to parenting, the larger family unit, and the acquisition of formal support; and to follow through with action—all components of self-management.

THE MECHANICS OF IMPLEMENTING THE INTERVENTION: A QUESTION OF FIT

Several lessons were learned from interactions with on-site personnel. In the Detroit area, project core staff met frequently during the first pilot year with on-site personnel. These meetings took place both on a site-by-site basis at each of the three sites and with representatives of the three sites at once to plan the year's activities and to try to assure understanding of project goals and consistency and standardization of the intervention.

There were also several interviewer training and facilitator "interaction" sessions. The going assumption was that, although one cannot teach or train the facilitators involved in this project—each of whom had his or her own style and considerable experience—one could share knowledge and advice regarding implementation. These sessions also allowed the facilitators to bring up questions, discuss nuances in content and presentation, and ask for clarification. Additionally, core staff members were in frequent ongoing discussion with individuals at the three sites throughout the 2-year pilot phase (Hirshorn & Van Meter, 1996).

Because the Columbia, South Carolina, pilot ran during the second year only, with just one site involved, core staff–on-site staff interactions were streamlined. Site staff interacted frequently with core staff and called on site staff in the Detroit area for advice as needed.

Some methods of recruitment worked; others did not. By the end of the 2-year pilot phase it was also clear that program recruitment is best done by partnering with community sites that had a ready-made client base from which to pull potential participants (e.g., a state or local government entity such as the county department of social services; a community-based mental health organization). Otherwise, recruitment could be an enormous challenge, forcing one to pull from the community at large. For example, project efforts to recruit participants through probate court records, fliers distributed with holiday packages and at community centers and churches, articles in newspapers, although generating publicity, resulted in few program recruits (Herskovitz, 1997).

In contrast, a recruitment pool of potential participants who were already involved in a client population (or were related to or concerned with someone who was) were by that time "in the system" somewhere (e.g., the services of a community mental health organization, a community substance abuse treatment program, or a therapeutic program for abused children). Although their lives may have been crisis-driven, they were already identified. Moreover, some were also members of a family system in which another member (e.g., a special needs grandchild, an incarcerated or substance-abusing daughter) was engaged in a change-oriented intervention (Hirshorn, Van Meter, & Sanders, 1997).

In the Detroit area during the first year of the pilot, challenges to recruitment included the interplay of, on the one hand, the geographically widespread distances of the sites and, on the other hand, an initial implementation design that required participants of only one specified ethnic group in the learning program at a particular site (one for Latino participants only; another for Whites only; and the third for African Americans). The distance that prospective participants of the inappropriate background for a site located in their part of town would have to travel to reach the site with the appropriate ethnic group was definitely discouraging. Consequently, potential participants in the neighborhoods of another site on the other side of town (35 miles away) could not participate in the nearby intervention yet, understandably, were unwilling to travel to the other end of the metropolitan area to enroll.

Other potential participants did not enroll because of personal or social context issues. Denial of the problem of substance abuse or of the proportions and dimensions of the problem was still a factor among many potential enrollees of *all* ethnicities. Still others, on initial intake interview, clearly admitted to the problem but were unwilling to admit to it publicly (and thus "air dirty laundry"). For this latter group of potential but unrealized enrollees it was clear that there was a big difference between, on the one hand, awareness and, on the other hand, a commitment to self to do anything about one's situation.

Still another potential but often unrealized group of enrollees were those who were frank about their situation but either unwilling or unable to marshal the resources (emotional/energy/time) to make the commitment to a morning a week for 10 weeks. In the worst cases this may have led to a self-selecting triage, where those most in need of the intervention never could circumvent the crisis-driven nature of their lives long enough to enroll or to do anything else requiring purposeful planning (Hirshorn, Van Meter, & Sanders, 1997).

We also learned the importance of cultural customization, yet this was mitigated by the need to seek common cause. Our preliminary (preproject) focus groups with grandparents raising grandchildren due to substance abuse concentrated on African American subjects. The design of our project took into consideration conversations with service providers, in neighborhoods with other ethnic concentrations, who had convinced us that this was a growing family structure with common attendant issues. This proved to be true. The basic curriculum was valid regardless of ethnic background.

Nevertheless, feedback from all of the first-year participant focus groups, held as a component of the process evaluation after exposure to the learning program, led to the conclusion that it makes sense from a group process standpoint to run the intervention with multi-ethnic groups. Participants indicated that "the great unifier" among them was that their lives had been reordered because of the impact of a substance-abusing adult child. Indeed, the participating grandparents themselves actually took comfort in learning theirs was not just a Latino problem or an African American problem. These grandparents maintained that they *wanted* to be with others of different backgrounds during the intervention process—both because of a need to be united through common cause and to verify, in their own minds, that their problems were indeed universal. In a few cases, moreover, grandparents were raising biracial grandchildren and wanted to interact with another specific cultural group for that reason.

Common cause also led to the formation of affectual ties and, thus, long-term social networks and friendships that succeeded the intervention period through the formation of a support group or ongoing friendships.

Finally, it is important to note that, periodically, site-based personnel would suggest the merit of the intervention for a wider range of grandparents raising grandchildren, not just those with substance-abusing adult children. This possibility has engendered some debate among site-based personnel, evaluators, and project investigators. Clearly, many other grandparents would benefit from insight into family boundary issues and from enhanced self-management skills.

However, applying this intervention without considerable alteration to other grandparents would create confusion for many participants. First, many of the topics in the intervention are approached from the perspective of families containing substance abusers and are thus, at best, marginally appropriate for other populations of grandparents. Moreover, mixing grandparent groups attenuates the experience for those dealing with substance abuse issues and would force those not dealing with substance abuse to focus on irrelevant issues and references. Finally, as the pilot experience demonstrated, participant self-validation came from interacting with others who were experiencing permutations of many of the same frustrations and challenges stemming from the substance-abusing adult child. Other populations of grandparents would be likely to threaten group solidarity. Thus, from both a clinical and a research perspective, to maximize the impact of the intervention on grandparent well-being, it is probably best not to mix participant groups (substance abuse involved and non-substance abuse involved) in this intervention.

It is also essential that clinicians heed closely the destabilizing impact of the substance-abusing middle generation on the inter- and intrapersonal dynamics in these family formations. Even in cases in which this adult child has died or is permanently incarcerated, thus providing some degree of homeostasis in the family system, the repercussions of this individual's behavior may be felt indefinitely by all generations in the family.

For grandparents raising grandchildren due to substance abuse in the middle generation, this intervention provided a much-needed vehicle for learning about boundary ambiguity, the appropriateness and acceptability of assertive behavior, new approaches to parenting, and how to problem-solve. It has merit both as an educational device and as a means for attaining self-validation across ethnic groups and geographic locale in the United States.

ACKNOWLEDGMENTS

This article is based on a project supported with funds provided by the W. K. Kellogg Foundation of Battle Creek, Michigan.

REFERENCES

Anglin, M. D. (1990). Drug-abuse treatment to ameliorate negative family and childhood effects of parental drug abuse. In *Raising children for the twenty-first century* (pp. 325–331). Washington, DC: American Enterprise Institute.

Boss, P. (1988). *Family stress management.* Newbury Park, CA: Sage.

Boss, P., & Greenberg, J. (1984). Family boundary ambiguity: A new variable in family stress theory. *Family Process, 23,* 535–546.

Boss, P., Greenberg, J. R., & Pearce-McCall, D. (1990). *Measurement of boundary ambiguity in families* (Station Bulletin 593-1990). St. Paul, MN: University of Minnesota, Minnesota Agricultural Experiment Station.

Burton, L. M. (1992). Black grandparents rearing children of drug-addicted parents: Stressors, outcomes, and social service needs. *Gerontologist, 32,* 744–751.

Deacon, R. E., & Firebaugh, F. M. (1981). *Family resource management: Principles and applications.* Boston: Allyn and Bacon.

Gross, I. G., Crandall, E. W., & Knoll, M. M. (1973). *Management for modern families* (3rd ed.). New York: Appleton-Century-Crofts.

Herskovitz, L. (1996). *Strengthening parenting across generations: A formative evaluation.* Detroit: Wayne State University.

Herskovitz, L. (1997). *Strengthening parenting across generations: A formative evaluation: Year two.* Detroit: Wayne State University.

Hirshorn, B. A., & Van Meter, M. J. (1996, June). Strengthening parenting across generation: A self-management learning program for grandparents raising grandchildren. A final report to the W. K. Kellogg Foundation. Detroit: Wayne State University Institute of Gerontology. (Unpublished)

Hirshorn, B. A., Van Meter, M. J., & Sanders, T. (1997, July). Strengthening parenting across generation: A self-management learning program for grandparents raising grandchildren. A final report to the W. K. Kellogg Foundation. Institute for Families in Society, University of South Carolina, Columbia, SC. (Unpublished)

McCubbin, H. I., & Patterson, J. M. (1983). Family transition: Adaptation to stress. In H. I. McCubbin & C. R. Figley (Eds.), *Coping with normative transition* (Vol. 1). New York: Brunner/Mazel.

Minkler, M., & Roe, K. M. (1993). *Grandmothers as caregivers: Raising children of the crack cocaine epidemic.* Newbury Park, CA: Sage.

Minkler, M., Roe, K. M., & Price, M. (1992). The physical and emotional health of grandmothers raising grandchildren in the crack cocaine epidemic. *Gerontologist, 32,* 5752–5761.

Minuchin, S. (1974). *Families and family therapy.* Cambridge, MA: Harvard University Press.

Saluter, A. F. (1996). Marital status and living arrangements: March 1994. In *Current Population Reports* (Series p-20, no. 478). Washington, DC: U.S. Government Printing Office.

Skaff, M. M., & Pearlin, L. I. (1992). Caregiving: Role engulfment and loss of self. *Gerontologist, 32,* 656–664.

CHAPTER 17

Goals for Grandparents and Support Groups

Robert D. Strom and Shirley K. Strom

S ome people have been identified as "the world's greatest grandmother" or as the "world's greatest grandfather." Their awards appear on T-shirts, hats, coffee cups, holiday greeting cards, and car bumper stickers. They are grateful for this show of affection and appreciate the assurance that such symbols represent. However, what grandparents want most is confirmation that their relatives see them as a favorable influence (Strom & Strom, 1997). In some ways this goal is easier to achieve now because people are living longer, enjoying better health, and retiring at an earlier age, and they have more leisure. These conditions present unprecedented opportunities to offer grandchildren continuity of affection, care, and guidance from birth through early adulthood.

Despite these advantages many grandparents believe the importance of their role is declining because of uncertainty regarding what should be expected of them in a technological society. Some acknowledge that changing times have caused them to lose touch with the way younger relatives see things. Others express disappointment because they are excluded from decisions about family affairs and lack enough time with loved ones. On the other hand, parents often assert that grandparents make only a minimal contribution to the family because they are preoccupied with self-interests. Most participants in our classes for parents report that they feel over-whelmed with how much they have to do and would appreciate more help from older relatives with the difficult task of raising children (Strom & Strom, 1997).

In stark contrast, a much smaller group of grandparents presents a different story (American Association of Retired Persons, 1997). They see their role as important because it involves taking care of grandchildren on a daily basis. Regardless of why younger relatives live with them, these grandparents are usually motivated to provide a stable and supportive environment (de Toledo & Brown, 1996). Their chances for success are improved when professionals enable them to recognize the adjustments they have to make, encourage goals consistent with their present circumstance, and improve the effectiveness of support groups.

GRANDPARENT GOALS

Knowing the goals of others makes it easier to understand them. We are less inclined to misinterpret their intentions and reach unfair conclusions about how well they are doing. For these reasons it is helpful to consider some of the goals that successful grandparents raising grandchildren appear to have in common. Specifically, they aspire to (a) be optimistic and adjust to the conditions of their role, (b) learn contemporary viewpoints about raising children and adolescents, (c) cooperate with the parent who shares some responsibility for child care, (d) monitor academic and social development of children, and (e) arrange periodic relief from daily responsibilities. Grandparents who realize the benefits of reaching these goals are more motivated to pursue them.

Be Optimistic and Adjust to the Role

It has been our observation that resistance to this goal is most often demonstrated by middle-income Caucasians. Their opposition comes from the belief that caring for a grandchild has cost them the freedom they sought for many years. They waited a long time for their children to grow up, supposing it would then be possible to give attention to personal interests and ambitions. Maybe they had plans to travel, become more involved in hobbies, and participate in special activities with their spouse or friends. Perhaps they imagined that being a grandparent would include fun visits, occasional baby-sitting, and indulging the grandchildren. However, these dreams never came true because daughters or sons needed them to help raise their children. The future seems uncertain when there is no way to forecast how long they will have to raise someone else's child. Generally they feel strained by the extraordinary demands on their time, energy, and finances (Jendrek, 1994; Kornhaber, 1996).

Grandparents frequently experience anger at being placed in a surrogate role with extensive responsibilities. Feelings of resentment toward the people who created the situation, guilt about things they might have done wrong as a parent, and doubts about whether they can actually manage by themselves are usual. Grandma Rose states her ambivalence, "I don't know if God thought I did a poor job and wanted to give me a second chance, or thought I did well enough to be given the task one more time. My daughter tells me she cannot handle her children anymore, but maybe I won't be able to manage them either."

Grandparents are beset with mixed emotions. They feel a sense of sadness for grandchildren and sense isolation from friends who seem unable to comprehend their mission. Some are depressed over having to relinquish their retirement goal of being relatively free of obligations to others. Despite these misgivings, most grandparents affirm that they would take the same path again to come to the assistance of grandchildren (Robertson & Johnson, 1997).

Grandparents who raise grandchildren need to adopt goals that match their surrogate function. Otherwise, they can remain locked in a state of disappointment for being unable to attain earlier aspirations that are no longer appropriate. A related danger is that the grandchildren may feel unwanted and think of themselves as an obstacle to grandparent happiness. Such youngsters are better off living with someone else, who can make them feel wanted and instill a sense of belonging. This means that sometimes foster care can be a healthier option than care provided in a grudging way by older relatives.

Children who are exposed to high levels of pessimism are at greater risk for depression and losing the creative capacity to see possibilities, including their own happiness. A sense of optimism demonstrated by family members is a vital asset to children and should be continually reinforced by grandparents who rely on it as their fundamental attitude toward life and daily affairs. Grandchildren should be regularly told by grandparents that helping them grow up is a source of great satisfaction (Seligman, Reivich, Jaycox, & Gillham, 1995).

Learn Contemporary Views About Children and Adolescents

Grandparents who underestimate what it takes to provide guidance are bound to disadvantage grandchildren. Suggestions that they enroll in a grandparent class should not be viewed as an insult. Rather, it is a compliment when people recognize our capacity to grow and desire to become successful. It should be expected that, as understanding about children and adolescents increases, better guidance practices will emerge. Grandparents should understand the contemporary goals for raising children, alternatives to corporal punishment, norms of behavior in elementary and high school, and teacher expectations for assistance from the family.

It is unreasonable to suppose that willingness to raise a grandchild and loving the child are the only qualities needed to fulfill this complicated role. Success always depends on good intentions, but it also requires knowing about the predictable difficulties children experience and ways to help them cope with personal problems. Older relatives who recognize the link between their own self-improvement and the well-being of grandchildren are eager to obtain the insights and emotional strength required to succeed.

Cooperate with the Parent Who Shares Responsibility for Care

In two-thirds of families where grandparents are the main caretakers, one of the grandchild's parents lives in the same household (American Association of Retired Persons, 1997). Usually, this situation arises when an unwed teenager has a baby and continues to attend school or is employed while the maternal grandmother acts as a surrogate (Cherlin, 1998; Clarke, Preston, Raksin, & Bengtson, 1999). Although they have the potential to form a partnership, there is often conflict between the two women as each of them attempts to build a satisfying relationship with the child.

An example of problems in the changing mother-daughter relationship is portrayed by Carmen, who got pregnant at age 16. Her mother, Esther, agreed to take care of Juan so that Carmen could get a general education certificate. That was 4 years ago, and Carmen still lives at home. Grandma Esther and her grandson Juan spend most of their time together and get along well. When Carmen returns home from work, she is tired out, routinely denies Juan's request for play, and yells at him for acting in ways she does not like. This response causes Juan to seek comfort from grandma Esther. Carmen admits that this behavior makes her feel jealous and guilty about being so impatient. Sometimes Carmen tries to regain Juan's favor by suspending Esther's rule about not having snacks after supper.

Carmen's behavior resembles that of noncustodial grandparents who spend too little time with grandchildren. They seldom have sufficient responsibilities for teaching or discipline, and they spoil grandchildren instead of encouraging them to mature by reinforcing the rules of parents for proper behavior. But in this family the roles have been reversed. It is Esther, Juan's grandparent, who is disappointed by the permissive behavior of her daughter Carmen. Esther believes that because she is the one who takes care of Juan most of the time, Carmen should show support for her rules instead of contradicting them.

Both women need well-defined responsibilities that they mutually agree on. Their complementary roles are essential so that Juan can benefit from a stable environment, knowing the women love him and share similar expectations of him. One way to increase this continuity is by establishing support groups for young parents who reside in grandparent-headed households. Efforts to unite the adult generations remain uncommon but have the potential to produce greater benefit than supposing grandparents are the only parties in need of support.

Monitor Children's Social and Academic Development

Children raised by surrogates may suffer from emotional problems. Feelings of rejection and abandonment by parents can trigger depression. Sometimes the dominant response is anger toward the people who are least likely to strike back—grandparents. Caretakers often fail to recognize when a child needs professional counseling to cope with the distress and maladjustment that often accompanies dysfunctional family relationships (Solomon & Marx, 1995).

Elementary students are inclined to blame themselves for the absence of a parent and may be fearful that grandparents will leave too. Hostility toward parents can be redirected to classmates. Children who are preoccupied by problems tend to daydream, so they do not pay enough attention to their lessons. As a result, falling behind in class is common, particularly in subjects such as mathematics, where knowledge is cumulative (Wallerstein & Kelly, 1996). Tutoring is usually necessary to catch up. Some grandparents worry that getting a poor report card and continued lack of self-control could be the beginning of serious troubles for their grandchild.

Most grandparents express uncertainty about how teachers expect them to support learning. Going to PTA meetings where parents are much younger than themselves reinforces the idea that grandparents do not belong. Conferring with a child's teachers can identify problems for mutual attention and can guide cooperative efforts. Administrators and faculty are wise to suggest that grandparent support groups meet at the school and offer to help identify educational resources for them. Our studies have produced guidelines for establishing grandparent education councils in schools (Strom & Strom, 1995).

Arrange Periodic Relief from Daily Responsibilities

Grandparents feel exhausted by their broad range of tasks. Instead of pacing themselves and accepting that certain chores may have to wait, some people overlook their own health and psychological needs. They do not recognize that their mental fitness and physical stamina must be preserved to remain an effective source of support for grandchildren. It is important to schedule rest, hobbies, and opportunities to learn. Regular exercise can counteract depression and reinforce a positive outlook. Learning to cope with continuous stress while feeling a sense of control in the important sectors of life can prevent grandparents from giving up or becoming abusive to children. In some cases, relief must take the form of individual counseling from a therapist.

Spending time alone while other trusted adults supervise grandchildren allows grandparents to recover their perspective and renew motivation. These goals to obtain relief are modest for the purpose of performing errands, attending a religious service, going to the hairdresser, or visiting with old friends. Nevertheless, some grandparents must forgo relief because no relatives are available to help, or those willing to act as caregivers are unreliable and cannot be trusted. Free respite care is an important service that churches and synagogues could consider as part of their community mission (Jendrek, 1994).

SUPPORT GROUP GOALS

Grandparents raising grandchildren are often encouraged to join a support group. Hundreds of these groups have been formed and are identified by names such as Grandparents as Parents, Second Time Around Parents, Grandparents Raising Grandchildren, Grandmothers as Mothers Again, and Raising Our Children's Kids. The support group usually consists of 5 to 20 members, with leadership assumed by grandparents themselves. Participants believe that spending time with peers who face similar challenges will reduce feelings of isolation, provide mutual comfort, and offer solutions for common problems. Sometimes the purposes include informing lawmakers about injustices to grandparents or urging introduction of welfare reforms involving custody and visitation. These initiatives have improved public awareness and the policies of courts and family agencies (de Toledo & Brown, 1995; Kornhaber, 1996).

The benefits for participants in support groups are poorly documented. These groups seldom receive external funding, so there are no demands to evaluate outcomes. National leaders of grandparent networks have identified their concerns (Slorah & Kirkland, 1993). Most difficulties can be overcome by implementing these goals: (a) encourage optimistic attitudes and constructive behavior, (b) establish growth expectations for all members, (c) acquire and practice group process skills, and (d) make education the basis for helping grandparents.

Encourage Optimistic Attitudes and Constructive Behavior

Support groups are often ineffective because of a format that encourages complaining but fails to offer opportunities for growth. Members suppose that it is therapeutic to make disappointments known to peers who will avoid judging them. Support group leaders recognize the dangers that flow from this behavior pattern: "I come home after meetings emotionally drained from listening to everyone"; "I disapprove of the inclination people have to pool their hostility"; "I have to limit the amount of time for sharing feelings to one in every three meetings or else the attendance drops off. People just can't take it more often than that"; "I'm uncertain about what to do with people who appear more interested in expressing endless complaints than making adjustments in their lives"; "Those who achieve success usually stop coming to meetings so we never get to talk about what it takes to be successful."

These observations of national support group founders illustrate why reform is necessary. It is vital to replace the outlook causing members to see themselves as victims who can benefit from taking turns presenting sorrows, listening to the disappointment of others, and reassuring one another that troubles are bound to end. Rather, the attitude that ought to permeate a support group calls on everyone to contribute hope by sharing their small victories, identifying short-term goals, recounting humorous things that happen, and reminding others of good things in their lives.

When a favorable outlook prevails, successful people do not stop attending support meetings to avoid listening to the complaints. They continue to come so they can share their strength and build confidence in others. The choice of attitude matters because, more than any other ingredient, attitude governs the expectations and behaviors a group can produce. Mental health depends on replacing corrosive emotions like anger, hatred, and bitterness as soon as possible with an outlook that is hopeful and healthy.

Establish Growth Expectations for all Members

At the outset, participants should be provided a written statement explaining the development sequence expected of everyone. This helps individuals set personal goals and guides their constructive involvement in the group. The recommended progression consists of three stages: (1) self-disclosure, (2) constructive self-evaluation, and (3) healthy adjustment.

Self-Disclosure

During the first stage, grandparents attempt to describe personal difficulties and listen carefully to peers who tell about the improvements in their family relationships. Initially, people usually express some anger, disappointment, blame, hopelessness, and self-pity. This tendency to portray oneself as a victim is quite common. Three or four sessions should be devoted to Stage 1 behavior and adjustment into the group.

Constructive Self-Evaluation

In Stage 2, people are expected to broaden their focus. The purpose is to go beyond just detailing unpleasant events and expressing discontent to begin activation of constructive self-evaluation. Individuals are expected to reflect aloud and identify factors they have the power to change. The reason for this shift is that it motivates people to turn away from the impression that circumstances cannot be altered in favor of a recognition that certain things are subject to self-control. Stage 2 people are expected to identify ways they handle problems rather than perpetually describe their difficulties.

At this stage other group members also do more than listen. They help generate options to broaden the basis of personal choice. Additional group functions are to monitor the logic of each individual, present objective ways of looking at situations, and remind one another about the productive use of energy. The duration of this stage is three or four sessions.

Healthy Adjustment

By the time most people attend from six to eight sessions, they are usually ready to enter Stage 3. Here the emphasis is on clarifying personal goals, sharing evidence of progress, describing setbacks, and formulating ways to revise efforts. These men and women are prepared to accept the full range of their responsibilities as surrogates and demonstrate healthy adjustment to daily challenges. They are no longer hindered by their earlier concentration on feelings of bitterness or regret. These individuals are living proof that conditions of adversity can be overcome by perseverance, creativity, and encouragement. Although some quit attending the support group, others remain as mentors for peers who struggle to progress beyond Stage 1 and Stage 2.

Some grandparents are unable to make the expected gains. Getting stalled often relates to depression (Goetzel, 1998). When people become depressed, they lose the perspective that is necessary to consider alternative courses of action. In such cases it is important to acknowledge that attending a support group is an insufficient way to produce improvement. Getting the person to contact a therapist and schedule individual sessions is more appropriate. Some older adults are reluctant to seek counseling because they grew up with misconceptions regarding this form of treatment. Accordingly, group members should be oriented to the nature and the benefits of clinical assistance. In addition, support group leaders need training to detect when individuals fail to make progress.

It is relevant to acknowledge that getting treatment for psychological illnesses like depression significantly reduce the cost of health care. Researchers studied 46,000 workers from six large companies over a 3-year period (Goetzel, 1998). Each person completed a survey about personal health habits, such as physical activity, exercise, alcohol intake, eating patterns, use of tobacco, exposure to stress, and experience with depression. About 20% of the workers reported high stress levels whereas only 2% indicated experience with depression. It was found that the depressed patients cost health care providers 70% more than did nondepressed patients. Health care costs of highly stressed patients were 46% greater than for those who reported lower stress levels. That grandparents raising grandchildren experience disproportionately high levels of stress, as well as depression, is a familiar observation.

Support groups should include participants from all three stages. Otherwise, the danger is that some members may become locked in Stage 1 and rendered incapable of making progress. When the support group is viewed as a forum to consistently express negative feelings, the constructive role of peers is minimized. Grandparents who make significant gains in their family relationships usually identify the focus on self-pity as their reason for leaving the support group. Most of them report that leaving was necessary to preserve their mental health (Slorah & Kirkland, 1993).

Acquire and Practice Group Process Skills

Leaders of support groups report difficulties in knowing how to deal with participants who monopolize conversations, rationing time so that all have an opportunity to express themselves, intervening when someone is critical of another member, keeping people focused on main issues, and ending arguments between factions seeking to impose their agenda on the entire group. Leaders wish that participants would assume more responsibility to make the group experience productive for everyone. However, interviews with participants reveal a fairly uniform impression that the leaders are supposed to handle all problems as they arise. These expectations exempt members from sharing the obligation to monitor group process and grow from the experience.

When today's grandparents were children, peers were less often seen as a significant source of guidance. Reading and listening to teachers were considered the important ways to learn. Conversation with peers in class was thought to be a waste of time; it was discouraged and treated as misbehavior. Consequently, grandparents did not acquire the group process skills that are routinely taught to students now. These skills are important because they enable dialogue among peers and stimulate respectful communication between the generations. Support groups should help members acquire and practice the social skills associated with sharing feelings and ideas, staying focused on a topic, yielding to other speakers, showing respect for opinions with which they disagree, challenging sources of information, reminding peers when their comments become repetitious, and relying on brainstorming to generate options for solving problems. Our studies have produced guidelines to help grandparents gain these skills (Strom & Strom, 1993a).

Assess Learning Needs and Evaluate Growth

Grandparents need a broader understanding of their role than can be provided by peers. A powerful way to stimulate individual growth is by including an education component to augment the emphasis on sharing experiences. This means scheduling half of each meeting for a learning activity or alternating the focus of entire sessions so that self-disclosure, feedback from the group, and education needs can be met.

Every support group should identify the areas of growth their members need most. This goal can be attained by having a school psychologist administer the Grandparent Strengths and Needs Inventory (GSNI) (Strom & Strom, 1993b). The GSNI helps people recognize their favorable qualities and detect aspects of their relationships for which further learning is needed. The common uses of the GSNI include finding out how grandparents are viewed by themselves and others, offering feedback about changes individuals should consider making, devising a focus for curriculum that fits particular grandparent groups, and evaluating how people change in response to intervention.

Grandparent effectiveness is measured by 60 Likert-type items, divided equally into six subscales that emphasize separate aspects of development. These subscales reveal the following:

Satisfaction: aspects of being a grandparent that are pleasing.
Success: ways grandparents successfully perform their role.
Teaching: scope of instruction expected from grandparents.
Difficulty: problems associated with grandparent obligations.
Frustration: grandchild behaviors that upset grandparents.
Information needs: things grandparents need to know about grandchildren.

The GSNI includes three versions: (1) grandparent version, (2) parent version, and (3) grandchild version. Persons who complete the grandparent version report on self-impressions. In the other two versions, grandchildren and parents make known their perceptions about a particular grandparent. The rationale for this multioperational approach is that a broader perspective of family interaction offers a more comprehensive picture of grandparent assets and learning needs. If grandparents are raising grandchildren on their own, these two generations can complete the instrument. Each grandparent receives a profile that shows their ratings for all 60 items, along with normative ratings from their grandchild's peer group. The children are assured that their personal responses will never be made known to their grandparents.

The GSNI was initially used in a national field test to determine whether grandparents could improve their influence when provided a curriculum designed to meet family learning needs. In this investigation for the American Association of Retired Persons, several hundred grandparents, parents, and children completed a pretest GSNI before the grandparents attended a 12-week instructional program and at the end of instruction as a posttest. It was found that, in the estimate of all three generations, grandparents significantly improved their behavior in response to intervention. When the GSNI was given a third time several months later, the gains each source had identified earlier were sustained. In contrast, a matched control group made no gains during the project. Replications have yielded similar results (Strom, Beckert, & Strom, 1996).

The GSNI has identified educational needs for African American, Asian American, Caucasian American, and Mexican American groups as well as overseas participants in national studies of Japan and the Republic of China (Strom & Strom, 1998; Strom, Strom, Collinsworth, et al., 1996; Strom, Strom, Shen, Li, & Sun, 1996). Further information can be found on the Arizona State University Office of Parent Development international Website <www.public. asu.edu/~rdstrom>.

CONCLUSION

Grandparents raising grandchildren know they are needed and should recognize that success depends on suitable goals and continued learning. Belonging to a support group can offer benefits when the emphasis is on linking optimistic attitudes and constructive behavior, when members are expected to progress through necessary growth stages, and when everyone gets practice in group process communication skills and acquires up-to-date lessons on raising children.

Some people reason that, until parent education becomes more common, grandparent learning can wait. However, this is not a matter of doing one thing before another; both must be done at the same time because family harmony requires adjustment of all generations. In a society of longevity, wisdom requires more than a knowledge of the past. Something of the present must be understood too, including an awareness of the needs of younger relatives and ways to help them attain their goals.

REFERENCES

American Association of Retired Persons. (1997). *Grandparents raising grandchildren: Statistics.* Washington, DC: Author.

Cherlin, A. (1998). Marriage and marital dissolution among Black Americans. *Journal of Comparative Family Studies, 39*(1), 147–158.

Clarke, E., Preston, M., Raksin, J., & Bengtson, V. (1999). Types of conflicts and tensions between older parents and adult children. *Gerontologist, 39,* 261–270.

de Toledo, S., & Brown, D. (1995). *Grandparents as parents.* New York: Guilford.

Goetzel, R. (1998). *Depression and health care costs.* Ann Arbor, MI: Medstat.

Jendrek, M. (1994). Grandparents who parent grandchildren: Circumstances and decisions. *Gerontologist, 34,* 206–216.

Kornhaber, A. (1996). *Contemporary grandparents.* Thousand Oaks, CA: Sage.

Robertson, J., & Johnson, C. (1997). Should grandparents assume full parental responsibility? In A. Scharlach & L. Kaye (Eds.), *Controversial issues in aging* (pp. 173–184). Boston: Allyn & Bacon.

Seligman, M., Reivich, K., Jaycox, L., & Gillham, J. (1995). *The optimistic child.* Boston: Houghton Mifflin.

Slorah, P., & Kirkland, B. (1993, March). *Problems encountered by grandparent support groups.* Paper presented at Generations United, Washington, DC.

Solomon, J., & Marx, J. (1995). To grandmother's house we go: Health and school adjustment of children raised solely by grandparents. *Gerontologist, 35,* 386–394.

Strom, R., Beckert, T., & Strom, S. (1996). Determining success of grandparent education. *Educational Gerontology, 22,* 637–649.

Strom, R., & Strom, S. (1993a). Grandparent education: Improving communication skills. *Educational Gerontology, 19,* 717–725.

Strom, R., & Strom, S. (1993b). *Grandparent strengths and needs inventory.* Chicago: Scholastic Testing Service.

Strom, R., & Strom, S. (1995). Intergenerational learning: Grandparents in the schools. *Educational Gerontology, 21,* 321–335.

Strom, R., & Strom, S. (1997). Building a theory of grandparent development. *International Journal of Aging and Human Development, 45,* 255–286.

Strom, R., & Strom, S. (1998). Education for grandparents in Taiwan and the United States. *Journal of Intercultural Studies, 25,* 119–166.

Strom, R., Strom, S., Collinsworth, P., Sato, S., Makino, K., Sasaki, Y., Sasaki, H., & Nishio, N. (1996). Developing curricula for grandparents in Japan. *Educational Gerontology, 22,* 781–794.

Strom, R., Strom, S., Shen, Y., Li, S., & Sun, H. (1996). Grandparents in Taiwan. *International Journal of Aging and Human Development, 42,* 1–19.

Wallerstein, J., & Kelly, J. (1996). *Surviving the breakup.* New York: HarperCollins.

Service Delivery and Public Policy Implications of Custodial Grandparenting

CHAPTER 18

Grandparent Education

Lillian Chenoweth

G randparents deserve help and support in raising their grand-children. One vital, often overlooked component of that help is grandparent education. The purpose of this chapter is to present elements of a model and to describe the components necessary for effective grandparent education. Although the literature is replete with parent education models, programs for grandparent education are as yet in their formative stages. There is crucial need for a model of the components for a nongeneric, targeted program specifically designed to help custodial grandparents raise grandchildren. This chapter represents a beginning effort at synthesizing the literature on grandparenting and parent education into a focus on custodial grandparent education. The chapter documents the unique role of grandparents as parents, presents their needs for education and support, recommends overall characteristics of the model, and then recommends program elements.

PARAMETERS OF GRANDPARENTING

This section explains the concept of grandparenting as a career, describing the antecedents of the career and the many variations. The uniqueness of the role of custodial grandparent also is portrayed.

Career Concept

It is imperative to acknowledge the whole environment of grandparenting, to focus on the context of the phenomenon rather than just the act of grandparenting. To date, society's knowledge of the parameters of the experience remains somewhat fragmentary. The concept of career broadens the focus to include the particular context in which grandparents assume custodial care. The boundaries of the role are defined by many variables, such as the number and age of grandchildren; length of time involved, from short to long term, intermittent to regular; number and gender of caregivers; reasons for assuming care; skipped-generation care or "double duty" of caring for child and grandchild; and many other variables. The many manifestations of the role and where the grandparent is in his or her own life career significantly influence the need for education. The grandparenting role must be examined within the context of other roles (Baydar & Brooks-Gunn, 1998).

Cherlin and Furstenberg (1986) described the "grandparental career" as a dynamic process, always evolving and changing. This career may include overlapping stages, such as caring for one's own children at the same time as assuming full-time care of grandchildren. Or grandparenthood may represent a separate stage of the family life cycle, with fewer roles and fewer obligations. Not unlike occupational careers, the grandparental career involves commitment of time and resources; there are distinct stages that change over time, with occasional forward progress and sometimes what seem like regressions. The career may be seen as a series of spirals rather than as a linear progression, always upward and forward. Grandparents experience different exigencies and constraints in their attempts to maximize their own satisfaction with the role and the good of the grandchildren over time.

The grandparental career encompasses different roles, positions, and relationships. Grandparent caregivers are frequently characterized by type, such as custodial (including those with legal custody as well as those whose grandchildren are living with them without legal custody) or "daycare grandparents" (Jendrek, 1994). The custodial grandparents are usually responsible for daily care without the assistance of parents. The day-care group may be able to return the children at night or on weekends, but they are still responsible for the majority of care decisions and for fulfilling many parental roles.

Grandparents may find themselves thrust back into the parenting role literally overnight, often without warning and with little or no preparation for this new role. The reasons for resuming parental roles also vary but frequently revolve around problem situations such as divorce, substance abuse, child abuse, teen pregnancy, death, incarceration, or mental health issues. Jendrek (1994) documented the fact that many grandparents assume custodial care because of problems in the grandchild's family. The grandparent is often attempting to bring some sense of stability and security into the child's life. According to Minkler and Roe (1993), unlike the usual 9-month transition to parenthood, custodial grandparenting may have several antecedents. Such a condition may be characterized by abrupt onset, with sudden, unanticipated new roles. Occasionally, this abrupt change results from incidences of "offtiming" or premature grandparenting (Aldous, 1995). The unexpected perceived off-time nature of the role can create stress regardless of the age or life stage of the grandparent. Perception of not being old enough or not being ready for the grandparent role can occur at any age.

There are variations in the relations between the grandparents and the grandchildren in this career as well. Cherlin and Furstenburg (1986) described grandparent-grandchild relationships as a continuum. Such relationships may range from remoteness to closely bonded; the continuum implies movement and change. The concept of relationship continuum is consistent with the nonstatic nature of a grandparental career. Sometimes discrete labels obscure the reality of individual differences and gradations. Program designers must be cognizant of the differences among grandparents as well as between parents and grandparents.

Uniqueness of the Role

Many grandparents have learned how to play the role from their own childhood experiences and observations of their own grandparents (King & Elder, 1997). They are prepared to reproduce that same role. This early socialization influences how they interpret and adapt to their grandparental career. The new role as full-time caregiver is often not the one for which they were prepared. Their assumptions about their lives, their children's lives, and their grandchildren's lives are in flux. The role remains incompletely institutionalized.

Although the role may not actually be new, for some cultures it is still often a "roleless role" that demands to be clarified (Burton & Dilworth-Anderson, 1991; Dressel, 1996; Emick & Hayslip, 1996; Hunter, 1997). Pruchno and Johnson (1996) assert that the role is weakly regulated and ambiguous; there are few normatively explicit expectations. Grandparents raising their grandchildren are unsure of what they are "supposed to do" in such a role. Society remains uncertain of the duties and requirements for successfully fulfilling this role. The predominant cultural image features grandparents as independent individuals whose most important developmental task has been to maintain autonomy (Gratton & Haber, 1996). The conventional role has become quite unconventional (Emick & Hayslip, 1996). Households formed by custodial grandparents are distinctively different in form and function from other grandparent households (Goldberg-Glen, Sands, Cole, & Cristofalo, 1998).

Two contradictory norms have been identified as influencing the role (Aldous, 1995). The societal norm of noninterference is seen as contrary to the norm of obligation. Society has taught the value of maintaining generational boundaries; the norm of family and the obligations of the situation require otherwise. Grandparents often feel obligated to rescue their grandchildren. Long-held patterns of reciprocity and mutual assistance may have to change (Johnson, 1993). Indeed, "current theories of adult development are inadequate in describing the challenges and needs" facing this population (Pinson-Millburn, Fabian, Schlossberg, & Pyle, 1996, p. 549). Past theories of development have often emphasized behavior as a function of the individual's age and stage of life. The tasks facing this group of grandparents go beyond those normally associated with aging, such as preparation for retirement, maintaining physical health, and coping with death of spouse. Jendrek (1994) describes the role as "time disordered" (p. 207). The lack of temporal congruence may violate existing norms and expectations.

The new role of grandparent as parent often comes with no set boundaries; its duration may be indefinite. Raising grandchildren may be a lifetime commitment, intermittent, or short-term in nature. Boundaries with other family members also may be unclear. Previously negotiated divisions of labor may have to be rethought, and responsibilities for other family members may have to be renegotiated. Indeed, custodial grandparents are forced to rethink, "What is family?" Rebuilding and redefining the family is a process, not a single step.

NEED FOR GRANDPARENT EDUCATION AND SUPPORT

Today's caregivers of all generations are forced to learn and develop skills to contend with increasing pressures facing family life. Multiple pressures have confronted families, resulting in a majority of parents reporting uncertainty about how to raise their children (Smith, Cudabeck, Goddard, & Myers-Walls, 1994). Families often lack adequate resources to deal with the myriad of problems (Norwood, Atkinson, Tellez, & Saldana, 1997). Second-time-around parents, especially custodial grandparents, are certainly not exempt from these challenges. Burton and deVries (1992) clearly articulated the challenge by asking, "Will we as a society create support for grandparents so that they can survive the challenges?" (p. 107). Research has suggested that grandparents will continue to serve vital roles in the lives of their grandchildren but will need support in filling these roles (Dilworth-Anderson, 1992; Dowdell & Sherwen, 1998).

Much of the research on custodial grandparents has emphasized the difficulties accompanying the role, which may include physical and mental health problems (Minkler, Fuller-Thomson, Miller, & Driver, 1997), fatigue, economic burdens, lifestyle and social changes, and legal barriers (Emick & Hayslip, 1996). Minkler et al. (1997) found that custodial grandparents were almost twice as likely as noncaregiving grandparents to be categorized as depressed.

Frequently, there are both physical and mental health issues surrounding the children and grandchildren (Hayslip, Shore, Henderson, & Lambert, 1998). Additionally, there may be traumas that precipitated the need for custodial care. For example, a parent may be jailed or be experiencing drug or alcohol problems. Grandparents must deal with their sadness, disappointment, or frustration. They may enter the new role of custodial grandparenting with feelings of failure and shame about their parenting role (Shore & Hayslip, 1994; Troll, 1983). Burton (1992) categorized the stressors facing custodial grandparents as contextual, familial, and individual. Contextual stressors include neighborhood dangers such as drug traffic. Familial stressors include providing care for multiple dependents and multiple generations. Individual stressors involve, for example, balancing multiple roles and meeting personal goals.

CURRENT APPROACHES TO GRANDPARENT EDUCATION

Grandparent education is one strategy for making the role less frustrating and more rewarding for grandparents. Such education follows the principle of parent education stating that parenting is extremely complex and that education can help persons perform their job more effectively (Wandersman, 1987). Although there is little consensus on the definition of parent education, one source described the process as an "organized effort with clear content, target population, and goals aimed at changing parental role performance" (Wandersman, 1987, p. 208). Brock, Oertwein, and Coufal (1993) similarly emphasized changing knowledge and skills but acknowledge the need to expand the focus beyond parents to a family system or child care system. Thus, extended kin could be included in parenting education. One goal of parent education is to strengthen and educate caregivers so that they are better able to facilitate the development of caring, competent, and healthy children (Smith et al., 1994). This broad objective encompasses grandparents as caregivers and is consistent with grandparental goals.

Parent education is distinguished from clinical approaches to helping families by its emphasis on family strengths rather than on problems. Parent education is also usually less confrontational and intrusive than family therapy or counseling (Fine & Henry, 1989). These distinctions do not mean that participating in parent education is not therapeutic or helpful. Well-designed, effective parent education and grandparent education can be extremely empowering and fill a vital support role.

Although there is little systematic, formal evaluation of parent education, many programs have been found to have a positive impact on family functioning and to assist families in coping with multiple stressors (see, e.g., Bogenschneider & Stone, 1997; Harachi, Catalano, & Hawkins, 1997; Norwood et al., 1997; and Repucci, Britner, & Woolard, 1997). The parent education model, which has frequently included grandparents as an audience, seems a particularly appropriate place to start to design an intervention to help grandparents. Surprisingly, few family life educators or family life education materials have included emphasis or focus on grandparent education.

Minkler, Driver, Roe, and Bedeian (1993) described community interventions and service programs for grandparent caregivers. In an examination of 124 programs, 24 were identified as comprehensive, beyond pure support groups. These programs included a range or services, such as individual counseling, parenting classes, respite care, and legislative advocacy. Unfortunately, the researchers found that all too often the programs were unfunded or underfunded, with little institutional support. Long-term programming was problematic, highlighting the need for broader-based support and integrated intervention efforts.

Strom and Strom (1984, 1989, 1990) have long and consistently advocated for grandparent education. They asserted that grandparents "deserve access to classes that help them adjust to their changing role and build satisfying family relationships" (Strom & Strom, 1990, p. 85). They have developed and implemented programs with numerous grandparents. The primary emphasis of their 12-week curriculum is to increase the involvement of grandparents in family affairs. The program developers denounce the "patronizing attitude toward grandparents" frequently found in other programs and instead recommend instructional programs to help grandparents continue to grow. Strom and Strom's 1990 report on 2 years of data collection revealed positive results in grandparent development. However, their curriculum and results are based only on noncustodial grandparents who self-selected one grandchild to evaluate changes. While Strom and Strom document results with traditional grandparents, few educational programs have been identified as specifically for custodial grandparents.

Watson (1997) surveyed more than 400 grandparents to assess their interest in a grandparent education course utilizing Strom's model. Only 8% of the sample were coresiding with grandchildren. Although grandparents who were raising their grandchildren were significantly more interested in a program than noncustodial grandparents were, 64% of this group were not interested in a 12-week program of standardized content.

DESIGN OF GRANDPARENT EDUCATION MODEL

This section describes general overall characteristics of an effective grandparent education model. The recommended design approach contrasts sharply with other, more standardized approaches. Program planners for grandparent education must exhibit much flexibility to meet the needs of participants. The basic premise is that program planners collaborate with participants. In this approach, the program is planned to focus on strengths, be culturally responsive, and serve a support function.

Strength-Based

Programs that understand and appreciate the unique strengths of the target audience of grandparents are crucial to success. Focusing on what caregivers can do well is more effective than emphasizing deficiencies or weaknesses. Accentuating strengths promotes empowerment and self-confidence. Hunter (1997) recommended viewing grandparent involvement as an intergenerational family strategy, a proactive choice about how to respond to family circumstances. Practitioners must adopt broader perspectives of what is normative for caregiving and validate various coping strategies. Programs for grandparents can follow a normative-adaptive approach; the realities can be noted without comparison to other family forms. To cite a familiar example, both apples and oranges can be valued—each has advantages.

Grandparents have long been valued for their roles in maintaining family connections, providing roots, and contributing a sense of groundedness. Grandchildren without parents can especially benefit from the family stories and traditions that can help to bond the families together. Grandparents can be taught to appreciate and utilize the natural skills they already possess. The model presented in this chapter recommends building on strengths such as intergenerational bonds rather than deficiencies.

Culturally Responsive

Many scholars have stressed the increasing importance of culturally responsive parenting programs (Cheng Gorman & Balter, 1997; Dilworth-Anderson, 1992; Harachi et al., 1997; Norwood et al., 1997). Such programs are seen as imperative in strengthening the abilities of grandparents to deal with problems and concerns. Knowledge, attitudes, and skills taught in such programs have been identified as effective in ameliorating the effect of societal and familial stressors. This approach makes no value judgments about the relative goodness of cultural groups or family structures. The aim is to preserve the dignity, integrity, and diversity of all groups. Each family is unique in cultural beliefs, values, and behaviors. If these elements are omitted during program development, the emphasis becomes families' weaknesses, causing a deficit orientation. This deficit model emphasizes the need to intervene in families' lives to mold, remediate, or fix what is "wrong." The deficit approach reinforces the ideology that certain types or groups of families are dysfunctional. An effective grandparent education program must not exhibit such stereotypical judgment.

To design a culturally responsive program, the program planner or educator must first and foremost be aware of his or her own cultural limitations and biases. The planner must also acknowledge the integrity and value of other cultures or compositions (McAdoo, 1993). Hildreth and Sugawara (1993) identified two dimensions that must be considered in designing culturally responsive programs: understanding needs, expectations, and strengths of the target audience and developing goals and objectives to match those unique needs, expectations, and strengths. Ideas from family life educators who have described culturally responsive program development can be adapted to focus on diverse family structures as well as ethnic groups.

Support Function

Typical parent education programs have focused on a broad spectrum of content. Fine and Henry (1989) described programs as having one or more of the following areas: information sharing, skill building, improving self-awareness, and problem solving. In addition to these areas, a fifth element of support is added. Support groups have been found effective for ameliorating the effects of numerous problems or circumstances, such as alcohol abuse, step-parenting, and grief. Support groups often help individuals keep their own problems in perspective. According to Minkler and Roe (1993), there are equivocal findings on the direct effects of belonging to a grandparent support group. However, participants generally perceive the groups as helpful, at least in the short term.

Strom and Strom (1993) suggested that grandparent support groups should encourage positive attitudes and sharing of small successes. The goal is to provide some cathartic release but to avoid becoming gripe sessions. The group format allows for mutual support and reduces feelings of isolation. Grandparents may feel separated from their friends and need to share with others in the same situation. In a book written primarily for grandparents, deToledo and Brown (1995) identified topics for grandparent support groups. Discussion topic ideas include stories about families, life changes, feelings, parenting issues, adult children and the rest of the family, and the bureaucracy.

In response to the need, there is a burgeoning development of support groups. A sample of such groups includes Grandparents Raising Grandchildren, Grandparents as Parents (GAP), and Raising Our Children's Kids (ROCK). There are also numerous groups sponsored by professional organizations or community agencies. Support groups alone cannot compensate for inadequate knowledge, but they can be the basis for learning about contemporary parenting. Education can be incorporated into the supportive atmosphere of a group.

PROGRAM ELEMENTS

Building on the collaborative approach described in the previous section, this section presents guidelines for needs assessment and ideas about the program elements of audience, content, and delivery. The planners must not presume to know all the answers in advance. Often educators mistakenly assume: "We know who needs help; we know what help they need most; and we know the best way to present this help." In a collaborative approach, the answers come from participants.

Needs Assessment

Prior to implementing any program, the educator should consider a needs assessment. A well-designed needs assessment provides information about the other design elements of audience, content, and delivery. More information is needed about what coping strategies and resources are most effective and helpful for custodial grandparents specifically. By assessing the kind of education and support participants need, from what sources, and when, the program developer can design a program to meet the participants' unique needs (Harachi et al., 1997; Repucci et al., 1997). An appropriate place to start meeting grandparental needs is by asking them directly. A standardized curriculum (Kornhaber, 1996) or packaged program is inappropriate.

Needs assessment can be conducted through interviews, by telephone or in person. Interviews could reach out to key leaders in the community, recognized leaders who are custodial grandparents. Other approaches include community forums or focus groups. Focus groups have been found especially effective in reaching Black extended family members (Armstrong, 1995) and Hispanic parents (Russell, 1994) interested in parenting education. Focus group participants frequently enjoy and benefit from the process as much as the organizers benefit from their input. Needs assessment could also be conducted through surveys, distributed through school or community organizations, sent out by mail, or conducted by telephone (see, e.g., Engelbrecht & Jacobson, 1994).

Audience

Programs that are planned and implemented for specific target audiences are more effective than those aimed at homogeneous mass markets. All grandparent groups will have some commonalities and common needs, but within the group there is much diversity. Some grandparents may be quite young and still involved in raising their own children; others may be much older and in very different life stages. Some grandparents may be involved in raising special-needs or high-risk children, whereas others face only "normal" challenges. Some grandparents will have parental participation; in other situations parents may be dead or absent for some reason, such as incarceration or substance addiction issues. Thus, in addition to being strength-oriented and acknowledging cultural differences in values and traditions, there are many other factors that must be acknowledged in program design.

The unique needs of adults as program participants must also be taken into account in program planning. For example, adults may feel uneasiness or anxiety in classroom situations. Their long absence from the classroom may create apprehension in this setting. Usually, an informal organization works better to provide social interaction and contact. Adults particularly need to feel that their time is well spent and that the program is relevant and practical. Adults want their broad background of experience to be recognized; grandparents have been parents and have acquired knowledge, attitudes, and skills. Grandparent education must be viewed as augmenting existing skills. A program designed or aimed at first-time parents would not be appropriate. Merely watering down the curriculum and changing the name to grandparent education is not enough. A newly designed curriculum to meet the needs of this specific audience is imperative.

Leaders ideally work toward blurring distinctions between members and leaders, as well as among members. Leaders who intentionally develop a sense of community and open sharing with all audience members will produce more effective programs (Norwood et al., 1997).

Content

Whatever specific topics are included, program planners must keep in mind the primacy of presenting information in the context of the culture. The needs assessment will facilitate identification of specific areas of interest. Rather than identify the set topics for any specified time period (e.g., the topics to be taught for a 12-week session), four content areas have emerged as important. These areas, based on previous grandparent research and parent education models, are self-care, communication, guidance, and advocacy. The areas represent a hierarchical approach to grandparent empowerment.

Self-Care

Before a caregiver can extend care to others, she may need to first learn to meet her own needs. Often self-care concerns must be addressed before grandparents can focus on the child or parenting issues. In research that asked culturally diverse groups of parents, "What keeps you from being the kind of parent you want to be?" parent perceptions of hindrances were identified (Armstrong, 1995; Russell, 1994). Responses cited most often included personal deficits: difficulties in managing time, money, physical exhaustion, balancing work and family, ability to help with homework. One parent poignantly commented, "I think the thing that keeps me from being the parent I want to be is that I get tired" (Armstrong, 1995, p. 62).

One parent education model (Smith et al., 1994) also included care for self as an integral part of the model. Norwood et al. (1997) found that allowing time to say prayers for each other and offer supportive hugs were elements of self-care that increased program effectiveness. Program topics might include time and stress management, learning how to ask for and accept help from others, and money management. Goal setting and taking one day at a time also would be topic ideas. Leaders can facilitate an awareness of community resources available to assist grandparents in such areas.

Communications

A second area would be topics related to communicating; this would include communications with spouse, grandchildren, children, extended family members, teachers, and other authorities. How to talk to teenagers born in a different world or how to talk to a teacher about homework issues are program suggestions. Information and communication skills can boost grandparents self-esteem and confidence.

Guidance

The area of guidance is always of much interest for caregivers. Most parents and grandparents want to teach their children and help them become the best they can be. Programs in this area might include how to set reasonable limits and consequences and how to understand contemporary childhood needs and tasks. Custodial grandparents may be stepping into parenting after patterns of behavior are developed; they need help in appropriate ways to guide behavior. Grandparents may want to focus on the balance between nurturing and controlling.

Many grandparents may hesitate to ask for help in this area for fear of being thought abusive or because their approaches are considered wrong. Denby and Alford (1996) cautioned that paramount consideration should be given to the aspect of dual socialization for some groups. Practitioners and educators must be aware of this element as it applies to discipline styles and parental goals. Cultural sensitivity is especially important for leaders in this area.

Advocacy

The fourth area focuses on grandparents as advocates. Some grandparents will have legal issues, questions about custody, or receiving financial support. Grandparents have to become knowledgeable about their rights and how to work within the system. Skills such as negotiating or letter writing could be the focus. Often grandparents must take action and become involved in processes they have previously ignored or denounced. Advocacy includes finding and using community resources and building relationships with neighborhood or community groups. These skills are crucial for grandparents who feel disenfranchised or for those with especially vulnerable grandchildren.

Delivery Systems

Despite the recent proliferation of parent education programs, little is really known about the most effective ways to deliver the information. As Bogenschneider and Stone (1997) have commented, it is "difficult to generalize about which strategies are effective, for what outcomes, and for whom" (p. 123). Program planners face the challenge of translating research-based knowledge into pragmatic advice for quite diverse groups. The efficacy of the delivery system depends at least in part on the personal preferences of the participants. Some grandparents may enjoy traditional modes of small-group instruction. Such instruction may feature videos, discussion, lectures, or some combination of these formats.

Little research identifies preferred locations. Educators have often assumed knowledge of appropriate locations. However, here also, program planners must allow for diversity. Some grandparents may desire a home-based program in which someone comes in to provide advice and listen to concerns. Others might prefer a child care center, church, senior center, place of employment, or school. The location must be a familiar place where participants feel safe and comfortable.

Reasons cited for nonparticipation in programs would hold true for custodial grandparents as well as parents: lack of time, lack of information about program details, child care, and transportation obstacles (Minkler & Roe, 1993). Program planners must work around these constraints. Many populations resist the concept of parent education or group support meetings because of values of self-sufficiency or sense of privacy. These real barriers require creativity to reach diverse audiences who may be more receptive to other delivery systems.

Other delivery methods include print media, such as newsletters or pamphlets. Bogenschneider and Stone (1997) found newsletters to be relatively inexpensive but effective. Print media have the capability of providing information at critical periods of need. Grandparents may receive the information and save it until the need arises; they can then refer to the written sources. Keller and McDade (1997) found preferences for print and video sources in recent research with culturally diverse populations. Although not a complete substitute for other delivery systems, print media can be complementary.

An increasing number of today's grandparents have Internet access delivered through a computer or through a television adapter (e.g., Webtv). Through the Internet, grandparents can be linked to numerous resources and timely information from chat rooms, listservs, discussion groups, and on-line courses. Numerous websites have been developed specifically for grandparents who are raising their grandchildren. Although such options may require new knowledge and skills, grandparents can often meet this challenge with minimal assistance. Indeed, the grandchildren themselves may be great in-house technical support. As is true with other types of delivery systems, the grandparents must judge the credibility of information through this venue. Electronic sources of ongoing networking may become more important in a society too busy for meetings.

RECOMMENDATIONS

Future grandparenting programs must focus on the grandparenting career and acknowledge the role within the context of other roles and relationships. Grandparenting must not be treated as an isolated act. Successful programs must incorporate information on ongoing transitions and changes, recognizing the dynamic nature of the role. Programs must move past offering canned curriculum with preidentified content. The efficacy of grandparenting programs must be evaluated with controlled research designed to assess differences over time. Longitudinal research is needed to determine both short- and long-term changes in grandparenting. Well-designed research can help establish the effectiveness of comprehensive grandparenting programs that go beyond one-shot efforts. Community-based, comprehensive programs with multiple delivery methods and approaches are desperately needed by grandparents to meet their growing needs.

SUMMARY

This chapter has presented essential elements for effective grandparent education. The need for unique, targeted programs was established. Grandparent education should build on existing strengths, be culturally responsive, and provide support for participants. The program design should be based on a needs assessment of the group. The elements of audience, content, and delivery systems were described, with specific recommendations for four content areas: self care, guidance, communications, and advocacy. Recommendations for future research, as well as program design and evaluation, also were presented. Implementing grandparent education programs on the basis of these suggestions can significantly empower grandparents and result in higher quality of caregiving.

REFERENCES

Aldous, J. (1995). New views of grandparents in intergenerational context. *Journal of Family Issues, 16*(1), 104–122.

Armstrong, J. J. (1995). *Parenting values, skills, practices, and education preferences of Black parents and extended family members.* Unpublished doctoral dissertation. Texas Woman's University.

Baydar, N., & Brooks-Gunn, J. (1998). Profiles of grandmothers who help care for their grandchildren in the U.S. *Family Relations, 47*, 385–393.

Bogenschneider, K., & Stone, M., (1997). Delivering parent education to low and high risk parents of adolescents via age-paced newsletters. *Family Relations, 46*, 123–133.

Brock, G. W., Oertwein, M., & Coufal, J. D. (1993). Parent education: Theory, research, and practice. In M. E. Arcus, J. D. Schvaneveldt, & J. J. Moss (Eds.), *Handbook of family life education* (vol. 1, pp. 87–114). Newbury Park, CA: Sage Publications.

Burton, L. M. (1992). Black grandparents rearing children of drug-addicted parents: Stressors, outcomes, and social service needs. *Gerontologist, 32*, 744–751.

Burton, L. M., & deVries, C. (1992). Challenges and rewards: African American grandparents as surrogate parents. In L. Burton (Ed.), *Families and aging* (pp. 101–108). Amityville, NY: Baywood Publishing.

Burton, L. M., & Dilworth-Anderson, P. (1991). The intergenerational family roles of aged Black Americans. *Marriage and Family Review, 16*(3/4), 311–330.

Cheng Gorman, J., & Balter, L. (1997). Culturally sensitive parent education: A critical review of quantitative research. *Review of Educational Research, 67*, 339–369.

Cherlin, A. J., & Furstenberg, F. F. (1986). *The new American grandparent.* New York: Basic Books.

Denby, R., & Alford, K. (1996). Understanding African-American discipline styles: Suggestions for effective social work intervention. *Journal of Multicultural Social Work, 43*(3), 81–98.

deToledo, S., & Brown, D. (1995). *Grandparents as parents.* New York: Guilford Press.

Dilworth-Anderson, P. (1992). Extended kin networks in Black families. In L. Burton (Ed.), *Families and aging* (pp. 57–64). Amityville, NY: Baywood Publishing.

Dowdell, E. B., & Sherwen, L. N. (1998). Grandmothers who raise grandchildren. *Journal of Gerontological Nursing, 24*(5), 8–13.

Dressel, P. (1996). Grandparenting at century's end: An introduction to the issue. *Generations, 20*(1), 5–6.

Emick, M. A., & Hayslip, B. (1996). Custodial grandparenting: New roles for middle-aged and older adults. *International Journal of Aging and Human Development, 43*(2), 135–154.

Engelbrecht, J., & Jacobson, A. (1994). A survey instrument: Assessment of education interests, experiences, learning preferences of parents of young children. *Resources in Education.* ERIC Reproduction Service No. ED361 092.

Fine, M. J., & Henry, S. A. (1989). Professional issues in parent education. In M. J. Fine (Ed.), *The second handbook of parent education: Contemporary perspectives* (pp. 3–20). San Diego, CA: Academic Press.

Goldberg-Glen, R., Sands, R. G., Cole, R. D., & Cristofalo, C. (1998). Multigenerational patterns and internal structures in families in which grandparents raise grandchildren. *Families in Society, 79,* 477–489.

Gratton, B., & Haber, C. (1996). Three phases in the history of American grandparents: Authority, burden, companion. *Generations, 20*(1), 7–12.

Harachi, T. W., Catalano, R. F., & Hawkins, J. D. (1997). Effective recruitment for parenting programs within ethnic minority communities. *Child and Adolescent Social Work Journal, 14*(1), 23–39.

Hayslip, B., Shore, R. J., Henderson, C. E., & Lambert, P. L. (1998). Custodial grandparenting and the impact of grandchildren with problems on role satisfaction and role meaning. *Journal of Gerontology, 53B*(3), S164–S173.

Hildreth, G. J., & Sugawara, A. I. (1993). Ethnicity and diversity in family life education. In M. E. Arcus, J. D. Schvaneveldt, & J. J Moss (Eds.), *Handbook of family life education* (vol. 1, pp. 162–188). Newbury Park, CA: Sage Publications.

Hunter, A. G. (1997). Counting on grandmothers: Black mothers' and fathers' reliance on grandmothers for parenting support. *Journal of Family Issues, 18*(3), 251–269.

Jendrek, M. P. (1994). Grandparents who parent their grandchildren: Circumstances and decisions. *Gerontologist, 34,* 206–216.

Johnson, C. L. (1993). Divorced and reconstituted families: Effects on the older generation. In L. Burton (Ed.), *Families and aging* (pp. 33–37). Amityville, NY: Baywood Publishing.

Keller, J., & McDade, K. (1997). Cultural diversity and help-seeking behavior: Sources of obstacles to support for parents. *Journal of Multicultural Social Work, 5*(1/2), 63–78.

King, V., & Elder, G. H., Jr. (1997). The legacy of grandparenting: Childhood experiences with grandparents and current involvement. *Journal of Marriage and the Family, 59,* 848–860.

Kornhaber, A. (1996). *Contemporary grandparenting.* Thousand Oaks, CA: Sage Publications.

McAdoo, H. P. (Ed.). 1993. *Family ethnicity: Strength in diversity.* Newbury Park, CA: Sage Publications.

Minkler, M., Driver, D., Roe, K. M., & Bedeian, K. (1993). Community interventions to support grandparent caregivers. *Gerontologist, 33,* 807–811.

Minkler, M., Fuller-Thomson, E., Miller, D., & Driver, D. (1997). Depression in grandparents raising grandchildren. *Archives of Family Medicine, 6,* 445–452.

Minkler, M., & Roe, K. M. (1993). *Grandmothers as caregivers: Raising children of the crack cocaine epidemic.* Newbury Park, CA: Sage Publications.

Norwood, P. M., Atkinson, S. E., Tellez, K., & Saldana, D. C. (1997). Contextualizing parent education programs in urban schools: The impact on minority parents and students. *Urban Education, 32,* 411–432.

Pinson-Millburn, N. M., Fabian, E. S., Schlossberg, N. K., & Pyle, M. (1996). Grandparents raising grandchildren. *Journal of Counseling and Development, 74,* 548–554.

Pruchno, R. A., & Johnson K. W. (1996). Research on grandparenting: Review of current studies and future needs. *Generations, 20*(1), 65–70.

Reppucci, N. D., Britner, P. A., & Woolard, J. L. (1997). *Preventing child abuse and neglect through parent education.* Baltimore: Paul H. Brooks Publishing.

Russell, L. R. (1994). *Focus group assessment of parenting education preferences of Hispanics and Whites.* Unpublished master's thesis, Texas Woman's University.

Shore, R. J., & Hayslip, B. (1994). Custodial grandparenting: Implications for children's development. In A. Gottfried & A. Gottfried (Eds.), *Redefining families: Implications for children's development* (pp. 171–218). New York: Plenum.

Smith, C. A., Cudabeck, D., Goddard, H. W., & Myers-Walls, J. A. (1994). *National extension parent education model.* Manhattan, KS: Kansas Cooperative Extension Service.

Strom, R., & Strom, S. (1984). Creative curriculum for grandparents. *Journal of Creative Behavior, 18*(2), 133–141.

Strom, R., & Strom, S. (1989). Grandparents and learning. *International Journal of Aging and Human Development, 29*(3), 163–169.

Strom, R., & Strom, S. (1990). Grandparent education. *Journal of Instructional Psychology, 17*(2), 85–92.

Strom, R., & Strom, S. (1993). Grandparents raising grandchildren: Goals and support groups. *Educational Gerontology, 19,* 705–715.

Troll, L. E. (1983). Grandparents: The family watchdogs. In T. H. Brubaker (Ed.), *Family relationships in later life* (pp. 63–74). Beverly Hills, CA: Sage Publications.

Wandersman, L. P. (1987). New directions for parent education. In S. L. Kagan, D. R. Powell, B. Weissbound, & E. F. Zigler (Eds.), *America's family support programs: Perspectives and prospects* (pp. 207–227). New Haven, CT: Yale University Press.

Watson, J. A. (1997). Factors associated with African American grandparents' interest in grandparent education. *Journal of Negro Education, 66*(1), 73–82.

CHAPTER 19

Legal Issues for Custodial Grandparents

Raymond Albert

C ustodial grandparents face significant legal issues, due largely to the law's conception of children's interests and norms surrounding grandparents' role in the life of their grandchild. The law typically treats the parent-child relationship as inviolate, and parents are presumed to have the primary claim on achieving and protecting their child's best interests. "Grandparents have always served as 'the family watchdogs' (Troll, 1985) and 'the second line of defense' for children (Kornhaber, 1985)," according to Roe and Minkler (1998). Indeed, citing Fuller-Thomson, Minkler, and Driver (1997), they argue that almost 11% of grandparents at some point raise a grandchild for at least 6 months.

That grandparents cope with the challenge of rearing a grandchild is a contemporary reality. The commensurate legal issues are driven by the array of parental deficits—drug or alcohol abuse; mental illness; foster care placement of children due to parental neglect, abuse, or abandonment; divorce; teen pregnancy; HIV/AIDS status of parents; poverty; family violence; or parental incarceration or death (Child Welfare League of America, 1998; Karp, 1996).

LEGAL CONTEXT OF GRANDPARENT INTERESTS

"The social interest is at its strongest," Andersen (1998, p. 955) argues "at the core of the nuclear family, in the relationships between spouses, child and parent, and siblings. But important bonds also exist with family members further from the center—grandparents . . . and more distant relatives." Alongside the state's interest in the parent-child bond, grandparents play a critical role in socializing children and, when necessary, becoming primary caregivers. The law recognizes and endorses this dynamic through a structure of relevant legislation and case law.

The legal context, then, begins with several pieces of federal legislation, including the Adoption Assistance and Child Welfare Act of 1980, the Indian Child Welfare Act, Title IV of the Social Security Act of 1935, and the Adoption and Safe Families Act of 1997 (ASFA; Pub. L. No. 105-89). (For illustrative purposes, the following discussion will be limited to the ASFA, an example of a state legislative initiative and a judicial decision that interpreted the ASFA.) Moreover, the U.S. Supreme Court decision *Miller v. Youakim* (1979) lays out the financial basis for enabling grandparents to receive foster care payments, provided certain requirements are met.

The Adoption and Safe Families Act of 1997

The goal of the ASFA—"to promote the adoption of children in foster care"—has important implications for grandparents who either seek or end up with custody of their grandchildren. Essentially, the legislation emphasizes kinship care options, including requiring (1) that the Department of Health and Human Services convene an advisory panel to review the state kinship care policies and complete a study on kinship care; (2) that notice of court reviews and an opportunity to be heard be sent to relatives (including grandparents) and other parties, such as foster care parents or preadoptive parents; (3) that states make the health and safety of the child the paramount concern in determining the extent to which "reasonable efforts" should be made to preserve and reunify families of children placed in foster care, but it also allows states to bypass the "reasonable efforts" provision in cases of child abuse or assault or where a parents have had their rights to another sibling involuntarily terminated; (4) that parent locator service be used to identify and locate parents or other relatives who may be interested in providing a permanent home for a child in foster care; and (5) that new time lines and requirements for filing termination of parental rights be instituted, some of which can be waived if the child in question is being cared for by a relative, such as a grandparent.

Clearly, the act's protectionist stance and goal of stabilizing foster care placement is exemplified in circumstances confronting grand-parents and is consistent with testimony supplied during the legislative history of the act (Robinson, 1995).

State Legislative Initiatives

State legislation rounds out the legal context. For example, the Pennsylvania General Assembly has announced, as a matter of public policy, that the commonwealth, pursuing the best interest of the child, has a stake in ensuring that a child maintain reasonable and continuing contact with a grandparent, when a parent is deceased, divorced, or separated (23 Pa. C.S. §5301). The grandparent may be granted reasonable partial custody or visitation rights, or both. The legislature intends that a court should consider the amount of personal contact between grandparents and the child prior to application (23 Pa. C.S. §5311). Moreover, grandparents may petition for visitation or custody, or both, if the child has lived with them for 12 months or more, or they may sue for custody if the child has been adjudicated dependent, pursuant to 42 Pa.C.S. Ch. 63, or if the child is at risk due to parental abuse, neglect, drug or alcohol abuse, or mental illness (23 Pa. C.S. §5313). All jurisdictions have enacted comparable legislation.

Other sources of grandparent authority exist. For example, Karp (1996) describes instances of so-called consent legislation, which allows a transfer of different sorts of authority with a showing of specified documentation. "Washington, DC," she notes, "[enacted] a law that allows parents, legal guardians, or legal custodians to authorize another adult to consent to medical, surgical, dental, or mental health treatment for children in their care. . . . California now has a similar but more far-reaching law" (p. 58).

Judicial Approaches

Judicial construction of state and federal legislation has implications for the scope of grandparent authority. This is especially the case for the ASFA, for which there is not much case law to date, but one Pennsylvania Superior Court decision offers a hint of how a court is likely to construe this new legislation. In *Lilley v. Lilley* (1998), a Pennsylvania court dealt with the involuntary termination of parental rights for a mother whose son had been placed with a foster family. Although the court upheld the trial court's termination of the mother's parental rights, the most revealing aspect of the decision was the court's enthusiastic endorsement of the potential of the ASFA, particularly the act's unequivocal goal of safety, permanency, and well-being. While recognizing that it is premature to predict the scope of the act's implementation, the court nonetheless proceeded to assert the viability of the act to resolve foster care issues in favor of expedited permanency, with preference likely to be given to relatives, including grandparents.

STRUCTURING GRANDPARENT-CHILD CAREGIVING RELATIONSHIPS

Flint and Perez-Porter (1997) argue that caregiving can take several forms, depending on the formality of the relationship, and not surprisingly, care along this continuum carries different legal obligations.[1] Grandparents may assume responsibility for a child on an informal basis for an indeterminate period of time, or they may pursue a more formal route, such as custody, foster care, adoption, or guardianship.

Informal Structures

Although grandparents may pursue informal arrangements when they assume responsibility for a grandchild, the parents typically retain parental rights unless the state has moved to terminate these rights. To guard against the creation of an "authority vacuum," grandparents may seek a more formal structure, including custody or guardianship, thereby ensuring that someone is able to make decisions for the child.

Day-to-day decision making on the child's behalf is critical to his or her well-being and sense of security. The child's interaction with myriad social institutions requires that grandparents be able to access medical and school records or medical treatment, and state legislation may vary regarding whether nonparents have the authority to grant such consent or obtain the requisite records. Parents may delegate certain responsibilities to another person, such as a grandparent, and thereby enable the caregiver to carry out these delegated tasks.

Formal Structures

More formal arrangements can be made, and these will spell out the scope of the grandparents' authority. A custody order, for example, will allow a nonparent to obtain physical possession of a child. Grandparents may petition for such orders, provided they can demonstrate that the child's parent is unfit. This level of proof is a heavy threshold to surmount; it requires more than a showing that the child's interest will be served by living with the nonparent. Even this award of custody has its limits, and while legal custody affords a measure of control over important decisions regarding the child, it does not extend to control over the child's property or other financial interests.

Guardianship offers another option, one that can be obtained if the child's parents are deceased, give their consent, or are deemed unsuitable. The scope of guardianship can be either expansive or limited, with the law providing for guardianship of the child's property or only her person or, if necessary, both. Unlike custody, however, the parents' rights are not terminated, and the nonparent is not financially responsible for the child. Moreover, the parent may petition for visitation. "A grandparent who has been appointed the legal guardian of a grandchild may be able to have the grandchild's medical care covered by the grandparents' health insurance policy," according to Flint and Perez-Porter (1997), and the grandparent guardian may even be able to designate a "standby or springing guardian who will assume the care of the child when the guardian is no longer able to do so" (p. 66).

Children removed from their home because of parental abuse or neglect may be placed with a relative, including a grandparent, for foster care. Grandparents may investigate the availability of foster care payments, which include

> . . . payments to meet the food, clothing, shelter, daily supervision, school supplies, personal and special needs of a child. Since foster care payment rates are much higher than public assistance . . . kinship foster care appears to be an attractive alternative for low-income grandparents. However, legal custody of the child remains with the official charged with the protection of children. . . . The grandparent, therefore, will not have the authority to consent to medical treatment, or make other decisions a guardian or custodian is empowered to make. (Flint & Perez-Porter, 1997, p. 66)

Notwithstanding, there are limits to grandparents' ability to obtain kinship foster care payments. Ultimately, foster care is a temporary arrangement, and grandparents risk losing their grandchild to an adoptive family if they decline adoption opportunities.

Finally, grandparents may elect to adopt their grandchild, a move that severs all parental rights and enables the grandparent to make all decisions concerning all aspects of the child's life. Termination of parental rights—voluntarily or via a showing of parental abandonment, neglect, or mental illness—is the sine qua non of grandparent adoption rights.

A COROLLARY PATH: GRANDPARENT VISITATION AND THE LAW

The demand for grandparents to care for their children's children is likely to increase. This trend is most apparent when one examines the phenomenon of grandparent visitation rights, a topic to which I shall now turn by exploring the contours of relevant case law. Grandparent visitation is worth examining at this point, because visitation is often a prelude to a shift to a more formal status, such as custody or adoption, and because it is frequently a logical extension of informal arrangements. Because all 50 states have enacted this type of legislation, I will limit the case law discussion to selected representative cases in just two jurisdictions: Pennsylvania and New Jersey. The details supplied in the discussion offer some sense of the diversity of fact situations regarding this area of law.

All 50 states have enacted legislation allowing grandparents to petition for visitation rights, but the considerations governing such petitions vary from state to state. Forty states currently use "best interest of the child" language, which requires grandparents to demonstrate that visitation is in the child's best interest. Others require that visitation not interfere with the parent-child relationship. The majority of states also only allow for visitation petitions to be filed when the child's parents are separated or divorced or one or both parents are deceased. However, 24 states have general visitation statutes that allow grandparents to seek visitation and do not limit the circumstances under which visitation may be sought (i.e., within intact families) (National Conference of State Legislatures, 1996). Judicial treatment of these statutes also varies. Some state courts have found grandparent visitation rights unconstitutional; others have expanded the scope of the rights.

The most controversial aspect of grandparent visitation rights is the expansion into intact families (i.e., where a married mother and father oppose visitation). The arguments in favor of expanding grandparents' rights to petition for visitation revolve around an emotional construct: theoretically, the state is increasing the amount of love and support received by the child. Family cohesiveness is strengthened, on the assumption that the grandparents' presence provides a safe and protective environment for the child. However, not every petition for grandparent visitation is successful. Opponents of the expansion of grandparent visitation rights argue that parental rights are superior to those of grandparents, and any legislation that attempts to interfere with the parent-child relationship is inherently suspect.

Pennsylvania Case Law

Pennsylvania recently debated expanding its state statute with regard to grandparent visitation rights. Currently, a grandparent may petition for visitation if the parents are separated or divorced or one has died or if the child lived with the grandparent for at least 1 year. (See 23 Pa.C.S. Sec. 5311-5313.) A bill aimed at expanding visitation rights into intact families was introduced in the 1998 Pennsylvania General Assembly; and although it successfully navigated the House of Representatives, it failed to emerge from the Senate Judiciary Committee.

Commonwealth ex rel. Zaffarano v. Genaro (1983)

In *Zaffarano v. Genaro* the grandparents, Zaffarano, initially petitioned for visitation and temporary custody rights. The trial court denied their petition, and on appeal to the Superior Court, the decision was reversed and remanded to order partial custody. On appeal again, the case ended up in the Supreme Court of Pennsylvania.

Prior to the mother's death in an accident, the grandparents often visited their grandchild. Subsequently, however, animosity arose between the grandparents and the child's father, Genaro. The trial court found that visits would not be in the child's best interest because of the friction between Zaffarano and Genaro. The Superior Court found their differences reconcilable and concluded that visits would be in the child's best interest and awarded partial custody. The Pennsylvania Supreme Court reversed, arguing that the burden of proof for partial custody was on the grandparents because parents have a prima facie right to custody unless convincing reasons rebut this presumption. In addition, the court held that the appellate court could not substitute its own findings of fact with regard to the parents and grandparents' hostility toward one another. The supreme court also reasoned that it did not require proof of harm, per se; rather, it was satisfied with the possibility of such harm pursuant to the animosity that existed between the parent and the grandparents.

Miller v. Miller (1984)

The grandparents in this case, R. and N. Miller, were granted visitation rights with their grandchild, and the case was appealed by the mother, C. Miller, who claimed that the hostility and tension between the parties would not make visitation in the best interest of the child.

The main issue before the court was whether the resulting level of family constituted a sufficient obstruction to deny grandparent visitation.

Relying on *Zaffarano v. Genaro* as a precedent to differentiate between custody and visitation, the court determined that the Millers had to show why it would be in the child's best interest to interrupt the parent's prima facie right to custody. Ultimately, the court found that the child would benefit from a relationship with the grandparents and that this would not interfere with the mother-child relationship.

Bishop v. Piller (1994)

In this case, the issue before the court was whether a paternal grandparent of a child born out of wedlock could be granted visitation when the father has no legal relationship with the child or the mother. The mother and father never cohabited or married, and the child was raised solely by the mother, Piller. The father and paternal grandmother, Bishop, filed a custody petition that included visits for the grandmother. The hearing court ruled that custody would remain with Piller but granted visitation with the grandmother. Piller appealed, and the Superior Court upheld the decision.

In order to decide this case, the Supreme Court had to interpret what the legislature meant when it included "separation" in the state statute. The Superior Court found that the term—which it defined, pursuant to Webster's, as an act or instance of dividing or an act or instance of parting company—applied to the parents in this case, and although it might be a stretch, it was legitimate. The court construed "separation" as beginning from conception—ample time to meet the 6-month statutory requirement. Piller disagreed, arguing that the visits could not be ordered under the statute unless the parents were married at one time or the parents had a long, cohabiting relationship. The court stated that the statute's intention was to grant visits to a grandmother whose child had died but not to one whose child did not marry or live with the other parent. The court held that grandchildren have a natural right to know their grandparents and that the statute's purpose is to provide for the child's best interest.

New Jersey Case Law

New Jersey's Grandparent Visitation Statute is the most accessible to grandparents. (See N.J.S.A. Sec 9:2-7.1.) It allows visitation petitions for all families, regardless of marital status. New Jersey courts have been relatively sympathetic to grandparent rights, compared to Pennsylvania.

Mimkon v. Ford (1975)

This case, which was decided before New Jersey expanded its Grandparent Visitation Statute, posed a complicated question: Is the maternal grandmother entitled to visitation when her daughter dies and the surviving spouse and his new wife refuse to permit visits?

The child's parents separated prior to the child's birth and subsequently divorced. The child lived with the mother and grandmother, Mimkon, until the mother died. The father, Ford, then took custody; he remarried, and his new wife adopted the child. Mimkon visited with the child, but upon denial of visits she petitioned for visitation.

The court noted that there was no judicial recognition of the rights of the grandparent, and in the past, the courts had been unanimous in denying visitation when the custodial parent objected. Notwithstanding, it also reasoned that a change in New Jersey's statute, to include visitation when one or both parents died, modified the state's common law rule regarding grandparents' rights by creating an independent ability to act without linking that right to the dead parent.

The child's adoptive status brought into focus the clash between the adoption statute, on the one hand, and the Grandparent Visitation Statute, on the other. Ultimately, the state supreme court reconciled this conflict in favor of the grandparent, reasoning that the Grandparent Visitation Statute did not clash with the underlying policies found in the adoption statute. The court concluded that the legislature did not intend for one statute to trump the other. Consequently, it ruled that it was proper for grandparents to enjoy visitation privileges over the objections of an adoptive parent, provided this arrangement represents the child's best interest. The lower court's decision was reversed and remanded to determine if visitation was in the best interest of the child.

Thompson v. Vanaman

Decided prior to the expansion of New Jersey's Grandparent Visitation Statute, this case revolves around the grandmother's (Thompson's) petition for visitation privileges over the parents' objections. Thompson used to care for the children while the parents were at work, but this practice was halted after a family dispute over money. Although the statute did not cover intact families, the court interpreted legislative intent in favor of grandparent visitation in cases involving death, divorce or separation.

Citing the Mimkon decision, which supported broad recognition of grandparent rights, the Superior Court found a positive preexisting relationship between Thompson and her grandchildren and thus ruled that there was no disadvantages to the visit. Unfortunately, the appellate division of Superior Court heard the appeal and held in favor of Vanahan, the parent, arguing that grandparents had no right to visit when the custodial parent objects. The court found it was not in the children's best interest to force them into the conflict between their parents and grandmother, despite her prior involvement in their upbringing.

R.T. and M.T. v. J.E. and L.E. (1994)

The parents in this case challenged New Jersey's Grandparent Visitation Statute, claiming it violated their Fourteenth Amendment rights in that it interfered with their fundamental right of liberty to raise their children as they saw fit. The grandparents, R.T. and M.T. petitioned for visitation after the parents denied it. After an unsuccessful attempt at mediation, the parents argued that the statute should not be applied to intact families. The court, while not unsympathetic to their view, argued that even constitutionally recognized rights are not without limits; and such relationships may be subject to legitimate regulation.

By creating a right for grandparent visitation, the court reasoned, the legislature sought to balance the competing interests of the grandparent, the parent, and the child. In addition, the statute gave the right to petition for visitation, not the absolute right to it. The statute also defined eight separate factors to be considered in determining best interest of the child. Ultimately, in holding the statute constitutional, the court concluded that it contained a refutable presumption regarding the benefit of a grandparent-child relationship; the legislature did not presume that all such relationships were automatically beneficial, and the grandparents bore the burden of proof.

CONCLUSION

Custodial grandparents face significant challenges, not the least of which are those framed by the law. Contemporary pressures on parents suggest that they will continue to turn to *their* parents for help with *their* children. Almost 4 million children now live with their grandparents, and the trend promises to continue unabated. Indeed, grandparent caregivers will continue to require legal authority for surrogate decision making and for coping with legal barriers to social programs.

Have pressures on the modern family transformed the grandparent role, from a benign supportive presence to an active decision maker and quasi-parent? The literature (Achenbaum, 1999; Andersen, 1998; Bostock, 1994; Burton, 1992; Hartfield, 1996; Mullen, 1996; Power & Malucchio, 1999; Quintal, 1995) and daily experience suggest that the traditional grandparent role has given way to a new conception of the grandparent as ultimate caregiver. The merits of this transformation are difficult to evaluate, but one might correctly suspect that the change does not portend well for the nuclear family—or for grandparents, either. That they are willing or able to take on the task is not the same as saying they will carry it out successfully. Against the backdrop of familial dysfunction or other parental difficulties that result in grandparents assuming caregiving responsibilities, the fact that they perform the role successfully is perhaps less important than that they stand ready to do it at all. Arguably, therein lies a conundrum: grandparents have either invoked the law for enlarged legal rights or have had the law thrust some responsibilities on them. The law has kept pace with the shifts in grandparent roles and competencies. Given the complexity surrounding the American family struggling to cope at the dawn of the new millennium, the law's competencies will certainly be challenged, but it seems clear that both the law and grandparents are the only game in town.

NOTE

1. This section draws heavily on Flint and Perez-Porter's (1997) wonderfully practical and informed discussion of the legal and economic issues confronting grandparent caregivers. My reliance is based on their comprehensive coverage of relevant state law.

REFERENCES

Achenbaum, W. A. (1999). The social compact in American history. *Generations, 23,* 2215–2218.

Andersen, E. G. (1998). Children, parents, and nonparents: Protected interests and legal standards. *Brigham Young University Law Review,* 935–1002.

Bishop v. Piller, 536 Pa. 41; 637 A.2d 976 (1994).

Bostock, C. (1994). Does the expansion of grandparent visitation rights promote the best interests of the child?: A survey of grandparent visitation laws in the fifty states. *Columbia Journal of Law and Social Problems, 27,* 319.

Burton, L. (1992). Black grandparents rearing children of drug-addicted parents: Stressors, outcomes, and social needs. *Gerontologist, 32,* 744–751.

Casper, L. M., & Bryson, K. (1998). Co-resident grandparents and their grandchildren. Grandparents maintained families. *Working Paper No. 26.* Washington, DC: U.S. Bureau of the Census.

Child Welfare League of America. (1998). Kinship care. [On-line]. Available: <http://www.igc.org/cwla/kinship/>.

Commonwealth ex rel. Zaffarano v. Genaro, 500 Pa. 256; 455 A.2d 1180 (1983).

Flint, M., & Periz-Porter, M. (1997). Grandparent caregivers: Legal and economic issues. *Journal of Gerontological Social Work, 28,* 63–76.

Fuller-Thomson, E., Minkler, M., & Driver, D. (1997). A profile of grandparents raising grandchildren in the United States. *Gerontologist, 37,* 406–411.

Hartfield, B. W. (1996). Legal recognition of the value of intergenerational nurturance: Grandparent visitation statutes in the nineties. *Generations, 20,* 53–56.

Karp, N. (1996). Legal problems of grandparents and other kinship caregivers. *Generations, 20,* 57–60.

Kornhaber, A. (1985). Grandparenthood and the "new social contract." In V. L. Bengtson & J. F. Roberts (Eds.), *Grandparenthood.* Beverly Hills, CA: Sage.

Lilley v. Lilley, 719A.2d 337 (1998).

Miller v. Miller, 329 Pa. Super. 248; 478 A.2d 451 (1984).

Miller v. Youkim, 440 U.S. 125 (1979).

Mimkon v. Ford, 66 N.J. 426; 332 A.2d 199 (1975).

Murray v. Marks, 1993 Del. Fam. Ct.

National Conference of State Legislatures (NCSL). (1996). *Third party custody and visitation.* Washington, DC.

Power, M., & Maluccio, A. (1999). Intergenerational approaches to helping families at risk. *Generations, 22,* 37–42.

Quintal, M. (1995). Court ordered families: An overview of grandparent visitation statutes. *Suffolk University Law Review, 29,* 840, n. 29.

Riley v. Quig, 1983 Del. Super.

Roe, K. M., & Minkler, M. (1998). Grandparents raising grandchildren: Challenges and responses. *Generations, 22,* 25–32.

Robinson, D. (1995, May). Testimony before Subcommittee on Human Resources, House Committee on Ways and Means.

R.T. and M.T. v. J.E. and L.E., 277 N.J. Super. 595; 650 A.2d 13 (1994).

Thompson v. Vanaman, 210 N.J. Super. 225;509 A.2d 304 (1986).

Thompson v. Vanaman, 21 N.J. Super. 596; 515 A.2d 1254 (1986).

Troll, L. E. (1985). The contingencies of grandparenting. In V. L. Bengston & J. F. Roberts (Eds.), *Grandparenthood.* Beverly Hills, CA: Sage.

CHAPTER 20

Organizational Advocacy as a Factor in Public Policy Regarding Custodial Grandparenting

Donna M. Butts

The dramatic increase in the number of grandparents and relatives raising children has sparked a public policy debate that will continue to escalate in the years to come. How the families are categorized, serviced, and supported is at the basis of an argument that has the potential to galvanize or alienate advocates concerned with issues affecting children, youth, and the elderly. At one time the issue was easy to ignore. Historically, extended families have always stepped in to care for younger members when their parents were unable to care for them, whether on a temporary or a permanent basis. But now the issue has taken on a new face. It is no longer someone else's family or a problem that can be isolated on the basis of race, geography, or economics. We can no longer ignore these families. For reasons discussed at length in other chapters, relatives are unexpectedly finding themselves called on to be parents, whether for the first time or, in the case of grandparents, for the second or third time around.

WHY ARE GRANDPARENTS AND OTHER RELATIVES RAISING CHILDREN?

In the mid-90s, Generations United (GU) was instrumental in helping to organize a Wingspread retreat to review the state of the intergenerational field and to create a working plan for the future. As a small organization and the only national coalition to focus solely on intergenerational public policy and programs, it was important to identify emerging issues that did not have an existing champion. The growing concern about grandparents and other relatives raising children appeared to have no broad, organized, national constituency.

The 1995 White House Conference on Aging was the first forum to bring the issue to national attention. However, a national umbrella for the growing number of individuals and organizations concerned about these unique families did not exist. Generations United, with more than 100 organizational members, was the natural coalition to fill this void.

Since 1986, GU has been the leading national organization fostering collaboration in support of intergenerational public policy initiatives, strategies, and programs. Although others have been involved in important work in the area of grandparents and other relatives raising children, GU was the first to frame the issues from the perspectives of what was needed by the caregivers as well as by the children in their care.

INTERGENERATIONAL APPROACH TO PUBLIC POLICY

An intergenerational approach to framing public policy issues is rooted in the understanding that interdependence and reciprocity characterize the relationship between the generations. Public policy initiatives are examined by looking at the impact across the entire life span. Questions include the following:

- What will this mean to our children and our children's children?
- How will this affect our elderly?
- Are children, youth, and the elderly viewed as assets?
- Is the policy sensitive to intergenerational family structures such as grandparents raising children?
- Is one generation being unfairly sacrificed to help another?
- Does it encourage division or interdependence between the generations?
- Does the policy encourage intergenerational transfers and interaction through shared care, services, and/or sites?

Grandparents raising children clearly fit the criteria for an issue with an intergenerational intersection affecting multiple ages.

WHY IS NATIONAL ORGANIZATIONAL ADVOCACY NECESSARY?

Gandhi once said, "I must hurry, for I am their leader and there they go." A national organization's unique role is that of a catalyst to help determine a shared agenda and action plan. National organizations have an obligation to be the conduits through which the collective wisdom found at the grass-roots level can flow, connect, and solidify into a shared, and therefore strengthened, national voice. National organizations can and do play a role in early issue identification, distillation, and broad dissemination, but the strength to carry out the agenda rests within the local-national partnership.

An organizational approach is vital. In the case of grandparents raising children the various stakeholders have organized to share their resources, based on a collective concern for the families. This includes groups whose traditional agendas are single-age focused. Together they can share resources and divide what could be overwhelming into a set of manageable tasks. In addition, the individuals and their associations bring credibility to the issue. Their specific networks and reputations lend endorsement to the critical nature of this issue.

The coalition also provides the voice of reason when the debate becomes unreasonable. For example, it can respond quickly to media reports that portray the families in a negative or stereotypical light.

WHO SHOULD BE INVOLVED?

Grandparents and relatives raising children is a complex issue that can and should involve a wide base of special interest groups. Because of the causal factors leading to this family structure, groups whose missions drive them to be involved in issues such as HIV/AIDS, incarceration, alcohol and drug abuse, mental health problems, poverty, teenage pregnancy, child abuse, and family preservation should be at the table. It is an issue that affects older and younger age groups. Therefore, organizations such as the AARP, the Child Welfare League of America, the National Council on the Aging, and the Children's Defense Fund are among the many colleagues active with the issue. Others whose work affects the families, such as health, housing, education, child care, welfare reform, employment, and legal rights should be involved. What is critical and often missing is the vehicle to connect the independent organizations to better support formal and informal kinship care families. Once convened, they may use the meetings to coordinate services, fill identified service gaps, and develop a public policy agenda.

FRAMING THE ISSUE

The Symposium and Our Intergenerational Action Agenda

Generations United offers a model for an organizational response. To begin, GU organized an invitational symposium in 1997 for a select group of national leaders to examine the growing number of grandparent- and relative-headed families. The 35 experts represented child welfare, aging, government, legal, and academic communities. In order to narrow the discussion, the focus was on (1) relative-headed households without a parent present and (2) informal caregivers who were providing care outside the formal foster care system and without legal custody. Background papers were prepared on the demographic and sociological contexts, public benefits, child welfare system, and supportive services.

After 2 days of presentations and discussions, the conclusions from the symposium were quite clear. Too little is known about the true circumstances of the families, their characteristics, and their genuine needs. Although the knowledge base is growing, it is still inadequate to fully understand the demographic and sociological characteristics of the families.

Two primary barriers emerged: (1) the inability of the families to access existing services and (2) the need for broad public education. The core issue with many public benefits and support services was that the grandparents simply did not know what was available to the child or to them as caretakers. Education was deemed critical because often the local caseworker or other front-line worker did not know that the grandparents or children in their care were eligible for services. Grandparents were told no and accepted the response without question. For example, grandparents said they could not access Head Start for the children in their care. After checking with Head Start, they found no prohibitions that would keep the grandparents from accessing services. Unfortunately, the myth that they could not had become accepted as fact.

The results of the symposium were published in a monograph, *Grandparents and Other Relatives Raising Children: An Intergenerational Action Agenda.* It includes key recommendations for policy makers, advocates, community organizations, and leaders. The report garnered the support of many diverse organizations and provided the first show of solidarity for the families. The coalition's membership helped to bring credibility to the issue. Politicians interested in their most vulnerable constituents—the elderly and the young—found an issue that bridged both age groups.

The report itself was divided into three broad areas: family supports, community education and media advocacy, and data collection. It was designed to describe the needs of the families, the need for accurate information dissemination about the families, and the need for additional data collection to learn more about the families. It was published as an invitation challenging professionals, policy makers, and community leaders to learn more and begin to address the identified problems within their reach. An overview of the three broad areas covered in the Action Agenda follows.

Family Supports. Often the relative caregivers step forward to provide care at great sacrifice to themselves. Many have planned and worked hard to build a comfortable retirement with enough resources to support themselves and not be a burden on their kin or the public. The additional financial strain created by children in the house can soon deplete the resources and even cause the caregivers to lose their housing, because of either zoning or occupancy limitations. The section on family supports provides an overview of economic supports, education, health care, child care, the child welfare system, legal issues, and supportive services.

Community Education and Media Advocacy. The public, including direct service providers and managers, is still largely unaware of the serious issues the families face and their sociological context. Comprehensive community education and media advocacy are needed to develop and dispense positive, accurate messages about the grandparents and the children in their care. Target audiences include federal and state policy makers, elected officials, advocacy organizations, and the business community.

Data Collection. Data collection and dissemination must be improved. It is integral to the development of effective public policies and important in any public education effort. There is a need for a national clearinghouse that works with research data, collects state and local information, and provides access to materials and resources located throughout the country. Support is needed for efforts to increase the quality and quantity of data collected and to identify specific areas calling for further research.

Release and Follow-Up

Working closely with key congressional leadership, GU planned a press conference to release the document. The event included key leaders of the coalition and testimony from grandparent caregivers and concluded with remarks from members of Congress. The news conference was held on Capitol Hill immediately following the National Council on the Aging and GU annual conference. Senator Jay Rockefeller (D-WV) and Representative Connie Morella (R-MD), both of whom have been early advocates on behalf of kinship care, sponsored it.

The document was further distributed during a subsequent briefing on Capitol Hill that educated more than 70 professionals on the issues, including innovative state responses. It also provided a perspective from a very articulate grandmother who, along with her husband, is raising her son's two sons. Her story was essential in adding a clear voice and a face to a session that otherwise focused on numbers and research. The grandmother's testimony is what people remembered.

Later the document was distributed to each congressional office with an invitation to a second briefing, highlighting housing and educational barriers confronting the caregivers.The coalition that GU works with continues to provide guidance for the agenda's dissemination. Additional Capitol Hill briefings, media contact, and federal agency symposiums are planned.

CONGRUENT FEDERAL EFFORTS

At the same time the Action Agenda was being created, Congress passed two related pieces of legislation. The Personal Responsibility and Work Opportunity Reconciliation Act of 1996 required that the year 2000 census include a question specifically designed to identify grandparent-headed households. This will mark the first census in which an attempt is made to gather data specifically about the families.

The Adoption and Safe Families Act of 1997 included a section on kinship care and was considered an important step in bringing the issues related to these families to the attention of Congress. In general the section called for a report to Congress on children in foster care who are placed with relatives, including a state-by-state breakdown of available numbers and policies affecting kinship care. A national panel was appointed by the Secretary of the Department of Health and Human Services to review the report prior to submission. Also of notable importance was the final section of the 1997 act, which outlines a "sense of Congress" that states should enact standby guardianship laws and procedures. The act does not address all the needs of kinship care families. However, most believe it is a good beginning and will provide the foundation from which to build in future years.

IMPLICATIONS FOR STATE AND LOCAL ACTION

The national movement in support of grandparents and relatives raising children is important for many reasons. The national coalition helps to gain recognition and visibility for the issue. It is helpful in solidifying an agenda and influencing federal policy-making and funding streams. Although the work of the national coalition continues, it has become quite apparent that the network and effort must grow at the local level. First, much of the advocacy effort and policy implementation on behalf of these families occurs at the state and local level. For example, housing has repeatedly been identified as a major problem, with local advocates citing case after case of grandparents being evicted from their housing when grandchildren come to live with them. In questioning representatives of the Department of Housing and Urban Development (HUD) it was learned that there are no national restrictions prohibiting grandparents from housing their grandchildren. However, as federal dollars are passed down to states, states create their own guidelines, which can terminate the eligibility status of a grandparent who takes in a child. Education is in a similar situation. State and local school authorities determine the policies and guidelines for their communities.

Looking to the future, informing and involving local policy makers and decision makers will become even more important. The current thrust toward devolution gives more and more power and decision making to local government. Efforts to deliver block grant funds directly to states increase the difficulty of advocating at the federal level. To succeed, the growing kinship care movement will have to focus its efforts on coordinated state and community-based advocacy.

Several states have developed legislation designed to support kinship care families. For example, in 1998, Florida passed the Relative Caregiver Program. It calls for relatives within the fifth degree of relationship by blood or marriage to receive up to 82% of the usual monthly foster care payment for each child they are caring for. The children are also eligible for family support and preservation services, Medicaid coverage, subsidized child care, and other safety net services.

During the same year, Kentucky passed a child custody bill that expands the legal rights of grandparents and other relatives and nonrelatives raising children. Under this law, if the court determines that the grandparent or other person satisfies the criteria for being considered a de facto custodian, that person is given the same standing as a parent in a custody proceeding. Therefore, they are given equal consideration with parents in determining custody based on the best interests of the child. Moreover, under this law the de facto custodian may be given joint custody of the child with the parents.

State and local groups are also working hard to increase familiarity and understanding of kinship care families. Washington state's governor proclaimed May 20, 1998, Grandparents Raising Grandchildren Day. Local grandparents involved with a support group wrote the document he signed.

The Brookdale Foundation has been the leader in providing funding for state and local programs designed to support grandparent caregivers in more than half the states. Small seed grants provide start-up funds for local and state agencies to develop support groups that provide respite for the grandparents and the children in their care. Several state networks have developed as a result of the support groups.

As grandparent support groups increase in numbers around the country, a growing kinship care movement is developing. Composed of grandparents, advocates, and other interested individuals, these groups are making progress with state legislation on behalf of grandparents. The networks are becoming more formal, and their ability to learn about other states' successes grows. Generations United's quarterly newsletter includes a special state legislative update section. Generations United also maintains a database of model legislation.

FINDINGS AND CONCLUSIONS

The public policy work must continue on the national level while expanding at the state and local levels. Many policies, such as those affecting housing, TANF (Temporary Assistance for Needy Families), and education are under state jurisdiction. Advocates for children and the elderly must work together to influence decision makers and educate them about the circumstances that surround these unique families. The compelling reason is quite simple. There are nearly 500,000 children in the formal foster care system and 3.9 million children in kinship care. As a country we need these brave caregivers to continue. They are the last bastion holding America's families together.

CHAPTER 21

Trends and Correlates of Coresidency Among Black and White Grandmothers and Their Grandchildren: A Panel Study, 1967–1992

Richard K. Caputo

This chapter reports findings of a panel study examining trends and correlates of coresidency among Black and White grandmothers and grandchildren. It shows trends of the odds that Black respondents were more likely to be coresident grandmothers than were White respondents. In addition, this chapter shows correlates of coresidency for two subsamples of this nationally representative sample of mature women: (1) ever-coresident grandmothers, that is, respondents who coresided with their grandchildren at any time between 1967 and 1992, and (2) coresident grandmothers in 1992.

LITERATURE REVIEW

As this volume attests, there is increasing scholarship and research in the area of grandparent caregiving. Much of the related research, however, has been based on small nonrandom samples in particular geographic areas (Aldous, 1995; Fuller-Thomson, Minkler, & Driver, 1997). An earlier national study of grandparents (Cherlin & Furstenberg, 1986) was based on interviews with the parents of a representative sample of children aged 7 to 11 years in 1976. Findings from such studies are not representative of the population of custodial or coresident grandparents.

Chalfie (1994) used data from the March 1992 *Current Population Survey (CPS)* and examined skipped-generation households, that is, those comprising grandparents and grandchildren with neither of the grandchild's parents present. Although Chalfie provided useful information about an important subset of grandparent caregivers, nearly two thirds of children residing with grandparents lived in homes in which at least one parent also was present. Hence, Chalfie's study did not provide nationally representative data on the broader population of grandparents who are raising grandchildren. Furthermore, Chalfie reported only results of bivariate analyses. Multivariate analyses are needed to account for the simultaneously relative influence of other variables on grandparent caregiving.

Using the second wave of data from the National Survey of Families and Households (NSFH), Fuller-Thomson et al. (1997) attempted to fill in some of these gaps. Their study, however, relied on data gathered within a relatively short time span, namely, 1992–1994. Information relevant to the study reported in this chapter, such as length of time spent as caregiving grandparents, was retrospective and therefore less reliable than if it had been gathered periodically at shorter time intervals. Likewise, by relying on *CPS* data, Chalfie (1994) was limited to a cross-section of the U.S. population interviewed in March 1992. Such studies did not have the benefit of information available in panel surveys that follow the same individuals over several decades. The availability of longitudinal data files such as the Panel Study of Income Dynamics and National Longitudinal Surveys (NLS) makes possible more accurate estimates of the incidence, duration, and prevalence of grandparent caregiving over the life course (Giarrusso, Silverstein, & Bengtson, 1996; Hunter & Ensminger, 1992).

The study reported in this chapter uses a nationally representative sample of mature women drawn in 1967 to fill some gaps in previous research. Specifically, it addresses the following questions of this cohort of women between 1967 and 1992:

1. To what extent did the odds of being a coresident grandparent vary over time by race?
2. How did the defining characteristics of coresident grandmothers and their grandchildren differ by race?
3. To what extent did predictors or correlates of coresident grandparent status vary by race?
4. Among coresident grandmothers, to what extent did predictors or correlates of residing within a three-generation versus a skipped-generation household vary by race?

METHODS

Sample and Data

Study data came from the National Longitudinal Survey of Labor Market Experience, Mature Women's Cohort, a nationally representative sample of 5,083 women who were aged 30 to 44 in 1967 when they were first interviewed. The most recent data available for this study reflected circumstances of respondents through 1992, resulting in a total of 15 survey years. Documentation about the sample was found in the *NLS Handbook 1995* (Center for Human Resource Research, 1995).

Measures

The labels and definitions of the study variables appear in Table 21.1. Respondents who reported at least one grandchild when asked about their relationship to each of the other household members at the time of the survey were classified as coresident grandmothers (CGM). Duration of coresidency (Duration) was determined by the

TABLE 21.1   Variables Used for the Analysis of Coresident Grandparents and Their Grandchildren

Variable	Label	Definition
Age	Age of respondent	Respondent's age at the time of the first interview in 1967 plus 25
CGC	Coresident grandchildren	The number of grandchildren living in the household
CGM	Coresident grandmother	1 = coresident grandmother, that is, a respondent who reported a grandchild when asked about their relationship to each of the other household members at the time of the survey; 0 = others.
Duration	Duration of coresidency	The number of years respondents reported at least one of their grandchildren lived in the household at the time of the survey
ED	Education level	Highest grade completed by respondent through 1989, the last year this data was reported
HT	Household type	1 = three-generation household, that is, those in which the grandmother resided with her own children and with her grandchildren; 0 = skipped-generation household, that is, those in which the grandmother resided with her grandchildren but without any of her own children.
Kids	Children	The number of respondent's own children living in the household
LOWINC	Income status	1 = low-income; 0 = other. Low-income families were those whose total annual family income reported for the previous calendar year was less than or equal to one-half the median family income based on the entire sample.
Race	Race	1 = Black, 0 = other.
Region	Region	1 = South, 0 = other.
Single	Marital status	1 = single (including separated, widowed, and divorced women); 0 = married, with spouse present.
WKSWRK	Work effort	The number of weeks worked (in units of 10) between survey years
YRSCGP	Duration of coresidency	The number of years in which respondents reported that at least one of their grandchildren lived in the household at the time of the survey

number of years respondents reported that at least one of their grandchildren lived in the household at the time of the survey. The marital status variable Single reflects previous research signifying that coresidency was more likely among single grandmothers.

Because the NLS defined household members in relation to respondents, data were not available to determine if a respondent's child who resided in the household was also the coresident grandchild's parent. For purposes of assigning values to the variable household type (HT), three-generation households were construed as those in which the grandmother resided with her own children and with her grandchildren. Skipped-generation households comprised those in which the grandmother resided with her grandchildren but without any of her own children. A related measure, CGC, comprised the number of coresident grandchildren in the household.

Procedures

Chi-square and Cochran-Mantel-Haenszel statistics were used to determine if Black respondents were more likely than Whites to have higher experimental mortality rates and to have grandchildren residing in the household in each of the 15 survey years in the study period (Cody & Smith, 1997). In addition, t-tests and chi-square statistics were used to determine the extent to which the eligible sample of respondents in survey year 1992 differed from the population sample in 1967 on selected demographic variables age, highest grade completed by respondents' mothers, and number of family members. Only those respondents for whom all relevant information was available were included in the two study subsamples defined below.

The first subsample comprised ever-coresident or caregiver grandmothers ($n = 745$; 422 Black, 323 White) between 1967 and 1992. Separate logistic regression analyses were used to compare correlates of coresidency versus noncoresidency in 1992 among Black and White ever-coresident grandmothers. Correlates or predictors were selected for inclusion in the regression model on the basis of theoretical significance and empirical findings of previous research. Black-White comparisons are made in light of culturally specific variations found in previous research on the role of grandmothers in family support systems (Kivett, 1993).

The second subsample comprised only coresident grandmothers in 1992 ($n = 279$; 198 Black, 81 White). Logistic regression analysis was used to compare correlates of those whose own children also resided with them in 1992 versus those whose own children did not live with them. This procedure distinguished three-generation from skipped-generation households. Coresident grandmothers who reported that no children of their own lived with them were construed as skipped-generation households. Separate regression analyses were used for Black and White coresident grandmothers.

LIMITATIONS

Use of the NLS, Mature Women's Cohort, limited this study to a nationally representative sample of American women between the ages of 30 and 44 in 1967. Because the cohort was not representative of all adult women and because the NLS data files contained no information about respondents' grandchildren living outside the household, generalizability about grandmothers was compromised. Also, to the extent that respondents who remained in the cohort in 1992 differed from the population sample in 1967, generalizability was further compromised. Despite these limitations, study findings provide a basis of comparison with previous research and thereby add to the growing body of knowledge about coresident grandparents and their grandchildren. Results are presented and policies recommended with these limitations in mind.

RESULTS

Comparison of Population Sample to Study Sample

Compared to the population sample in 1967 ($n = 5083$), those remaining in the cohort in 1992 ($n = 2953$) tended to be younger (37.6 years of age compared to 37.0, $t = -5.1$, $p < .001$), to reside in larger families (5.00 family members compared to 4.42, ($t = 9.5$, $p = .001$), and to have mothers with higher levels of education (8.86

years compared to 8.40, $t = 3.7$, $p = .001$). Differences were also found in regard to experimental mortality by race for 3 of the 15 survey years, with a 95% confidence interval about the odds ratio in 1986 (0.763 to 0.988), 1987 (0.769 to 0.993), and 1989 (0.768 to 0.989). Although proportionately fewer Blacks than Whites were likely to have been interviewed in these three survey years, the oversampling of Blacks for the initial 1967 survey makes this loss less problematic than might have been the case otherwise. In addition, no differences in experimental mortality by race were found in any of the other survey years, including 1992, the last year of available data.

Bivariate Analyses: Trends and Characteristics

In each of the 15 survey years, Black respondents were more likely than Whites to have grandchildren living in the household with them. Figure 21.1 shows the trend in the likelihood that the grandparents were Black rather than White. In 1967, Black respondents were more than 14 times as likely as Whites to be coresident grandparents. By 1992, however, the odds decreased by half.

Figure 21.2 shows trends in the percentages of Black and White respondents who were coresident grandparents between 1967 and 1992. The percentage of coresident grandparents among Blacks increased from a low of 7.34 in 1967 to a high of 17.84 in 1982, decreasing slightly thereafter. Among Whites the percentage of coresident grandparents increased within a narrower range than

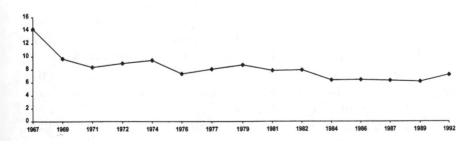

FIGURE 21.1   **Odds ratios of coresident grandparents being Black vis-à-vis White.**

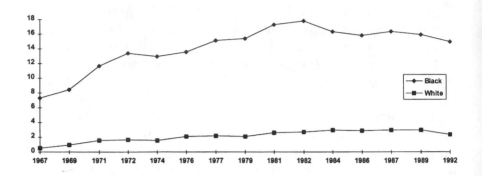

FIGURE 21.2   Percentage of Black and White respondents who were coresident grandparents by year.

that of Blacks, from a low of 0.55 in 1967 to a high of 3.00 in 1987, with a slight decrease in 1992. These results reflect the younger age at which Black women are more likely than other women to become first-time parents (Glick, 1988; McElroy & Moore, 1997). They suggest that despite a narrowing of differences over time, young Black mothers nonetheless remain far more likely to be coresident grandparents than Whites as they mature.

Table 21.2 shows defining characteristics of coresident grandmothers and grandchildren. Coresident grandmothers are far more pervasive among Black respondents than among Whites. Nearly 60% of Black respondents reported having resided with at least one grandchild between 1967 and 1992, compared to only 15% of Whites. Black respondents were also coresident grandmothers for longer periods of time than Whites were. A sizable majority (65.7%) of ever-coresident Black grandmothers had grandchildren living in their households for 5 years or more, whereas ever-coresident White grandmothers were twice as likely to have their grandchildren living with them for 2 years or less (43.2% compared to 21.2%). Nonetheless, 29.6% of ever-coresident White grandmothers lived with their grandchildren for 5 years or more.

Table 21.2 also shows that in 1992 slightly more than half of Black and White coresident grandmothers lived with one grandchild, and coresident Black grandmothers were 2.7 times more likely to be living with four or more grandchildren. Sizable proportions of Black

TABLE 21.2 Defining Characteristics of Coresident Grandmothers and Grandchildren

Variable	% Blacks	% Whites
Lifetime incidence		
Percentage of population sample ever coresided with a grandchild (n = 422 of 716 Black, 323 of 1,979 White)	58.9	14.8
Duration of coresidency among coresident grandmothers in 1992 (n = 198 Black, 81 White)		
1–2 yr	21.2	43.2
3–4 yr	13.1	27.2
5–9 yr	40.4	22.2
10–15 yr	25.3	07.4
Number of grandchildren among coresident grandmothers in 1992 (n = 198 Black, 81 White)		
One	50.0	51.9
Two–three	39.9	44.4
Four–six	10.1	03.7
Age of coresident grandmothers in 1967 (n = 56 Black, 12 White)		
30–35	12.5	00.0
36–40	51.8	16.7
41–44	35.7	83.3
Age of coresident grandchildren in 1967 (n = 81 Black, 17 White)		
1 yr old or less	44.4	35.3
2–4 yr	25.9	47.1
5–12 yr	29.7	17.6
Age of coresident grandmothers in 1992 (n = 198 Black, 81 White)		
55–60	50.5	49.4
61–65	31.3	32.1
66–69	18.2	18.5
Age of coresident grandchildren in 1992 (n = 361 Black, 137 White)		
1 yr old or less	06.6	06.6
2–4 yr	12.2	13.1
5–12 yr	39.9	43.1
13–18 yr	29.4	25.5
19–21 yr	08.3	06.6
22–41 yr	03.6	05.1

(39.9%) and White (43.1%) grandchildren in 1992 were between the ages of 5 and 12, whereas nearly one-fifth of the grandchildren of both races were less than 5 years old. In addition, about half of Black and White coresident grandmothers were between the ages of 55 and 60, and nearly one-fifth of each race were between 66 and 69 years old.

A small number of respondents ($n = 78$) were coresident grandmothers in 1967, when they were between 30 and 44 years of age. About one-eighth of coresident Black grandmothers in 1967 were relatively young, between the ages of 30 and 35, but all of the coresident White grandmothers were 36 years of age or above. Black grandmothers were 1.7 times as likely as Whites to have grandchildren of grammar school age.

Multivariate Analyses

Based on the subsample of ever-coresident grandmothers ($n = 745$), Table 21.3 shows the odds associated with correlates of being a coresident grandmother in 1992. Age, number of own children, and number of prior years of coresidency predicted being a coresident grandparent for both Black ($n = 422$) and White ($n = 323$) respondents; education was a good predictor for Blacks. Number of own children and years of coresidency were positively related to being a coresident grandmother, and age was inversely related to being a coresident grandmother in 1992. Each additional year of coresidency between 1967 and 1989 increased the likelihood of being a coresident grandmother in 1992 by about 15% for both Blacks and Whites. In 1992 each additional child of one's own increased the odds of being a coresident grandmother nearly four times for Whites and more than two times for Blacks.

Among Blacks, in 1992 the odds of being a coresident grandmother increased by 11% with each additional year of education. Marital status approached statistical significance ($p = .06$), so single ever-coresident grandmothers were more than 1 1/2 times as likely to become coresident grandmothers in 1992 than their married counterparts. No relationship was found between income status or work effort and coresidency in 1992 for either Blacks or Whites,

TABLE 21.3   Logistic Regression Odds Ratios of Coresident Grandmothers vs. Noncoresident Grandmothers in 1992, Among Ever-Coresident Grandmothers by Race

	Odds Ratios	
Correlates	Black (n = 422)	White (n = 323)
Age	0.94*	0.89**
Children (no. of own)	2.10***	3.89***
Education	1.11*	0.98
Income status (1 = low income)	0.71	0.45
Marital status (1 = single)	1.54	1.17
Region (1 = south)	1.42	1.04
Weeks worked (10^{-1})	0.99	0.96
Years coresident grandparenthood	1.16***	1.15***
R^2	0.16	0.21
Hosmer and Lemeshow Goodness of Fit Statistic	3.4498	2.8455
	(df = 8)	(df = 8)
	p = .9031	p = .9437

*$p < .05$.   **$p < .01$.   ***$p < .001$.
df, degrees of freedom.

although 11% of White and 38% of Black coresident grandmothers in 1992 lived in low-income families.

Based on the subsample of coresident grandmothers in 1992 ($n = 279$), Table 21.4 shows the odds associated with correlates of living in a three- versus skipped-generation household. Marital status was the only predictor of three-generation households for both Blacks and Whites. The odds of being single and living in a three-generation household increased by nearly six times for Whites and more than two times for Blacks.

Among Blacks, income status and number of coresident grandchildren also were predictors of three-generation households in 1992. The odds of living in a three-generation household declined by 68% for low-income families.

In a subsequent analysis of low-income Black families, no differences were found in regard to the presence or absence of adults other than one's spouse among three-generation and skipped-generation

TABLE 21.4 Logistic Regression Odds Ratios of Three-Generation vs. Skipped-Generation Households in 1992, by Race

	Odds Ratios	
Correlates	Black ($n = 422$)	White ($n = 323$)
Age	0.93	0.96
Coresident grandchildren (no.)	1.44*	0.93
Education	1.00	0.81*
Income status (1 = low income)	0.32**	0.61
Marital status (1 = single)	2.07*	5.98**
Region (1 = south)	1.15	0.66
Weeks worked (10^{-1})	0.99	0.98
Years coresident grandparenthood	0.95	0.83*
R^2	0.12	0.19
Hosmer and Lemeshow Goodness of Fit Statistic	6.9954	5.6563
	($df = 8$)	($df = 8$)
	$p = .5371$	$p = .6857$

*$p < .05$. **$p < .01$.
df, degrees of freedom.

households, nor in regard to the number of such adults in skipped-generation households. Low-income three-generation households, however, had fewer such adults than skipped-generation households (1.57 compared to 1.98, $t = 2.80$, $p < .05$). These findings suggest that coresident Black grandmothers who live in skipped-generation households are also likely to reside with a greater number of other low-income adults than are those who live in three-generation households.

Table 21.4 also shows that the number of coresident grandchildren among Blacks was positively related to the likelihood of living in a three-generation household. Each additional coresident grandchild increased the likelihood of living in a three-generation household by 44%. To the extent that coresident Black grandmothers had more of their grandchildren living with them, at least one of their own children—presumably a parent of a grandchild and contributor to family income—was also likely to reside in the household.

Among Whites, in addition to marital status, education and number of years of coresidency were inversely related to the likelihood of residing in three-generation households in 1992. The odds of residing in a three-generation household decreased by 19% for each year of education and by 17% for each year of coresidency. No relationship was found between household type and age, region, or work effort for either Blacks or Whites.

DISCUSSION

Findings revealed that the prevalence of coresident grandparenting may be more pervasive than previous estimates, particularly among Blacks, and they corroborated research indicating that many caregiving grandparents were so for sustained periods (Fuller-Thomson et al., 1997). The study also found that disproportionate numbers of coresident grandmothers were between 55 and 65 years old and had school-age grandchildren living with them. Blacks tended to become coresident grandmothers at younger ages and to have more grandchildren living with them than Whites did. In addition, among Blacks, better educated and, to a lesser extent, single mothers, who often have less income than their married counterparts, faced increased prospects of residing with a grandchild.

For younger mothers, these findings imply that their future potential as wage earners may be compromised, as they are likely to care primarily for the preschool children or, to a lesser degree, the grammar school children of their own relatively young children. For older mothers, findings signify caregiving responsibilities—primarily of grammar school and, to a lesser degree, high school–age grandchildren—for a substantial proportion of coresident grandparents during preretirement and, to a lesser degree, retirement years. The decreased proportion of coresident grandmothers between the ages of 66 and 69 suggests that retirement-related factors such as lower income and ill health may prevent many mothers from assuming responsibility for their grandchildren despite need (Caputo, 1997; Cherlin & Furstenberg, 1986; Doeringer, 1990; Morris & Caro, 1995; Schulz, 1995).

Somewhat unexpectedly, no relationship was found between income status and coresidency in 1992 for either Black or White evercoresident grandmothers, but longer duration of coresidency increased the likelihood of being a coresident grandmother among both groups. These findings suggest that once a mother assumes the role of coresident grandmother, she is more likely to do so again after she has relinquished this responsibility, regardless of her level of income. These findings also corroborate the Fuller-Thomson et al. study (1997) of custodial grandparents versus noncustodial grandparents in the 1990s. Although they did not find poverty to be a significant predictor of custodial grandparenthood when accounting for other factors, Fuller-Thompson et al. nonetheless report that a sizable proportion of such caregivers (22.9%, compared to 13.7% of noncaregiving grandparents) had family incomes below the poverty line. The higher percentage (38%) found for Blacks in this study remains a cause of concern, particularly in light of the increased likelihood of low-income coresident Black grandmothers being single and living in skipped- versus three-generation households.

In the absence of wage-related or other cash income from other adults in the household, these low-income families are most in need. They require resources, and as discussed below, changes in existing welfare legislation, though apt and necessary for some, may be either inappropriate or insufficient for many coresident grandparents, particularly because work effort was found to have no relation to household type.

The study also found that the likelihood of becoming a coresident grandmother at any given time for ever-coresident White grandmothers was contingent to a greater extent on the woman's having more of her own children in the household than was the case for Blacks. This finding varied with that of Fuller-Thomson et al. (1997), that there was no significant relationship between the overall number of children and caregiving. Although the NLS provided information only about household members in relation to the respondent, it is reasonable to infer that for many coresidents grandmothers the children reported as household members included one or both of the grandchild's parents. Findings of this study suggest, by extension, that this may more likely be the case for Whites than for Blacks.

POLICY RECOMMENDATIONS

Efforts should be made to increase the capacity of skipped-generation caregiving grandparents to obtain greater resources. Revisions to the foster care program to permit kinship care or to the Social Security program to ensure promised benefits to low-income grandmother caregivers are appropriate (Karp, 1996; Kingston & Quadagno, 1995; Morris & Caro, 1995; Mullen, 1996). Such efforts would assist coresident Black grandmothers, who tend to be disproportionately needier, more than they would help Whites (Burton & DeVries, 1992; Rappaport, 1995).

Another way of improving the economic plight of skipped-generation households is to modify provisions in the Personal Responsibility and Work Opportunities Reconciliation Act of 1996. In particular, this act specified that only families with a minor child who resided with a custodial parent or other adult relative or a pregnant women could receive assistance from the grant (*CQ Almanac*, 1996). In many instances, this restriction on aid means that the minor child will reside with her mother, thereby increasing the number of three-generation households.

In the short run, findings of this study support this policy. The job training and placement emphasis of the legislation may translate into increased family income. To the extent, however, that such job requirements preclude the prospect of additional education, whose positive correlation with economic well-being remains strong, the 1996 act may be at cross-purposes with itself. Modifying the legislation to include academic education in the training package of job-enhancing skills would be a step in the right direction.

Several guidelines also are in order to assist states further now that they have primary responsibility for indigent families. First, it is less costly to provide small cash grants and Medicaid benefits to grandchildren in their grandparents' care than it is to provide foster care. Second, states should readily exempt coresident grandparents from whatever welfare-related time limits they impose. Third, elderly and ill grandparents should automatically be exempt from work requirements. And fourth, states should develop child-only Food Stamp grants while streamlining application procedures for cash assistance and related programs.

REFERENCES

Aldous, J. (1995). New views of grandparents in intergenerational context. *Journal of Family Issues, 16*(1), 104–122.

Burton, L., & DeVries, C. (1992). Challenges and rewards: African American grandparents as surrogate parents. *Generations, 17*(3), 51–54.

Caputo, R. K. (1997). Psychological, attitudinal, and socio-demographic correlates of economic well-being of mature women. *Journal of Women and Aging, 9*(4), 37–53.

Center for Human Resource Research (1995). *NLS Handbook 1995.* Center for Human Resource Research. The Ohio State University. Columbus, OH.

Chalfie, D. (1994). *Going it alone: A closer look at grandparents parenting grandchildren.* Washington, DC: American Association of Retired Persons.

Cherlin, A. J., & Furstenberg, F. F. (1986). *The new American grandparent: A place in the family, a life apart.* New York: Basic Books. (Reprint, Cambridge, MA: Harvard University Press, 1992).

Cody, R. P., & Smith, J. K. (1997). *Applied statistics and the SAS programming language* (4th ed.). Upper Saddle River, NJ: Prentice-Hall.

CQ Almanac. (1996). Welfare overhaul. Washington, DC: *Congressional Quarterly.*

Doeringer, P. B. (Ed.). (1990). *Bridges to retirement: Older workers in a changing labor market.* Ithaca, NY: IRR Press.

Fuller-Thomson, E., Minkler, M., & Driver, D. (1997). A profile of grandparents raising grandchildren in the United States. *Gerontologist, 37,* 406–411.

Giarrusso, R., Silverstein, M., & Bengtson, V. L. (1996). Family complexity and the grandparent role. *Generations, 20,* 17–23.

Glick, P. C. (1988). Demographic pictures of Black families. In H. P. McAdoo (Ed.), *Black families* (2nd ed., pp. 111–132). Newbury Park, CA: Sage Publications.

Hunter, A. G., & Ensminger, M. E. (1992). Diversity and fluidity in children's living arrangements: Family transitions in an urban Afro-American community. *Journal of Marriage and the Family, 54,* 418–426.

Karp, N. (1996). Legal problems of grandparents and other kinship caregivers. *Generations, 20*(1), 57–60.

Kingston, E., & Quadagno, J. (1995). Social security: Marketing radical reform. *Generations, 19*(3), 43–49.

Kivett, V. R. (1993). Racial comparisons of the grandmother role. *Family Relations, 42,* 165–172.

McElroy, S. M., & Moore, K. A. (1997). Trends over time in teenage pregnancy and childbearing: The critical changes. In R. A. Maynard (Ed.), *Kids having kids: Economic costs and social consequences of teen pregnancy* (pp. 23–53). Washington, DC: Urban Institute Press.

Morris, R., & Caro, F. G. (1995). The young-old, productive aging, and public policy. *Generations, 19*(3), 32–37.

Mullen, F. (1996). Public benefits: Grandparents, grandchildren, and welfare reform. *Generations, 20*(1), 61–64.

Rappaport, A. M. (1995). Employer policy and the future of employee benefits for an older population. *Generations, 19*(3), 63–67.

Schulz, J. H. (1995). *The economics of aging.* Westport, CT: Auburn House.

CHAPTER 22

A Comparison of Low-Income Caregivers in Public Housing: Differences in Grandparent and Nongrandparent Needs and Problems

Steve Kauffman and Robin S. Goldberg-Glen

G randparent caregivers who reside in public housing present a variety of unique challenges to the social service community. The population confronts all of the normative life-span subject matter associated with aging and parenting but with the added burdens imposed by poverty and/or residence in the distressed communities that commonly typify the public housing setting. As such, personal, interpersonal, and institutional problems may be magnified and new levels of complexity created. At the same time, it is unclear whether social workers and others in the helping professions have the necessary resources and established referral networks to systematically address the commingled issues.

For the purposes of beginning to understand the problems encountered by low-income grandparent caregivers who reside in public housing, this chapter examines the problems and unmet needs of a sample of public housing residents from Chester, Pennsylvania. The chapter presents the data drawn from a random sample of public housing residents ($n = 82$) and supplements the discussion with additional comparative statistics provided by a variety of federal, state, and local sources. The goal of the chapter is to present a taxonomy of the special needs of this population and to begin the process of developing a strategy for problem remediation through policy, program development, and direct practice interventions. Specifically, the chapter (1) presents a brief description of public housing and the community context, (2) describes the city of Chester and the public housing services in that community, (3) examines the unique problems and unmet needs of this group through a comparison of grandparent caregivers, parent caregivers, and non-child households, and (4) offers practice suggestions for this population.

PUBLIC HOUSING AND THE COMMUNITY CONTEXT

Public Housing in America

Federal public housing initiatives in America have a relatively short history. The first low-rent public housing projects in the United States were constructed during the depression of the 1930s. Subsequently, the Federal Housing Acts of 1937, 1949, and 1954 created the urban renewal programs of the 1950s, publicly owned housing, and Section 8 programs still in operation today (U.S. Social Security Administration, 1997). More recently, a series of block grants to state and local governments have been established to allow a degree of flexibility in housing approaches. All of these programs are intended to help the poor to afford shelter.

The public housing programs are generally under the control of approximately 3,350 local public housing authorities (PHAs) and Indian Housing Authorities (IHAs). Funding for the programs of the PHAs and IHAs comes largely through grants from the U.S. Department of Housing and Urban Development (HUD), a cabinet-level department created in 1965. Funding for all HUD housing programs in fiscal year 1998 amounted to more than $23 billion, with $6.3 billion dedicated to public housing (Citizen's Housing and Planning Association, 1997). In 1997, HUD public housing programs resulted in service to about 1.25 million households.

The two primary low-income housing assistance programs operated by the P/IHAs are publicly owned housing complexes and a system of housing vouchers commonly known as Section 8. Generally (though with some important exceptions), the publicly owned sites are large apartment complexes to which the renter pays rent based on income. The amount of rent the tenant pays for housing (called the total tenant payment [TTP]) is based on income, less HUD-approved deductions. In 1995 the median income of public housing residents was $6,420, and the average monthly rent was $169 per month for living in one of 13,741 housing developments (U.S. Department of Housing and Urban Development, 1995).

The Section 8 system, however, depends on the private rental market. In this system, an I/PHA client receives a voucher that can be used to rent an apartment (or house) approved by the I/PHA. The amount of the voucher is determined by client income and prevailing rental market costs. Similarly, the quality of Section 8 rental stock varies greatly. The choice allotted by Section 8, however, makes the system quite popular among I/PHA clients.

Unfortunately, the number of both public housing rental units and available Section 8 vouchers is much smaller than the total demand. The number of rental units, for example, has substantially decreased in recent years (Lazere, 1995). As many as 800,000 individuals are on waiting lists (Atlas & Dreier, 1994) for an average 17 months between a request for assistance and service (Waxman, 1995).

Further, for residents already living in public housing, the quality of the housing stock is mixed. Although many of the PHAs are capable of effective management "some older public housing developments have deteriorated over the years, becoming magnets for crime and roadblocks to efforts to revitalize the surrounding area" (Cuomo, 1998, p. 1). Moreover, 200,000 units of public housing are operated by housing authorities that have performance problems. Among performance problems common to public housing are a lack of preventive maintenance (Atlas & Dreier, 1994) and slow implementation of unit development for the elderly and disabled (U.S. General Accounting Office, 1998).

The Community Context

One of the criticisms most often leveled at public housing and one clearly linked to the concentration of the poor both in public housing and as typically found in areas around such housing sites are high rates of crime and substance abuse. Former secretary of HUD, Henry Cisneros, presented these problems in the form of research conducted by the Research Triangle Institute.

> Overall, about one in five housing residents said they felt unsafe in their developments and neighborhoods. Nearly two out of five residents of high-rise buildings said they felt unsafe. Twenty-two percent of residents in high-rises reported that serious crime—gunfire, burglary, robbery, assault—was a major problem, compared with about half that percentage in all other types of public housing. Furthermore, 8.6 percent of high-rise residents reported that they or a household member had been a victim of violent crime in the six months preceding the survey, compared to about four percent of all public housing residents. (Cisneros, 1995)

The primary issue is that the income base necessary for high-quality community services in many areas where public housing are located are inadequate. Services such as public safety, education, infrastructure, and governance depend largely on revenues generated by personal, property, and business taxes, supplemented by fees, grants, and credit. In communities populated by large percentages of low-income wage earners and/or characterized by a weak business sector, the taxes and fees generated may be limited.

Further, political and social fragmentation are common consequences in such communities. This fragmentation results from competition over scarce resources and disagreements over problem prioritization. It is undoubtedly difficult to argue effectively that one social problem is more important than another when a vast array faces a poor community. Thus, as increasing crime rates; higher rates of substance abuse; deteriorating schools, transportation, and recreational infrastructure; and a decline in the accessibility of high-quality medical care all affect the quality of life, finding common priorities is difficult.

Moreover, as city services deteriorate and taxes increase, individuals and families who can afford to move from the community and the public housing sites often do. This negatively affects the tax base and also loses the political strengths and the presence of important role models from the community. It could be argued, for example, that a primary cause of concentrated inner-city poverty and the development of what has been called the "underclass" was the movement of the middle and professional class from such communities in the wake of the "war on poverty."

There are other consequences of poverty in these poor and disempowered communities, and one only recently recognized is the problem of environmental justice. Poor and disempowered communities, partly because of a desperate need for employment and partly because of the intentional targeting of such communities by business, tend to be magnets for types of business that are generally undesirable. These include prisons, factories that discharge large amounts of pollutants, and various forms of waste management industries. Although it is true that poor communities need employment opportunities, the concentration of these types of businesses may result in a variety of negative social and health effects on the community—effects ranging from lowered property values to disagreeable odors to increased rates of respiratory diseases and even cancer.

CHESTER: A DISTRESSED COMMUNITY

The urban problems discussed above establish the context in which many grandparent caregivers living in public housing must exist. The city of Chester, Pennsylvania, from which much of the following data will be drawn, presents a classic case of this context. The city has a population of approximately 42,000 and is located approximately one-half hour south of Philadelphia, along the Delaware River. The city of Chester once housed a thriving manufacturing base, producing ships, steel, iron, cloth, pottery, paper, and refined oil.

The economic changes of the post–World War II era, however, strongly affected Chester. The City lost 32% of its jobs between the

1950s and the 1980s. The economy collapsed, and much of the middle class moved away. Moreover, the city's problems were compounded by several decades of poor (and corrupt) political leadership. Beginning in 1910 and continuing into the last decade, a political machine controlled public resources and distributed them in ways not always beneficial to the city as a whole. The economic change and political inefficacy have created a variety of socio-economic problems for the community.

Housing

One such problem confronted by Chester residents involves the availability of quality housing. Housing values, occupancy rates, the condition of housing, and the state of public housing in Chester are all poor relative to the county and the state. The Chester Housing Authority (CHA) operates five public housing sites, with a total of 1,455 units (840 occupied), and provides additional assistance through Section 8 certificates or vouchers to around 700 households. The 1,707 public housing units represent approximately 10% of all housing units and is quite high relative to any city in the state.

After several years of financial and administrative problems (resulting in federal court receivership, *In re Velez v. Cisneros et al.*) the CHA has, in the past 3 years, undertaken a series of initiatives to improve the conditions of its public housing facilities and the quality of life of its residents. Improvements have been identified in most aspects of the housing authority, and the CHA is no longer considered a troubled PHA. Moreover, significant funding has been successfully sought for facilities and services improvement.

Beyond public housing, large percentages of Chester residents are severely cost-burdened by housing. The housing market in Chester faces severe problems: very few new homes have been constructed in Chester in the past decade, and almost 80% of all homes in Chester were built before 1959; 40% of all homes were built before 1940. Vacancy rates, median home value, and the percentage of homes requiring maintenance all compare quite unfavorably with surrounding Delaware County. Many homes in the community also have high lead levels because of the age and lack of upkeep of the housing stock.

Chester does, however, have a large number of potentially nice homes if the funding could be found to rehabilitate the housing stock and assist low-income families with maintenance costs.

Grandparent Studies

Although recent research has recognized the vital role that grandparents play in preserving family integrity for children who have lost their parents, studies examining grandparent caregivers living in public housing are nonexistent. This study compares grandparent to parent caregivers and nonchild households in an attempt to highlight the unique problems of grandparent-headed families living in Section 8 Housing, who are likely to represent the most poverty-stricken groups addressed but are singularly overlooked in recent studies.

METHODS

Population and Sample

A random sample ($n = 150$) was drawn from the population of leaseholders of a public housing site ($N = 350$) owned by the CHA. The purpose of the study itself was to develop baseline data for an ongoing evaluation of several of the programs of the CHA. The housing site from which the sample was drawn is in a redevelopment phase because of extreme degradation. The site is surrounded by an area with high crime and drug use rates and is characterized by high unemployment and poor schools.

Each leaseholder who agreed to participate was interviewed by a team of two social work students. The students (both MSW and BSW) received approximately 3 hours of training in interviewing techniques prior to actual data collection. All leaseholders signed consent forms at the time of the interview. The total number of participants was 82, for a response rate of 54.6%.

Instrument and Analysis

The interview instrument was quite long (approximately 250 questions), and interview times ranged from 50 minutes to 1 1/2 hours.

Questions on the instrument covered a wide assortment of substantive areas, including family composition, economic issues, attitudes, and service needs. The large number of interviews completed is the result of the support given by the tenant association, which "spread the word" in advance of the study. Nevertheless, many residents refused to participate because of the time commitment or the sensitive nature of some of the questions on the survey.

Depending on the type of question, the analysis presented below will compare the service needs and attitudes of two or three groups. The selection is determined by the presence of children. If the question (or series of questions) on the instrument does not depend on the assumption of a child in the house, the comparison includes three groups: grandparent caregivers, other caregivers, and nonchild households. If children are assumed, the comparison includes only grandparents and other caregivers. Descriptive statistics and ANOVAs or *t*-tests are used to demonstrate the comparisons.

Measures

Several measures that examined resident problems associated with various aspects of living in public housing were included. A partial list of those problems includes poverty, homelessness, AIDS/HIV, substance abuse, unavailability of aging services, unemployment, adult crime/violence, cost of housing, diet/nutrition, inflation, race relations, alcohol abuse, drug abuse, juvenile crime/gangs, family violence, mental illness, illiteracy, lack of availability of recreation or leisure resources, welfare dependency, health insurance, and unavailability of child care.

Also included were questions that asked about barriers to service that the residents had experienced. These barriers included child care, waiting lists, cost, eligibility, and service availability. Finally, questions were asked about experience with a variety of family problems, including unemployment, adult crime, juvenile crime, family violence, mental illness, managing teenagers, debt, money strain, and whether a family member had recently been arrested. Respondents also were asked about their general health. In most cases, questions were dichotomized as yes/no answers.

FINDINGS

Demographic Characteristics

Virtually all participants in the study were female and African American. Of the 82 households, 43 (52.4%) had children present, and 17 (20.73%) reported the grandparent as the primary caregiver. This latter percentage is possibly an overrepresentation of the total number of grandparent caregivers when compared to the total population, although official housing authority statistics are not clear on this point.

In the sample, the grandparents worked an average of 17.5 hours per week, compared to 21.77 for the other caregivers and 9.91 for the childless group. Though not statistically significant, the grandparents had a greater percentage of incomes above the poverty line (59%) than the other caregivers (46%) and the childless group (29%). No statistically significant differences existed for TANF (Temporary Assistance for Needy Families) and OASDI (Old Age Survivor and Disability Insurance) utilization, assets, or automobile ownership, although the grandparents had on average greater assets than the other groups. Grandparent caregivers did, however, have higher average Food Stamp utilization (53%) than did the childless households (32%), though it was lower than that of the other caregivers (63%). These results are presented in Table 22.1.

TABLE 22.1 Demographics and Income Characteristics

Variable	No Children Present	Grandparent Caregivers	Other Caregivers	F Ratio (or t)	p Value
Hours worked per week	9.91	17.50	21.77	3.116	.050
Income (% with income above poverty line)	29	59	46	2.459	.092
TANF recipients (%)	NA	24	38	$t = -.93$	.356
OASDI recipients (%)	37	29	25	.483	.619
Food stamp recipients (%)	32	53	63	3.302	.042
Automobile ownership (%)	39	53	33	.807	.450
Financial assets (%)	22	35	33	.751	.475

Problems and Social Service Needs

When service needs are examined, a very mixed picture results relative to the three groups. In several areas it appears that the grandparent caregivers had fewer problems than the other groups. A higher percentage of the grandparent caregivers (88%) than the other caregivers (50%) and the childless group (68%) reported that their transportation needs were met. Similarly, the grandparents had less concern about unemployment, juvenile crime, family violence, money strain, and mental illness in the family than did the other caregivers. Further, in terms of barriers to service, grandparents perceived waiting lists and child care as less of a barrier than did other caregivers. They also perceived service availability as less of a problem than did other caregivers. There were no statistically significant differences in perceptions of cost and eligibility requirements.

On the other hand, there were specific problem areas where the issues faced by the grandparent caregivers were significantly greater. The grandparents, for instance, had significantly poorer health than either of the other groups, with a greater number of reported problems. There was also a statistically significant greater problem of conflict among children in grandparent caregiver households than in other households. The grandparents reported more difficulties in managing teenagers than did other caregivers. In addition, they reported more concerns about recent debt than did the other caregivers, and they more often reported the arrest of a family member. These results are reported in Table 22.2.

DISCUSSION

The information provided from the surveys strongly suggests that the grandparent caregiver experiences both the same types of problems as the "typical" public housing resident and some unique problems. To begin with, they are slightly better off financially than the other resident groups, perhaps because they are slightly older and more settled. Moreover, they are slightly less affected by some of the common problems in accessing services, such as child care or waiting lists. In these respects, the grandparent caregiver might be

TABLE 22.2 Reported Problems and Service Needs

Variable	No Children Present	Grandparent Caregivers	Other Caregivers	F Ratio (or *t* value)	*p* Value
Transportation (% reporting transportation needs adequately met)	.68	88	50	3.482	.036
Service barriers					
Waiting lists (%)	24	35	75	9.809	.000
Cost (%)	27	53	38	1.841	NS
Availability (%)	17	29	46	3.245	.044
Child care (%)	NA	05	37	*t* = −2.43	.020
Eligibility (%)	15	35	29	1.796	NS
Family Problems (% responding a concern)					
Unemployment	NA	65	83	6.84	.013
Adult crime	NA	59	71	1.991	NS
Juvenile crime	NA	59	79	6.285	.013
Family violence	NA	11	25	5.041	.030
Mental illness	NA	11	25	5.041	.030
Managing teens	NA	37	14	4.10	.050
Debt	NA	13	.05	14.89	.000
Money strain	NA	38	53	10.56	.002
Family member arrested	NA	29	.05	5.96	.019
General health (reported problems)	11.16	11.20	8.82	3.849	.027

somewhat better at coping with urban life than younger, less experienced caregivers.

On the other hand, they clearly face some unique problems. Their health is not as robust as that of members of the other groups, which could prove problematic for the care of the children in the event of potential disability. Similarly, the grandparents seem to face greater difficulties in managing the children than do the other caregivers. Both of these problem areas would seem to imply the need for some form of supportive, respite-like services in acute situations, as well as ongoing supports, such as counseling, for the general management issues.

Moreover, although the degree to which debt is a serious burden to the sample is unclear, it may be an area of concern for future research. Many of the grandparents are at a life stage in which saving is a critical concern; but with the addition of new family members, the potential risk of needed alternative housing and the increased expenses may make saving difficult or impossible. Therefore, financial supports to reduce this burden are essential—perhaps through the addition of new tax breaks. As suggested by the study, their Food Stamp utilization is already higher than for the other groups, and therefore it is perhaps desirable to increase allotments as well.

Finally, it is suggested in this study that the additional child-rearing responsibilities are caused by the arrest of the parent. If this is the case, it would appear that supports for the grandparent in the form of counseling also may be of utility. The grandparent not only has to take on the responsibility for the children but also may face additional responsibilities for the parent when she or he gets out of jail. This additional burden lies in the future, but if this turns out to be a wide-scale phenomena, the low-income grandparent caregiver living in subsidized housing may face a whole new set of responsibilities in the next few years. This possibility bears further examination, and if such additional responsibilities seem likely, supportive structures should be prepared now to deal with this eventuality.

One way of enhancing the lives of caregivers and their grandchildren would be to improve their housing opportunities. Two programs have recently evolved in the United States. The Grandfamilies Program of Boston: Aging Concerns Young and Old United is one of the first housing programs in the United States for grandparents raising grandchildren. Designed to meet the intergenerational needs of grandparent caregivers, Grandfamilies House offers 26 apartments and a variety of services for the children and the grandparents. Grandfamilies House was developed in response to the problems and policies that place barriers and prevent accessibility to safe and affordable housing for these newfound family forms. Their mission is "to provide the highest quality intergenerational housing and related services to assist people in need, especially elders" (BAC-YOU, 1999). Additionally, Massachusetts was the first state to provide 100 Section 8 certificates designed for grandparent caregivers. This demonstration project, called Raising the Next Generation, provides low-rent housing primarily for grandparents aged 62 or older and then for those aged 50–61.

The Hope for the Children project also provides services, stipends, and low-rent housing for adoptive and foster families. Forty-seven rental units are mixed in an Illinois neighborhood and provided at a discount to older adults who are willing to provide 6 hours of assistance to children. Fourteen units are provided to families that make a lifetime commitment to raise children who are not likely to return home. Although specifically designed to serve grandparent caregivers, surrogate grandparents are not excluded from this program.

These programs represent an important trend toward using housing as an intervention for relatives whose family composition has been compromised. Each program illustrates an important thrust in recognizing that grandparents play a pivotal role in children's lives; therefore, we must attend to opportunities for these older families members to maintain the continuity of their family lineages, especially those who either reside in or can benefit from low-income housing.

ACKNOWLEDGMENTS

Based on a paper presented at the 52nd Annual Scientific Meeting of the Gerontological Association of America, Philadelphia, November 1999. The research described in this chapter was funded by the Chester Housing Authority as part of an evaluation of the Lamokin Village Hope VI Revitalization Program.

REFERENCES

Atlas, J., & Dreier, P. (1994). *Public housing: What went wrong?* National Housing Institute, Shelterforce [On-line]. Available: <http://www.nhi.org/online/issues/77/pubhsg.html>.

Cisneros, H. (1995). *Public housing design examined* [On-line]. Available: *Isdesignet* <http://www.isdesignet.com/isdesignet/Magazine/Sep'95/Sep'95Index.html>.

Citizens' Housing and Planning Association. (1997). *Summary of FY'98 HUD budget bill* [On-line]. Available: <http://www.chapa.org/policy_factsheet-15.htm>.

Cuomo, A. (1998). *Clinton administration awards $498.3 million to transform public housing nationwide* [On-line]. Available: <http://www.hud.gov/pressrel/pr97-250.html>.

Lazere, E. (1995). *In short supply: The growing affordable housing gap.* Washington, DC: Center on Budget and Policy Priorities.

U.S. Department of Housing and Urban Development. (1995). *Characteristics of households: PD&R Recent Research Results.* Washington, DC: Author.

U.S. General Accounting Office. (1998). *Public housing: Impact of designated public housing on persons with disabilities* (Letter Report, 06/09/98, GAO/RCED-98-160). Washington, DC: Author.

U.S. Social Security Administration. (1997). *Social Security programs in the United States.* (SSA Publication No. 13-11758). Washington, DC: Author.

Waxman, L. (1995). *A status report on hunger and homelessness in America's cities, 1995.* Washington, DC: United States Conference of Mayors.

Epilogue

Robin S. Goldberg-Glen and Bert Hayslip Jr.

T he past decade has witnessed a burgeoning of literature describing custodial grandparents and the circumstances that provided the impetus to become primary caregivers for their grandchildren. *Grandparents Raising Grandchildren: Theoretical, Empirical, and Clinical Perspectives* brings together the ideas of researchers, practitioners, educators, and professionals. Their discussions attest to the need to continue recognizing that grandparent-headed families represent family systems than reflect a variety of diverse issues. Moreover, all contributors acknowledge the shortage of available empirically tested programs, treatment interventions, educational opportunities, and policies—important today, as grandparent-headed families are likely to increase in the future because of social factors, including poverty, substance abuse, incarceration, domestic abuse problems, homelessness, crime, teen pregnancy, untreated mental health conditions, or AIDS.

The idea for the book emerged as a consequence of several symposia conducted at the Gerontological Society of America's annual scientific meetings. Early in the 1990s, few individuals were exploring the field of custodial grandparenting. Soon a grandparent interest group evolved at which it was announced that Springer Publishing Company had also recognized this emerging area and was seeking a book prospectus. We are especially grateful to Helvi Gold and Bill Tucker for their invaluable comments, support, and assistance in the completion of this book.

THE DEMOGRAPHICS OF CUSTODIAL GRANDPARENTING

In the gerontology and child welfare literature, grandparent-headed families have been conceptualized as groups of persons whose caregiving patterns are complex and involve individuals at opposite ends of the family life cycle. Such families have not been included in family life cycle paradigms, nor have the primary caregivers been considered in relation to individual age-stage schemas.

Research in the early 1990s focused on developing a picture of grandparent caregivers. Samples were cross-sectional, small, and purposive; many times they reflected little diversity. This literature was, however, useful in that it allowed us to begin to profile grandparents who raise their grandchildren and acknowledge that these nontraditional family systems do indeed exist.

This evolving picture has led to more refined studies, which now employ longitudinal designs, comparative methods, cross-cultural samples, qualitative data analysis techniques, and an emphasis on special populations. Clearly, researchers are expanding their interests to advance our understanding and describe the heterogeneity of this population. For example, three chapters in this collection conducted a secondary analysis of nationally representative longitudinal data to (1) delineate a national profile of America's grandparent caregivers (Fuller-Thomson & Minkler), (2) describe how coresidency increases one's chance of becoming a grandparent caregiver in the United States (Caputo), and (3) discern the link between custodial grandparent caregiving and depression (Minkler, Fuller-Thomson, Miller, & Driver). Several chapters use a comparative design to examine the concept of health (Solomon & Marx; Fuller-Thomson & Minkler), whereas others have used cross-sectional methods to contrast different racial, ethnic, and cultural groups (Hayslip,

Silverthorn, Shore, & Henderson; Toledo, Hayslip, Emick, Toledo, & Henderson), as well as the influence of gender, housing arrangements, hours of care provided, perceptions of the transmission of values, and the impact of AIDS (Goldberg-Glen & Sands; Joslin; Kauffman & Goldberg-Glen; Kopera-Frye & Wiscott; Solomon & Marx). In contrast to quantitatively oriented work, qualitative methods are used to shed light on African American custodial grandparents (Baird, John, & Hayslip) and to examine family social interactions that shed light on the dynamics of grandparent-headed households (Sands & Goldberg-Glen).

Finally, chapters by Butts and by Connealy and DeRoos each urge us to carefully use theoretical frameworks for advancing family policy and encourage national advocacy in heightening our awareness regarding the impact of policies. Moreover, they urge us to bridge the gap between researchers, policy makers, and practitioners, particularly with regard to the emotional, mental, social, and physical health of custodial grandparents (Minkler, Fuller-Thomson, Miller, & Driver; Fuller-Thomson & Minkler; Solomon & Marx).

Both cross-sectional and longitudinal findings suggest that a large proportion of custodial grandparents are depressed and unhappy, enjoy life less, and are less satisfied with their houses, neighborhoods, physical health, jobs, and life as a whole (Caputo; Fuller-Thomson, & Minkler; Minkler et al.). Significantly, grandparent caregivers often report that they have fewer people to rely on for assistance, to turn to in emergencies, and to confide in (Solomon & Marx). Custodial grandparents of the 1990s are more likely than noncaregiving grandparents to be unmarried, young, African American or Hispanic, female, not high school-educated, living in the South, and below the poverty line (Fuller-Thomson & Minkler). Unfortunately, they are also more likely to have had a child die in the preceding 5 years. This may alternatively strengthen their commitment to raising a grandchild as well as make them more vulnerable to loss. Indeed, Caputo's longitudinal data suggest that the prevalence of coresident grandparenting may be more pervasive than previously thought, particularly among Blacks, who tended to become coresident grandmothers at younger ages than Whites and had more grandchildren living with them.

SPECIAL POPULATIONS OF CAREGIVING GRANDPARENTS

In developing a profile of grandparent caregivers, we have underestimated the importance of "special" populations. Typically, fleeting reference is given to distinct racial groups, including Asian and Native American grandparent caregivers. As Fuller-Thomson and Minkler point out, only one study has examined the Latino population. We have also assumed that grandparents from different ethnic groups have corresponding parenting and grandparenting styles. Not surprisingly, many contributors in this book have identified several specific grandparent caregiver groups with distinct characteristics and needs.

The Goldberg-Glen and Sands, Joslin, and Kauffman and Goldberg-Glen chapters describe the attributes that are unique to overlooked custodial grandparent populations: secondary caregivers, grandfathers, grandparents living in subsidized housing, and grandparents whose grandchildren are affected or infected by AIDS. Significantly, although secondary caregivers, especially males, have been overlooked in the literature, recent census data indicate that households where children were also cared for by their grandfathers grew by 39% between 1990 and 1997 (Casper & Bryson, 1998). Only 6% of these grandfathers where primary caregivers. This void is underscored by the chapter by Goldberg-Glen and Sands, who indicate that this newly acquired role, with its added responsibilities, may actually be more difficult for the secondary than the primary caregiver.

Kauffman and Goldberg-Glen's examination of the needs and problems of grandparent caregivers and noncaregivers in public housing highlights the importance of recognizing custodial grandparents' heterogeneity. They surprisingly found that grandparents tended to be less disadvantaged in many respects than other caregivers and those without children. Yet grandparent caregivers reported poorer health and more conflict among children, experienced more difficulties in managing teenagers, and were more likely to report the arrest of a family member.

Joslin points out that the physical and psychological well-being of grandparents raising HIV-affected and orphaned children is compromised by recent bereavement, a finding also observed in the study by Minkler et al. on grandparent care giver depression. Yet Joslin acknowledges the strengths of this special population, alluding to the emotional resiliency of older relatives who are willing to care for their grandchildren under such painful conditions, recognizing that only a resilient individual would "compromise" his or her lifestyle and be willing to experience raising grandchildren who may die at any early age, before the grandparent. Collectively, many chapters here reveal that grandparent caregivers are indeed a diverse group, and in many respects their circumstances can be viewed in both a positive and a negative light.

GRANDCHILDREN

Foremost in this volume is the emphasis on the important role grandparents play in their grandchildren's lives. Kopera-Frye and Wiscott explored how grandparents forward cultural values to their grandchildren and how grandchildren interpret this cultural transference. Whereas most research on African American and Native American grandparents enumerates how grandparents play the role of keeper of their culture, studies exploring the transmission of culture within Caucasian populations are nonexistent. Overall, their findings document that grandparents, regardless of whether or not they were primary caregivers, influenced their grandchildren's belief formation, religion, family, education, work, morality, and personal identity. This differential pattern of intergenerationally shared activities found among minorities is quite relevant to the custodial grandparent context, given the number of African American grandparents raising grandchildren. Kopera-Frye and Wiscott call attention to how grandchildren's belief formations may be influenced by their grandparents and suggest that the formation of cultural beliefs may have a future influence on the values the grandchildren bring to their own offspring. The study is particularly important because the author's sample involves an ethnically homogeneous group of grandparent caregivers. The findings of Hayslip, Shore, and Henderson echo this need to understand grandchildren's perspectives on their relationship to their grandparents. Such research, however, focuses on traditional grandparents and consequently needs to be extended to custodial grandparent households.

The chapters by Baker, Chenoweth, Silverthorn and Durant, Rogers and Henkin, and Strom and Strom provide a rich source of information for implementing programs designed to support the grandparent-grandchild family unit. The authors' discussions accentuate the need to work with grandparents as a direction for bettering the grandchildren's livelihoods. These chapters are encouraging for practitioners in providing many ideas for intervention in the context of both the family and the larger social system, ideas that were not readily available in the past.

Grandparent families today are more likely to seek out professional help now that service providers have recognized them as legitimate sources of assistance. Grandparents and service providers also have available to them more avenues for becoming informed about available services. National organization such as the Child Welfare League of America and Generations United (Butts) sponsor yearly conferences addressing kinship care provider programs. This is in distinct contrast to a decade ago, when researchers were just beginning to discern the importance of this issue.

On the other hand, programs and interventions offered to these families are rarely empirical in nature. Hirshorn, Van Meter, and Brown's contribution to this volume is her recognition of the need for an empirically tested treatment models, focusing on the grandparent's needs. Recognizing that role ambiguity and fluid boundaries within grandparent-headed family systems can have a negative impact on the family unit and other available systems, Hirshorn's program helps grandparents develop self-management skills in the context of systems theory.

PSYCHOSOCIAL CONSIDERATIONS IN CUSTODIAL GRANDPARENTING

The chapters by Kopera-Frye and Wiscott and by Hayslip, Shore, and Henderson should alert us to the fact that not only are grandparents viable influences on their grandchildren's lives before the assumption of the caregiving role but that, indeed, grandparents were at one time parents—a fact that is lost on many grandparents and adult children. Thus, their experiences with both their children and grandchildren in a more traditional, age-normative role context have an influence on their subsequent experiences as custodial grandparents. This suggests that studying such experiences, which both precede and follow the assumption of the surrogate parenting role in middle or later life, is necessary to understand that role adequately. Thus, it is important to frame custodial grandparenting in the context of aging, illness, death, and grief, as well as in light of one's experiences as a parent, spouse, or traditional grandparent. To date, prospective, longitudinal research of this nature has yet to be carried out.

This perspective can be generalized to those grandparents who happen to be raising a child with behavioral, emotional, school, or physical difficulties (Baker and Silverthorn & Durant). Thus, a grandparent's particular experiences as a parent or as a traditional grandparent, regarding the extent of knowledge about a given problem (i.e., depression, ADHD), likely influence the degree of adjustment difficulties that interacting on a daily basis with such children creates, as well as the extent to which they recognize the problem as amenable to some form of intervention (Hayslip, Silverthorn, Shore, & Henderson), whether at the level of the grandchild, the grandparent, the grandparent-grandchild dyad, the school, the community, or society. Consequently, individual or family therapy, program or curriculum development, parental skills training, advocacy, community support services, or public policy avenues of change may all be viable alternatives not only in dealing with one's impending parental responsibilities but also with regard to coping with the demands of active custodial grandparenting on a daily basis.

More also needs to be learned about the how and why of social support for grandparents who raise their grandchildren; some grandparents are obviously more successful in soliciting help from friends or other family or in gaining access to needed community services than are others. Some may be more interpersonally skilled or have convoys of support that are more dense and/or stable. In this respect, Carstensen's notion of socioemotional selectivity or that of psychological resiliency/hardiness by Kobasa (Joslin and Solomon & Marx) may be important avenues to pursue. Likewise, more fully understanding why some grandparents are able to deal with their new responsibilities, whereas others are not, might be facilitated by greater attention to factors such as grandchild peer relationships, gender differences in both grandchildren and grandparents, marital satisfaction in middle and later life, and importantly, parental style (i.e., authoritative, laissez-faire), a concept proposed by Diana Baumrind nearly three decades ago. Moreover, attachment theory also might be valuable, wherein the construct of attachment styles (those of the grandchild and grandparent) that may or may not complement one other might explain why some custodial grandparents adjust well and others do not.

Many grandparents do indeed continue to manage their personal, marital, and social lives well in the face of the burdens of raising a grandchild. In this light, we may learn a lesson from those Mexican-born grandparents in the Toledo et al. chapter, who reported greater grandparental meaning than did their United States counterparts, despite being in poorer health and living in more drastic financial circumstances.

INTERVENTION MODELS

Although researchers have detailed the many needs of grandparent-headed families, intervention models are nonexistent. Four chapters in this book have reconceptualized intervention models to suit the grandparent caregiving context (Chenoweth; Rogers & Henkin; Silverthorn & Durant; Strom & Strom). Each acknowledges the uniqueness of the grandparent's newfound role and responsibilities, in that they do not fit into the traditional paradigms of individual development or the family life cycle, and discusses the complexity of the grandparent's relationship to his or her grandchildren and to the larger social system. Each identifies education as a principal component of an intervention model, wherein each is aimed at improving the parenting performance of grandparent caregivers and stresses the need to be culturally sensitive. Chenoweth focuses on a strengths perspective and on designing culturally responsive programs that target family diversity; Strom and Strom underscore the goals that "successful" grandparents have in common in the context of a strengths model. Rogers and Henkin approach grandparent-headed families' needs from a macro level. Their program on school-based interventions for children in kinship care are testament to the need to work with the larger (macro/exo system) environment. These authors recognize that schools are untapped resources, yet typically unprepared to address the distinct needs of both the school-children and grandparents themselves.

METHODOLOGY IN THE STUDY OF CUSTODIAL GRANDPARENTING

Several methodological recommendations can be made regarding the grandparent literature. Although there is now an emphasis on large data sets, we cannot underestimate the contributions of qualitative data and the importance of taking a micro perspective on grandparent-headed families. Of central importance is consistency in operational definitions of critical variables. For instance, many studies define family units differently. Households where the grandparents are the primary caregivers may or may not include the biological parent, may include other kin or boarders and/or may include significant others in the care of the grandchild. Different labels and constellations of the family unit can interfere with the generalizability of findings. Furthermore, "primary caregiving" has numerous meanings. Several authors have referred to primary caregivers as either those who continue providing care after a given period of time, the grandparent who has self-identified as the primary caregiver (what we term the "functional caregiver"), and/or the grandparent who has chosen to become the foster parent or legal guardian. Similarly, many variables referred to in many chapters may mean the same thing but use different measures or have been operationalized differently (i.e., emotional well-being, well-being, social well-being, social isolation, grandparent needs). Utilizing clearly stated, common operational definitions ensures that policy makers' efforts to develop appropriate programs would not be compromised by research design methodological shortcomings.

Although research focusing on broad issues and aggregated data is important, these methodologies cannot aid in helping us understand the variables and interactions that are unique to grandparent-headed families. Microanalysis and focus groups allow researchers to raise questions about subject matter, nonverbal cues, body language, and the environments that are unique to each family.

Baird, John, and Hayslip utilize the focus group method to expand the existing knowledge base regarding minority grandparents. The grandparents in the Baird et al. chapter expressed confidence in their parenting skill yet identified the need to modify their parenting styles. Grandparents also reported being "cut off" from community supports. As this theme has been overlooked in the grandparent literature, the erosion of community supports of both a formal and informal nature should raise concern for policy makers attempting to ameliorate grandparents' stressful life conditions. Interestingly, this chapter also identifies great-grandmothers as parenting resources for grandchildren. Given where these relatives are in their life cycle, it is clear that we should not be aggregating them with grandparent caregivers, who on average are middle-aged and less likely to be dealing with issues revolving about integrity versus despair or "grandgenerativity."

Sands and Goldberg-Glen use a microanalysis of a videotaped interview to understand the dynamics of a grandparent-headed household. This study emphasizes the need to train interviewers in both clinical and research domains to know how to probe and elicit responses and to anticipate unexpected data. Again, most literature based on broad issues does not attend to the clinical issues that might enhance therapeutic practice with these family systems.

ADVOCACY AND CUSTODIAL GRANDPARENTING

Advocacy efforts by grandparents in the early 1990s have made great strides within their states and the nation with regard to grandparental legislation. National grandparent support groups' efforts have also reinforced the notion that grandparents should and will adhere to the concept of filial responsibility and voluntarily provide care even if support services are not offered. Paradoxically, as the chapter by Albert points out, caregiving grandparents have evoked the law or have had the law thrust some responsibilities on them.

Nevertheless, grandparents' endeavors have continued to help develop legislation, yet such legislation often conveys confounding information. Connealy and DeRoos outline how family preservation has evolved from focusing on family pathology to emphasizing family resilience. This chapter details the importance of child welfare programs considering contextual issues in grandparents' and grandchildren's lives. It forces policy makers and practitioners alike to develop solutions that modify the environment rather than removing children from their relatives. Moreover, their judicious review of the benefits of family preservation indicate that legislation should focus less on theoretical foundations and more on a strengths perspective.

Regardless of the above observations, many still ponder whether or not grandparents are appropriate replacement parents. Unlike the elder care literature, care for grandchildren is viewed as nonnormative. This perspective raises numerous questions regarding whether grandparents should be granted the right to have legal custody, to become foster parents, or to adopt their grandchildren. Grandparent caregivers are skeptically assessed and reassessed, their privacy invaded, and their home environments inspected. Grandfathers are suspiciously viewed as potential "child molesters," and grandmothers' parenting of their own children is questioned. The fact that we assume that grandparents need parenting classes over courses on self-management, increased access to services, or even information on dealing with problems specific to their needs is clear evidence of how suspicious we are. Moreover, we have assumed that grandparents are divorced from the culture their grandchildren are in and that they have forgotten how to provide care.

Unlike that of Connealy and Deroos, Albert's analysis indicates that legal proceedings still focus on the best interests of the child and many times reinforce the above assumptions about grandparents. Although the legal context can at times send a message that discourages willing grandparents from providing care to their grandchildren, family preservation suggests that the whole family is important and that the welfare system will empower grandparents to obtain the resources needed for maintaining their homeostasis.

One way of overcoming this confusion is to rely on national coalitions to wade through the conflicting messages found within legislation and service programs. The Butts chapter suggests that organizations such as Generations United are needed to concretize a public policy grounded in considering the needs of the family throughout the family life cycle. Butts's chapter offers an action-oriented approach to intergenerational advocacy and clearly shows how it is a useful vehicle for improving the well-being of grandparent-headed families.

CONCLUSIONS: WHERE DO WE GO FROM HERE?

One refreshing aspect of this volume is the authors' consistent recognition of how resilient grandparent caregivers are in the face of adversity. Many authors note that despite such circumstances, grandparents willingly provide support for their grandchildren in hopes that they can minimize the "cut-offs" in their family system. The fact that, despite the slow development in policy and provision of services, grandparents have been able to provide for their grandchildren and keep their families somewhat unaltered emphasizes the importance of preserving family lineages and relationships.

In acknowledging the commitment of grandparent caregivers, society will be required to consider the special challenges of multi-generational households. Although certainly not exhaustive, the contributions to this book provide useful information to those interested in grandparent-headed families. As a whole, we believe that the discussions provide direction for future research, policy, and clinical development.

Framing these processes in the context of aging, illness, death, and grief, as well as in light of one's experiences as a parent, spouse, or traditional grandparent, can help educators, service providers, clinicians, and those who set public policy to understand more accurately the concerns of custodial grandparents and consequently target more precisely community or school-based services to those grandparents in the greatest need of help and support.

A FINAL WORD

What is less evident in this book are collaborative approaches to knowledge building. Hess and Mullen (1995), in their book *Practitioner-Researcher Partnerships*, make an appeal for more effective partnerships between the worlds of research and practice (p. ix). If we reflect on the chapters in this book and articles on grandparent caregiving in general, we arrive at similar conclusions. Indeed, the contributors to this volume have worked in isolation from one another. McCartt and Mullen's call is instructive in that it forces gerontologists to consider forging multidisciplinary institutional arrangements that would effectively unite the gerontology research community with the practice community in developing knowledge for service provision to grandparent-headed families. Many of the chapters in this volume could assist agencies in their consideration of developing programs, and service providers and agencies could inform scholars and funding agencies regarding research agendas. Overall, we must recognize that rapprochement of the research, practice, policy, and funding communities could help us reach our real goal: improving the welfare of grandparents and the grandchildren they care for.

REFERENCES

Casper, L. M., & Bryson, K. R. (1998). Co-resident grandparents and their grandchildren: Grandparent maintained families. *Population Division Working Paper No. 26.* Washington, DC: U.S. Bureau of the Census.

Hess, P. M., & Mullen, E. J. (Eds.). (1995). *Practitioner-researcher partnerships: Building knowledge from, in and for practice.* Washington, DC: National Association of Social Workers. (NASW Press).

Index